ANTICANCER MEDICINAL HERBS

Author of Chinese Edition
Chang Minyi
Translator in Chief
Bai Yongquan
Translators
Wang Ke   Li Zhaoguo
Ai Runlian   Jiao Wenxu

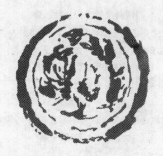

Hunan Science and Technology Publishing House

ANTICANCER MEDICAL HERBS

ISBN7—5357—1023—9/R·220

Author of Chinese Edition：Chang Minyi

Translator in Chief：Bai Yongquan et al

First edition 1992

Hunan Science and Technology Press

3 Exhibition Hall Road，Hunan Changsha 410005，China

Distributed by China International Book Trading Corporation

35 Chegongzhuang Xilu，Beijing 100044，China

P. O. Box 399，Beijing，China

Printed in Second Xinhua Printing House of Hunan Province，China

抗 癌 本 草

常敏毅 编著

白永权 主译

*

湖南科学技术出版社出版

（中国湖南省长沙市展览馆路 3 号）

邮政编码 410005 湘新登字 004 号

湖南新华印刷二厂印刷

中国国际图书贸易总公司发行

（中国北京车公庄西路 35 号）

北京邮政信箱第 399 号 邮政编码 100044

1992 年（16 开）第一版

（英）

ISBN7—5357—1023—9/R·220（外）

02820

14—E—2672D

FORWARD

Dr. Chang Minyi was my student. With ten years' painstaking effort, he has finished the compilation of an excellent book, "Anticancer Medicinal Herbs", which is a heartening achievement and deserves congratulation.

The book was finished in 1979 and I was fortunate to be invited to write a forward for it and was pleased to recommend it to certain publishers for publication. Thereafter, I was transferred to a different hospital and I was disappointed to learn that my departure had brought failure to the publication of the book. But, in the past four years, Dr. Chang has revised the draft of the book four times by adding discriptions of pharmacological experiments and clinical prescriptions to each herb listed in the book. Learning from others' experience and guided by the theories of traditional Chinese medicine, he developed a complex prescription known as the "Anticancer Single Blade Sword" which has been administered to 5000 patients since 1981. Most of the patients who had taken the prescription have commented that it is definitely effective in relieving the pain caused by cancer and improving the condition and the survival period of the patients. Many of overseas Chinese have come to him for help because they admire this eminent physician who has earned respect of the medical community. Dr. Chang has included his theory of and experience with the Anticancer Single Blade Sword in the book and this has increased the practical value of the contents.

I am delighted to be invited again to write a new forward for the book on the occasion of its publication 12 years after its completion.

Xin Shao-zhou
Deputy Chairman, Adviser
and Associate Professor
Chinese Antisenility Research Institute
March 8, 1986, in Harbin

PREFACE

Malignant tumors are the worst enemy endangering the lives of human beings. But we are confident that with the joint efforts of tumor researchers and health professionals, we will certainly conquer them one day.

At present, each of the tumor therapies such as the surgical, chemical, radiative and immune, has its own indications and contraindications, because of the variation in pathology, location and progressive stages of tumors. Generally speaking, combined therapies, that is to say, integrated Western and traditional Chinese medicine and combined external and internal therapy, have proved to be relatively satisfactory.

Is the goal in the treatment of tumors to resist the cancer directly by attacking the tumor itself or indirectly by promoting the immune functions of the body? Researchers are working hard on questions like this. For some of these questions, the answer is clear, but for others, a definite answer is still being sought. In traditional Chinese medicine, the clinical anticancer therapies are based on principles such as clearing away heat and toxic materials, treating toxifying diseases with poisonous agents, activating blood to remove stasis, softening and resolving hard lumps and invigorating qi. According to my experience, the above principles should be applied after careful consideration of an overall analysis of symptoms, signs, causes, nature and location of the illness, and the patients's condition. In accordance with these principles, Longhua Hospital of Shanghai Traditional Chinese Medical College treated 300 cases of primary cancer simply with medicinal herbs and the total effective rate was found to be 51%, with the longest survival period being 11 years. Judged by pathological classification and observation at different stages, squamous cancer had the highest effective rate——55.86%. In addition, the hospital selected 60 patients with advanced squamous cancer and randomly divided them into two groups of 30 patients, a group treated with traditional Chinese medicinal herbs and a group treated with chemotherapy. The survival period of the herbal group was 465 days while that of the chemotherapeutic group was 204 days, and the survival rates after 12 and 24 months were 66.7% and 13.3% for the herbal group and 33.3% and 3.3% for the chemotherapeutic group respectively, according to a report in *Journal of Integrated Western and Traditional Chinese Medicine* (Vol. 2, 1985). Based on the above facts, I think that treatment of tumors with traditional Chinese medicine has boundless prospects.

Chang Minyi is full of confidence and determination in his efforts to solve the cancer mystery and this is a praiseworthy spirit. He has already made gratifying achievements in the prevention and treatment of cancer with traditional Chinese medicine, and in this book, he introduces 236 kinds of herbs that have been carefully selected in the light of the scientific standard, and describes the practical value of anticancer herbs and herbal prescriptions used commonly both at home and abroad. It is a good book with substantial contents arranged in an aesthetic format for popularization and improvement of the prevention and treatment of tumors with traditional Chinese medicine. I, hereby, recommend this volume to clinical practitioners, teachers, researchers and people who are engaged in the prevention and treatment of tumors, as a book of reference.

Pan Chen-lian
Advisor and Research Fellow
Zhejiang Research Institute of
Traditional Chinese Medicine
March 20, 1986, in Hangzhou

TRANSLATOR'S NOTES

Anticancer Medicinal Herbs is a translation of *Kangai Bencao* in Chinese edition. During translation, every effort has been made to keep its meaning as exact as its original, though the theory of traditional Chinese medicine is different from that of Western medicine and so are the technical terms, which have been translated directly if they have equivalent or similar terms in Western medicine, indirectly or literally with supplementary and comprehensive explanations if they have no equivalent expressions in Western medicine. The following are what we want to explain to readers.

1. For those terms such as" *qi, yin, yang, ying and wei*", we have translated them with italic Chinese *pinyin* because they are the unique terms in traditional Chinese medicine and have a very broad concept even if they all are a single Chinese character.

2. The herbs in the book have been listed according to its Chinese edition, which had been set in an order according to the number of stokes of Chinese characters, but to facilitate easy reference to a particular herb or drug, we have worked out an index and put it at the end of the book under the title "Appendix Three: Index of Anticancer Medicinal Herbs".

3. Some names of the formulas or prescriptions in traditional Chinese medicine are too long when translated into English, so we used italic Chinese *pinyin* instead of its long English equivalents, and added an explanation immediately after them whenever we think it is necessary as far as understanding is concerned.

4. The names of books and journals quoted in the book, and the latin names of plants have been typeset in an italic form so as to distinguish the former from normal text and the latter from English.

5. With permission, some alterations have been made in this edition so as to make its contents more concise and easier to be comprehended by doctors of Western medicine.

We are very grateful to Professor Lu Juxian, Dean of the Faculty of Pharmacology, Xian Medical University, for her allowing us to use her reference books and dictionaries.

We are also grateful to Mr. Michael Hale, Mr. Allen Tompkins and Mrs. Marry Morgan for their proofreading.

In the interest of all patients and users of Anticancer Medicinal Herbs, readers are kindly requested to communicate any errors, that may have occurred, to the author, editor or us, in order that they may be corrected in the subsequent edition.

Bai Yongquan
Dean and Professor
Xian Medical University
November, 1991

TABLE OF CONTENTS

HERBA SOLIDAGINIS

It is reported in *Jiangxi Journal of Medicinal Herbs* that: "The drug is bitter and sweet in taste and neutral in nature. It reduces heat, clears away toxic material and relieves pains through promotion of the blood circulation."

Herba Solidaginis is the dried herb of goldenrod, *Solidago decurrens* of the family *Compositae*, which is found growing all over China and mainly contains chlorogenic acid, caffeic acid, quercetin, rutin, astragalin and tannic substances. Its decoction inhibits staphylococcus aureus, pneumococcus, pseudomonas aeruginosa and bacillus dysenteriae, to various degrees.

ANTICANCER PHARMACOLOGICAL FUNCTIONS

1. In tests against ascitic sarcoma-180 with total cellular volumetric method, the substance extracted with methyl alcohol is found to have a strong antineoplastic action when given to an affected guinea-pig under a dosage of 100mg/per kilogram of body weight through injection once daily for five days. The inhibitory rate was 82%. The ethyl alcohol extract from this herb also has an antineoplastic action with an inhibitory rate of 12.4%.

2. Screening tests with bacteriophages in vitro show an active antineoplastic effect.

3. The drug also promotes the phagocytic function of leukocytes.

EXPERIMENTAL FORMULAS

For tumor of the thyroid:

        Herba Solidaginis 15g
        Herba Scutellariae 12g
        Herba Kalimeris 12g
        Herba Lysimachiae 24g

A dose a day for 20 days makes a therapeutic course. Each dose is simmered and then the broth is divided into three portions to be taken in the morning, afternoon and evening. The formula is continued for 1 to 3 more courses after the tumor mass has disappeared. *Fujian Journal of Medicinal Herbs* reported that the Qiu Lu Clinic in Pu Tian, Fujian Province tried this formula on 53 cases of thyroid tumor and 28 of them were cured after taking the formula for a year, 36 after 2 years and 1 after 10 years.

For cancer of the tongue and the larynx:

Research Data of Traditional Chinese Medicine (Vol. 6, 1978) reported that 15 grams of Herba Solidaginis was boiled in 500ml of water and the broth was administered through gargling daily.

HISTORICAL COMMENTS

Jiangxi Journal of Medicinal Herbs reported that: "For the treatment of lumbodorsal carbuncle, acute mastitis and bubo, 21 to 30 grams of Herba Solidaginis is simmered in wine. This decoction is taken orally and the dregs ground into paste to be applied on the lesions."

In An Illustrated Book on Plants, it is said that: "Washing with a decoction of this herb can cure pathogenic infections."

Hunan Journal of Medicinal Herbs points out that: "The herb functions to dispel pathogenic wind, remove poisonous substances, control fever, promote blood circulation, subside swelling and relieve pain."

Quangdong Journal of Medicinal Herbs commented that: "The herb is good for removing blood stasis and obstructions and is effective for various traumatic injuries, skin itches and herpes zoster. But, the herb can not be decocted for a long period of time as broth decocted for too long may cause vomiting."

THE AUTHOR'S NOTE

Domestic animals show a toxic reaction to this herb. Thus consideration must be given to the fact that long-term administration and over dosage of this herb may cause gastrointestinal bleeding. Usually, the recommended dosage for oral administration is 6 to 15 grams. If the herb is fresh, the dosage can be increased, but no more than 30 grams.

FOLIUM MAHONIAE

Revised Reference of Processed Medicinal Herbs reported that: "Folium Mahoniae is bitter in taste and cold in nature, cures pulmonary tuberculosis and removes fever of the deficient type."

The herb is the dried leaf of Chinese mahonia, *Mahonia japonica*, *Mahonia bealei* and *M. fortunei* of the family *Berberidaceae*. *Mahonia japonica* mainly contains palmatine while *Mahonia bealei* and *M. fortunei* have berberine in them, and both of the chemicals have certain antineoplastic functions.

ANTICANCER PHARMACOLOGICAL FUNCTIONS

1. In screening tests with bacteriophages, it has been verified that *Mahonia bealei* inhibits the activity of bacteriophages and hence it is suggested that the herb has the same effect on cancer cells.

2. Palmatine derived from *Mahonia japonica* has been found to inhibit the cells of ascites carcinoma in mice.

EXPERIMENTAL FORMULAS

For pulmonary carcinoma with metastasis to the brain:

Folium Mahoniae 15g
Rhizoma Arisaematis 30g
Herba Galii Aparinis 30g
Concha Haliotidis 30g
Bombyx Batryticatus 9g
Ramulus Uncariae Cum Uncis 9g
Scorpio 6g

The formula is taken one dose daily in decoction. (Reported in *Shanghai Journal of Medicinal Herbs in March 1979*)

For cancer of the liver:

Folium Mahoniae 30g
Herba Solani Nigri 30-60g

The formula is decocted and the broth is divided into two portions and taking twice a day. (Reported in *Handbook of Herb Medicine*)

HISTORICAL COMMENTS

In *An Illustrated Book on Plants*, it is described that: "The plant has a firm, upright and black stem, with opposite, hard, bright and serrate leaves. Long spikes grow at the terminal of the stem and bear the seeds that look like those of *Sarcanda glabra* of the family *Chloranthoceae*. Folk doctors use the plant for the management of vomiting blood and the juice squeezed out of its roots is used as a gargle for toothaches."

Chinese Medicinal Herbs Growing on the Mountains and Plains commended that: "The herb is good for purging pathogenic fire and reducing fever, so it is used for the management of fever, vexation, diarrhea and acute conjunctivitis of epidemic febrile disease."

Jiangxi Journal of Medicinal Herbs reported that: "The decoction of 9 grams of Folium Mahoniae is taken daily for toothache due to pathogenic wind-fire and the dosage can be doubled if the condition is very serious."

Contemporary and Practical Herb Medicine said that: "The herb, like Fructus Ligustri Lucidi, is a tonic cool in nature, indicative for afternoon fever, hectic fever due to *yin*-deficiency, soreness and weakness in the loins and knees, dizziness and tinnitus."

FOLIUM ET RAMULUS SARCANDRAE

New Jiangnan Medicinal Herbs says that: "The herb is bitter and acrid in taste and slightly warm in nature. It eliminates pathogenic wind, promotes blood circulation, reduces swelling and relieves pain."

Folium et Ramulus Sarcandrae is the dried leaves and branches of sarcandra, *Sarcandra glabra (Thunb.) Nakai*, which is found mainly containing flavonoid glycoside, volatile oil, astilbin and isofraxidin.

ANTICANCER PHARMACOLOGICAL FUNCTIONS

1. The dried extract of the herb has an inhibitory rate of 30.5-56.7% on sarcoma-180 and Walker's cancer of mice.

2. The extract has an inhibitory rate of 30-50% on spontaneous cancer-615 of mice.

3. The rate for prolonging the survival time of mice with spontaneous leukemia ascites-771 is 160%.

4. Isofraxidin extracted from the herb shows a strong inhibition on lymphatic leukemia.

5. Volatile oil shows an inhibitory rate of 30-40% on Ehrlich ascites carcinoma, Walker's cancer and sarcoma-37.

6. The volatile oil also shows a strong cytotoxicity in vitro, reduces the size of the tumor mass when injected into it and prolongs the survival time of the experimental animals.

7. The extract and its separated substances from the herb do not have cytotoxicity, but they can promote cytophagy and immune functions of the experimental animals.

8. In animal immune tests, Folium et Ramulus Sarcandrae has manifested a similar function as Radix Ginseng, that is, a small dose increases immune function greatly and a large dose decrease it.

9. Tests with the decoction of the herb in vitro showed an antiphagocytic function, hence indicating an antineoplastic activity.

10. The volatile oil of the herb inhibits macrophage phagocytic function in a similar way as cyclophosphamide, so it suggests that the herb should be boiled for a long time to remove the volatile substances before use.

EXPERIMENTAL FORMULAS

For cancer of the digestive tract:

Practical Oncology reported that Folium et Ramulus Sarcandrae is made into tablets, each being 0.3 gram. The patients are asked to take 4 to 6 tablets each time, three times a day.

For cancer of the pancreas:

Journal of Medicinal Herbs says that flavone extracted from the herb and made into tablets or injections can improve the symptoms of the patient and reduce the size of the tumor mass. Each tablet contains 200mg, and each injection 25mg. The tablets are taken three times a day and each time 100 to 400mg according to the condition of the patient. The injection is given twice a day and each time 25mg.

HISTORICAL COMMENTS

Mingdong Journal of Medicinal Herbs reported that: "The drug invigorates the function of the spleen, promotes blood circulation, quenches thirst and controls swelling. It is indicative for postpartum external infection and alternate attacks of chills and fever".

Chinese Medicinal Herbs Growing on the Mountains and Plains commended that: "The drug is good for bone-knitting, removing blood stasis and lumps, and relieving pain."

In *Quizhou Journal of Medicinal Herbs*, it is said that the decoction of 15 grams of the drug is effective for stomachache.

In the *Dictionary of Chinese Medicinal Herbs*, it is said that: "The leaves of the herb has a strong antibacterial power, and the fresh root is better than the dried ones. The drug also has certain effect on bacteremia caused by staphylococcus aureus in rabbits."

THE AUTHOR'S NOTE

As the drug has both anticancer and antibacterial activity, it is indicative for cancer complicated with infection. According to the literature, 17 hospitals in Shanghai treated total 373 cancer patients with the herb preparation and found the effective rate of the preparation was 53.9%. Among the 113 cases treated only with the herb preparation, the remarkable effective rate was 22.1% and the effective rate was 62.8%. A hospital in Zhejiang Province gave the herb preparation to 70 cancer patients alone for a month and 6 of the cases showed remarkable effect and 49 cases showed improvement, with a total effective rate of 78.57%. As far as the curative effect is concerned, the preparation seems more effective for stomach cancer, liver cancer, adenocarcinoma of the pancreas, carcinoma of the esophagus, leukemia and lymphocytic reticulosarcoma. After the administration of the preparation, the symptoms of the patients were relieved, their appetite becoming increased and their lives prolonged. In some patients, the drug can relieve fever and reduce tumor mass. The preparation do not cause any local or general reactions and are safe to use. Pharmacological experiments showed that the herb has a remarkable anti-fatigue and sedative effect, and also can improve the frigidity remarkably in animals with both of their adrenal glands removed. All these are beneficial to the treatment of cancer patients.

RADIX ZANTHOXYLI

Canon of Materia Medica says that: "The herb is bitter in taste and warm in nature. It is effective for arthralgia due to wind-cold dampness, severe and migratory arthralgia and cold limbs".

It is the root or leaves of shiny prickly ash, *Zanthoxylum nitidum* (*Rutaceae*), which grows in the bushes on hills and mountain slopes in Quangdong, Quangxi, Sichuan and Yunnan provinces. The root contains nitidine, oxynitidine and diosmin, while the leaves and the nuts mainly contain volatile ail.

ANTICANCER PHARMACOLOGICAL FUNCTIONS

1. LD_{50} data of the cellular culture of ascites sarcoma-180 show that the drug contains a mixture of alkaloid, benzol and nitrogen, which resists the activity of cancer.

2. Test with rats showed that the total alkaloid of the herb inhibits Ehrlich's ascites carcinoma.

EXPERIMENTAL FORMULAS

For nasopharyngeal carcinoma:

Radix Zanthoxyli 30g

Rhizoma Imperatae 30g

Periostracum Serpentis 30g

Radix Cynanchi Paniculati 15g

Rhizoma Dioscoreae 15g

Rhizoma Ligustici Chuanxiong 15g

Radix Rehmanniae 24g

Herba Rubi Parvifolii 60g

The herbs are taken in decoction and a dose daily.

HISTORICAL COMMENTS

Origin of Materia Medica says that: "When decocted after being removed off the outer layer, the herb is effective for subcutaneous nodule and acute laryngeal infection".

Chinese Medicinal Herbs Growing on the Mountains and Plains points out that: "The herb is good for relieving pain and stasis".

Handbook of Common Chinese Medicinal Herbs says that: "The extracted fluid of the herb with alcohol at a ratio of 1 to 1 inhibits hemolytic streptococcus and staphylococcus aureus more powerfully, while the water solution seems less powerful. The herb is poisonous and it may cause abdominalgia and diarrhea. It is contraindicates sour food."

RADIX GINSENG

Classification of Chinese Medicinal Herbs says that: "The taste of the herb is good, neither bitter nor acrid, with mild nature."

It is the dried roots of Panax ginseng of the *Araliaceae* family, which grows in Northeast China and North Korea. Its allied species, *P. quiqueform L.*, is cultivated in the United States, and *P. ginseng* grows in Japan.

ANTICANCER PHARMACOLOGICAL FUNCTIONS

1. Ginsenosides and polysaccharide of the herb have certain inhibition on Ehrlich's ascites carcinoma in rats.

2. The steride of the herb inhibits sarcoma-180 and adenocarcima-755.

3. The infusion of the herb showed an inhibitory rate of 99.9% on cancer cell-26 of human uterine cervix.

4. When administered together with Radix Astragali seu Hedysari and Gaboderma Lucidum, the herb shows a higher inhibitory rate on cancer cells than when it is used alone.

5. When the extract of the herb is injected into guinea pigs with leukemia, the curable rate reaches 99.9% and the survival time increases twice as much as that of the control group.

6. Lately a substance called prostisol has been derived from the herb and it can promote the formation of ribonucleic acid, protein and lipid, improve immunity and help to cure cancer as an adjuvant.

7. The ether extract of the herb is found inhibiting sarcoma-180 and adenocarcinoma-755 in mice.

EXPERIMENTAL FORMULAS

For cancer of the esophagus:

Talks on Medicine says that: "Equal amount of the juice of Radix Ginseng, Arillus Longan, Rhizoma Phragmitis, sugercane, pear and milk is put together, added with a little juice of ginger and stewed into a soft extract for taking slowly."

For lung cancer:

Precious Mirror of Hygiene reports that the following herbs are ground into fine powders and taken 6 grams each time with honey water:

Radix Ginseng 60g

Poria 60g

Flos Fritillariae Thunbergii 60g

Semen Armeniacae Amarum 150g

Cortex Mori Radicis 90g

Rhizoma Anemarrhenae 30g

For advanced cancer of the stomach:

Prescription for Diseases due to Three Pathogenic Factors relates that equal amount of the following herbs is made into small pills for oral administration 50 pills each time with rice water:

Radix Ginseng

Poria

Cortex Magnoliae Officinalis (processed with ginger)

Baked Fructus Aurantii

Roasted Rhizoma Sparganii

Prepared Rhizoma Pinelliae

Cortex Mori Radicis

Rhizoma Atractylodis Macrocephala

For cancer of the uterus:

Proved Recipes of the Experienced Doctors of Traditional Chinese Medicine says that: "18 grams of Radix Ginseng, 18 grams of dried Carapax Trionycis and 9 grams of Pericarpium Zanthoxyli are ground into fine powder and divided into 6 portions. One such portion is taken each night with boiled water and 24 portions make a therapeutic course. Abdominalgia usually disappears after taking 3 portions.

For cancer of the breast:

Explanation on the Clinical Prescriptions of Traditional Chinese Medicine says that: "The following prescription is taken in decoction."

Radix Ginseng 3g

Radix Angelicae Sinensis 3g

Rhizoma Ligustici Chuangxiong 3g

Cortex Moutan Radicis 3g

Ramulus Cinnamomi 3g

Lignum Sappan 3g

Radix Platycodi 3g

Rhizoma Atractylodis Macrocephalae 2g

Radix Astragali seu Hedysari 2g

Radix Aucklandiae 2g

Radix Linderae 2g

Cortex Magnoliae Officinalis 2g

Fructus Aurantii 2g

Semen Arecae 2g

Radix Ledebouriellae 2g

Radix Glycyrrhizae 2g

Summary of Internal Diseases says that: "The following herbs, when taken in decoction, are also effective for breast cancer."

Radix Ginseng 5g

Poria 5g

Baked Rhizoma Atractylodis Macrocephalae 5g

Radix Bupleuri 2.5g

Rhizoma Ligustici Chuangxiong 2.5g

Baked Fructus Crataegi 2.5g

Baked Cortex Moutan Radicis 2.5g

Baked Radix glycyrrhizae 2.5g

Radix Rehmanniae Praeparata 30g

Radix Angelicae Sinensis 30g

Taking 3 grams of Radix Ginseng daily can prevent and treat the side effects of radiotherapy for cancer in the head and neck region.

HISTORICAL COMMENTS

Zhong Zang Jing compiled by Hua Tuo said that: "Radix Ginseng, Cacumen Biotae and Herba Schizonepetae are burned to ashes to be scattered on the face of the patient to treat derangements of *qi* and blood such as bleeding from the nose and the mouse."

Illustrated Herbs compiled by Su Song said that: "To try the effect of Radix Ginseng, get two persons to walk along for a distance of 3 to 5 *li*, one with Radix Ginseng in his mouth, and the other without. In the end you will find that the one without Radix Ginseng in his mouth will gasp for breath and the one with Radix Ginseng in his mouth will breath normally."

True Materia Medica compiled by Huang Gongxiu said that: "The herb is effective in relieving thirst and upsetness, activating the channels and the pulse, removing phlegm stasis, curing vomiting, regurgitation, cough and short breath due to deficiency, chronic lingering diarrhea, stranguria and other illnesses due to the deficiency of *qi* and blood."

THE AUTHOR'S NOTE

Traditionally it is known that Radix Ginseng and Faeces Trogopterorum are incompatible. In September 1980, a scholar published in *Prescriptions of Traditional Chinese Medicine*, Research on Using Radix Ginseng and Faeces Trogopterorum Together, which reports that the use of these two drugs together did not turn out poisonous reaction in the animals experimented and the anti-fatigue function of Radix Ginseng did not become weak. The combination of these two drugs was also recorded in ancient literatures and may be beneficial to the treatment of cancer.

Research Institute of Biologically Active Substances in Russia reported that they found Radix Ginseng could inhibit the growth of induced cancer in rats and guinea pigs, with an inhibitory rate of 48%. Another inspiratory research in Russia on cancer of human lips found that in their controlled study, patients with cancer of lips responded so well to radiotherapy when they had been given a certain dose of Radix Ginseng daily before the therapy, and that no relapse and metastasis occurred on follow-up. *Japanese Journal of Chemistry* reported in 1981 that Radix Ginseng could increase immunity remarkably. After a mouse was first injected with red blood cells of goat as antigen and then with 5 micrograms of panaxoside Rb1, they found the total number of cells produced by antibody was 4.5 times as much as that of the controlled group.

FRUCTUS AKEBIAE

Dietetic Materia Medica says: "The herb, cold and nontoxic in nature, is effective for loss of appetite due to evil heat and regurgitation of food from the stomach."

It is the dried fruit of akebia, *Akebia quinata (Thunb.) Decne.*, which mainly contains sugar.

ANTICANCER PHARMACOLOGICAL FUNCTIONS

1. The herb is found active in inhibiting sarcoma-180 and sarcoma-37 in rats.

2. The inhibitory rate of the herb on JTC-26 is 50 to 6o per cent.

EXPERIMENTAL FORMULAS

For cancer of the stomach:

Shanghai Journal of Traditional Chinese Medicine reported in August, 1984 that the decoction of the following herbs was indicative for the disease:

> Fructus Akebiae 30g
> Folium Cycadis Revolutae 30g
> Herba Hedyotis Diffusae 30g
> Herba Scutellariae 30g
> Nidus Vespae 9g
> Rhizoma Atractylodis Macrocephalae 9g
> Pericarpium Citri Reticulatae 9g

For cancer of the Liver:

Handbook of Common Anticancer Drugs recommends the decoction of the following herbs daily:

> Fructus Akebiae 30g
> Fossil of Cyrtiospirifer sinensis (Graban.) 30g
> Herba Verbenae 30g

HISTORICAL COMMENTS

Dietetic Materia Medica says that: "The herb can make the muscles of the digestive tract grow thicker, hence increasing the evacuation of the lower portion of the digestive tract and helping to increase the appetite of the patients. It is also good for clearing the twelve regular channels."

Ri Hua Zi Materia Medica says: "The herb is effective for mass in the hypochondrium."

Dictionary of Chinese Materia Medica says: "The herb soothes the liver through regulating the circulation of *qi*, abates pain through promoting blood circulation, relieves restlessness and alleviates water retention. Thus it is indicative for stomachache due to emotional depression and the attach of hyperactive liver *qi*, indigestion due to the stomach-heat, polydipsia, dysentery, lumbago, costalgia, hernia, dysmenorrhea and tenesmus of the uterus."

Supplementation to Compendium of Materia Medica reports that: "The herb removes excessive body fluid and relieves dysphoria with smothery sensation. After taking it, you may feel ease-minded, thirst-relieved and the adverse *qi* flows downward."

THE AUTHOR'S NOTE

This herb is mainly indicative for tumors of the digestive tract, but when combined with other anticancer drugs, it is also indicative for other types of cancer. According to *Treatment and Prevention of Common Types of Cancer in Qinghai*, taking 60 grams of each of Fructus Akebiae, Rhizome Rhodomyrti Tomentosae and Herba Hedyotis Diffusae daily in decoction is effective for chorioepithelioma. The author has also found that, as an adjuvant, 20 grams of Fructus Akebiae and 4 grams of Radix Ginseng, when cooked together with rice into gruel, can modify the symptoms of cancer patients if taken daily.

RHIZOMA DYSOSMAE PLEIANTHAE

Miao Xiyong, a physician in the Ming Dynasty, wrote: "The plant is pungent in flavor, warm in property and poisonous. It can prevent and treat snake or insect bite."

It is the dried root of *Dysosma pleiantha (Hance) Woodson*, which mainly grows in the Yangtze River Valley. *Dysosma veitchii (hemsl. et Wils)* and *Podophyllum emodi Wall. var Chinese Sprague* are its homogeneous plants and can be used to substitute the drug when it is in shortage.

ANTICANCER PHARMACOLOGICAL FUNCTIONS

1. Its main substance, podophyllotoxin, can inhibit metakinesis of cells.

2. Podophyllinic acid-2-ethyl hydrazide, a commercial product derived from podophyllotoxin, is widely used as an anticancer drug.

3. It has been proved that podophyllotoxin, being very poisonous, has a strong inhibition on many tumors, Walker's carcinoma and sarcoma-180.

EXPERIMENTAL FORMULAS
For cancer of the skin and uterine neck:
Handbook of Practical Anticancer Drugs recommends external application to the lesion with 10-20% solution of the herb.
For lung cancer:
Handbook of Practical Anticancer Drugs suggests taking 1.5g of the powder of the herb daily.
For malignant lymphoma:
Journal of Fujian Folk Herbs reports that 30 to 60 grams of Rhizoma Dysosmae Pleianthae and 60 grams of millet wine are decocted together in water and taken a dose a day.
For cancer of the esophagus:
Zhejiang Tumor Journal says that: "30 grams of each of Rhizoma Dysosmae Pleianthae, Folium Euonymi Fortunis, Herba Dianthi and Folium Indocalami Tessellati, 9 grams of Rhizoma Atractylodis Macrocephalae and 6 grams of Pericarpium Citri Reticulatae are decocted into a syrup to be taken in several times in a day. This formula has a quick effect."
Therapies Based on Differentiation of Symptoms and Signs remarks that: "For patients with cancer of the esophagus, 9 grams of Rhizoma Dysosmae Pleianthae is boiled and taken as tea daily."

HISTORICAL COMMENTS
Compendium of Materia Medica compiled by Li Shizhen reads: "The herb is able to eliminate pathogenic factors, lessen all kinds of poisoning, remove the dead fetus and cure pernicious malaria."
Dictionary of Chinese Medicine says that: "The herb is very potent and combats poison with poison."
Supplement to Compendium of Materia Medica says that: "If you really understand *Dysosma pleiantha (Hance) Woodson*, you are not afraid of sleeping together with poisonous snakes. The herb can combat all kinds of poison, soften hard masses and evacuate pus."

THE AUTHOR'S NOTE
According to a report of *American Journal of Medicine* in 1982, resin derived from its homogeneous plant, *Podophyllum emodi Wall. var. Chinese Sprague*, reacts with podophyllotoxin to form an artificial substance similar in function as narcissine and terminates metakinesis of cancer cells. Experiment on 250 cases of acute monocytic leukemia, acute granulocytic leukemia, malignant lymphogranulomatosis, malignant lymphoma and breast cancer showed the substance has certain effect. Since 1973, the herb has been used clinically for the treatment of parvicellular bronchopulmonary cancer and carcinoma of testis, and has showed remarkable effect.

RADIX WIKSTROEMIAE INDICAE

Chinese Medicinal Herbs says: "The herb is bitter in taste and cold, pungent and poisonous in nature. It relieves swelling and hard masses and removes phlegm through eliminating dampness."

It is the dried root or root bark of wikstroemia, *Wikstroemia indica* (*Thymelaeaceae*), which mainly grows in the region south of the Yangtze River. Resin extracted from it has a strong purgation and contains an unknown substance which causes strong stimulation to the skin.

ANTICANCER PHARMACOLOGICAL FUNCTIONS

1. Its water decoction shows an inhibitory rate of 45.4% on lymphosarcoma-1 of ascites type in mice.

2. The water decoction of the herb is also found inhibiting cervical cancer-14 and sarcoma-180.

3. The methanol extract of the herb manifests a remarkable anticancer activity, with an inhibitory rate of 97% to Ehrlich's ascites carcinoma and a T/C value of 180% to lymphocytic leukemia-388.

EXPERIMENTAL FORMULAS

For cancer of the breast:

Collection of Proved Recipes in Hunan reports that 30 to 60 grams of Radix Wikstroemiae Indicae, after being ground into fine powder and mixed with boiled water or millet wine, is taken daily.

For malignant lymphoma:

Fujiang Folk Medicinal Herbs says that 30 grams of Radix Wikstroemiae Indicae is decocted for 4 hours to remove its toxin and the broth is taken orally."

For carcinomatous ascites:

Treatment of Cancer with Medicinal Herbs reported that: "Radix Wikstroemiae Indicae 12g, Herba Lobeliae Radicantis 30g and Pericarpium Lagenariae 30g are decocted and taken daily."

For cancer of the lung and liver:

It is reported in *News Bulletin of Medicinal Herbs* that 60ml of the water solution of Radix Wikstroemiae Indicae is taken once daily, and a therapeutic course lasts for 20 days.

For various cancers of the body surface:

Chinese Herbology reported that 1500 grams of the fresh leaves of the herb is decocted and the decoction is further boiled into a paste to be mixed with 100 grams of sebum and 200 grams of vaseline, for application to the lesion.

For different types of cancer:

The injection prepared from the herb is injected intramuscularly twice a day, each time 2-5ml.

HISTORICAL COMMENTS

Lingnan Herbology commended that: "The herb is indicative for venereal diseases and malignant sore."

Chinese Medicinal Herbs Growing on Mountains and Plains says: "The herb reduces fever, alleviates water retention and removes stasis."

Guangxi Medicinal Herbs evaluated that: "The herb destroys parasites and removes toxic substances and is effective for leprosy, malignant sore and gonorrhea."

THE AUTHOR'S NOTE

The herb is poisonous and needs 3 to 4 hours' boiling to remove its toxin. Its poison may turn up symptoms such as severe nausea, vomiting, diarrhea and dizziness. If poisoning occurs not long after taking the herb, the patient is first given gastrolavage and then thick tea and activated carbon or tannalbin. He may also be given a lot of salty water to drink and intravenous drip with 5% glucose saline. The decoction of 3 grams of Cortex Cinnamomi, 6 grams of Radix Glycyrrhizae and 6 grams of Radix Ledebouriellae is effective for poisoning caused by the herb. According to *Poisonous Plants in South China*, eating frozen rice porridge can relieve poisoning caused by the herb.

RADIX NOTOGINSENG

According to Huang Gongxiu in the Qing Dynasty, "The herb, being bitter in flavor and warm in nature, can remove blood stasis. When put in pig blood, the herb can turn the blood into water."

This is the dried root of notoginseng, *Panax pseudo-ginseng Wall. var. notoginseng (Burkill) Hoo and Tseng*, which grows in Guangxi and Yunnan provinces and mainly contains various arasaponin.

ANTICANCER PHARMACOLOGICAL FUNCTIONS

1. The hot water extract of the herb inhibits cancer effectively with an inhibitory rate of over 90% on JTC-26 in vitro.

2. Experiments in vivo showed that the herb also inhibits sarcoma-180 in mice. Mice with sarcoma-180 were fed with glucose derived from the herb with a dose of 2.5mg per kilo of their body weight and after two weeks, the size of the tumor mass became reduced and after five weeks, the tumor mass disappeared completely in six out of the ten mice.

3. In tests with phagological scanning for anticancer drugs, the herb was found antiphagologic.

EXPERIMENTAL FORMULAS

For cervical cancer:

Practical Oncology recommends external application of the powder of the following herbs:

Radix Notoginseng 3g
Realgar 3g
Venenum Bufonis 15g
Rhizoma Bletillae 12g
Prepared Arsenicum Trioxidum 1.5g
Alumen 60g
Sal Ammoniaci 0.3g

For cancer complicated with blood in the sputum, urine and stool:

Records of Integrated Western and Traditional Chinese Medicine recommends the powder of the following herbs for oral administration twice a day with boiled water:

Radix Notoginseng 6g
Ophicalcitum 9g
Crinis Carbonisatus 3g

For cancer of the esophagus:

Collection of Proved Recipes in Anhui Province recommends the powder of the following herbs for oral administration with honey water three times a day and each time 6 grams:

Radix Notoginseng 18g
Rhizoma Pleionis 120g
Sargassum 60g
Bulbus Fritillariae 60g
Pruina Kaki 60g
Prepared Rhizoma Pinelliae 30g
Flos Carthami 30g
Prepared Resina Olibani and Myrrha 15g

HISTORICAL COMMENTS

New Compilation of Materia Medica by Wu Yiluo commended: "The herb, being sweet and bitter in taste and warm in nature, can disperse blood and relieves pain."

Compendium of Materia Medica says: "The herb can stop bleeding, disperse blood stasis, relieve pain, and hence it is indicative for hematemesis, epistaxis, metrorrhagia, dysentery with blood stool, profuse menstruation, retention of putrid blood after birth, dizziness and pain due to blood stasis, acute conjunctivitis, carbuncle and snake or animal bite. For wound caused by sharp metal weapons and tools or flogging trauma, applying the powder or paste of the herb to the lesion can stop bleeding immediately."

Collections of Simplified Recipes of Binhu says: "For innominate inflammatory swelling with persistent pain, grind the herb into a paste and apply it to the swelling. The swelling and the pain will be relieved at once. The powder of the herb is used if the swelling becomes ruptured."

Essentials of Materia Medica says: "The herb is very effective for incised wound caused by sharp metal weapons or tools, particularly for flogging trauma. The herb is similar to Bletilla striata and Rehmannia glutinosa in appearance and a bit sweet like Radix Ginseng. Its powder, when mixed with blood of pigs, can change the blood into water."

THE AUTHOR'S NOTE

Yunnan Pulvis Medicinalis Albus, a white medicinal powder consisting of pulverized notoginseng root and other ingredients, has been proved to inhibit sarcoma-180 in rats.

People's Hospital in Fuzhou City tried to cure cancer of the esophagus and the liver with Yunnan Pulvis Medicinalis Albus. They asked the patients to take the powder after meals, three times a day, each time 1 to 2 grams. Each course constituted two weeks and between courses, the powder was ceased for a week. The drug can be administered on a long term basis. In his practice, the author has found that the drug has an unpleasant taste of pepper and some patients do not like it. The best way of taking it is to mix it with food. To treat hematemesis in stomach cancer and epistaxis in lung cancer, the author found the following recipe, taken a dose daily, is very effective:

> Herba Agrimoniae 40g
> Radix Ginseng 9g
> Yunnan Pulvis Medicinalis Albus 0.5g

According to report by *American Journal of Drugs*, the analysis made on Yunnan Pulvis Medicinalis Albus by American National Research Institute of Cancer proved that the two kinds of arasaponin derived from the herb had a definite inhibition on lymphatic leukemia-388 and leukemia-1210 and nasopharyngeal epithelial cancer.

RHIZOMA SPARGANII

Luo's Medical Classics commended: "The herb is bitter and acid, promoting the circulation of *qi* in the blood and removing all kinds of blood stasis."

The drug is the dried tubers of *Sparganium stoloniferum (Sparganiaceae)* or *Scirpus yagara Ohiwi.*

ANTICANCER PHARMACOLOGICAL FUNCTIONS

Screening tests with animals in vitro showed that the herb inhibits the growth of tumors.

EXPERIMENTAL FORMULAS

For cancer of the abdominal cavity:

Supplement to the Essential Prescriptions Worth a Thousand Gold says that: "Five kilos of the herb is decocted first and the broth is further boiled into a thick syrup to be taken twice a day, each time 4 grams."

For thyroid adenoma:

Jiangsu Journal of Traditional Chinese Medicine offers the following prescription. Collect all the herbs and grind them into fine powders to be made into pills about the size of green bean:

> Rhizoma Sparganii 50g
> Fructus Aurantii 50g
> Radix Curcumae 50
> Radix Angelicae Sinensis 50g

Radix Salviae Miltiorrhizae 50g
Radix Paeoniae Alba 50g
Pericarpium Citri Reticulatae 50g
Semen Sinapis Albae 50g
Prepared Squama Manitis 50g
Thallus Laminariae seu Eckloniae 100g
Sargassum 100g
Spica Prunellae 100g
Flos Carthami 25g
Rhizoma Zedoariae 150g
Herba Taraxaci 150g
Concha Ostreae 150g

For cancer of the uterus, the ovary and the liver:

Liaoning Journal of Traditional Chinese Medicine recommended intravenous or local injection of the 150% solution derived from Rhizome Sparganii and Rhizoma Zedoariae once daily or once every other day, each injection contains 20 to 60ml.

HISTORICAL COMMENTS

Kei Bao Materia Medica says: "The drug is mainly used for hypochondriac lump and mass in the abdomen."

Origin and Development of Medicine reads: "The drug is indicative for cardio-diaphragmatic pain."

Luo's Medical Classics says: "The herb reduces vital energy, so it is always used together with Radic Ginseng."

CEPHALOTAXUS FORTUNEI

Pharmacopoeia of People's Republic of China says: "The seed of the plant is sweet, acrid and astringent, while its branches and leaves are bitter, astringent and cold."

It is the dried leaves, seeds or bark of *Cephalotaxus fortunei Hock. f.*, or *C. sinensis (Rehd. et Will) Li, C. wilsoniana Hayata* and *C. harringtonia.*

ANTICANCER PHARMACOLOGICAL FUNCTIONS

1. The herb is found to have certain inhibition on sarcoma-180 and Walker's carcinoma-256.
2. The herb has a remarkable inhibition on lymphocytic leukemia-338 in rats.
3. Harringtonine derived from the herb shows a remarkable inhibition on lymphocytic leukemia in rats.
4. The herb is a broad-spectrum anticancer drug, which has certain effect on carcinoma-14 of the uterine cervix, reticulosarcoma, cerebroma-22 and leukemia-615.

EXPERIMENTAL FORMULAS

For various malignant tumors:

One gram of cephalotaxine crystal is added to 100ml of water for boiling to dissolve the crystal completely and the boiled solution is filtered before being loaded into ampules with 2ml of the filtered solution in each containing 20mg of the crude drug. The preparation can be given intravenously after disinfection for 30 minutes. If administered intramuscularly, benzyl alcohol is added to prevent pain.

THE AUTHOR'S NOTE

Harringtomine of the herb has a good immediate effect for acute granulocytic leukemia and acute monocytic leukemia. Its cephalotaxine has certain effect on pulmonary cancer, lymphatic sarcoma, eosinophilic lymphogranuloma, gastric cancer, supramaxillary cancer, Hodgkin's disease, leiomyoma of the uterus, cancer of the esophagus, prostatic cancer and synoviosarcoma. But caution should be given to the fact that it inhibits the hematopoietic system.

According to *Journal of Chinese Medicine* (Vol. 3, 1978) and *Bulletin of Chinese Medicinal Herbs* (Vol. 12, 1977), No. 187 Hospital of the People's Liberation Army administered harringtonine to treat 72 cases of leukemia and found 24 cases were cured and 38 relieved, with a total effective rate of 86.1%. It was also reported that when used together with other anticancer drugs, harringtonine had a better effect. *Treatment and Prevention of Cancers* reported in 1974 that Quangzhou Association of Female Cancers used harringtonine to treat malignant trophoblastic tumor and the effective rate was found to be 37.8%.

RHIZOMA BOLBOSTEMMAE

New Materia Medica says that: "The herb has a bitter taste and cures external pathologic phlegm."

It is the dried rhizoma of *Bolbostemma paniculatum (Maxim.) Franquet (Orchidacea)*, which grows in Hunan and Shaanxi Province. Its rhizoma mainly contains mannose and sucrose.

ANTICANCER PHARMACOLOGICAL FUNCTIONS
1. Through scanning tests in vitro, it is found that the herb inhibits the activity of tumor.
2. The injection prepared with the herb can reduce morbidity of cervical cancer induced by methylcholanthrene.

EXPERIMENTAL FORMULAS
For breast cancer:

        Bulbus Bolbostemmae 15g

        Herba Taraxaci 15g

        Squama Manitis 15g

        Semen Aurantii 15g

        Flos Lonicerae 15g

        Spica Prunellae 15g

The formula is taken a dose a day in water decoction, half of the broth in the morning and another half in the evening. The formula is very effective for febrile pain due to reddish swelling. (*Anticancer Medicinal Herbs*)

Yao Xizhou's *Proved Recipes for Breast Cancer* recommended the decoction of the following herbs either in water or in wine:

        Bulbus Bolbostemmae 9g

        Fructus Forsythiae 9g

        Flos Lonicerae 9g

HISTORICAL COMMENTS
Mirror of a Hundred Herbs recorded: "The herb is good for scattering carbuncles, removing pus, dispelling wind and damp pathogenic factors and resolving phlegm."

Supplement to Materia Medica said: "15 grams of Bulbus Bolbostemmae, when added to *Yanghe Tang* Formula, is very effective for breast cancer. At the early stage of acute mastitis, the mixture of an equal portion of the powder of Bulbus Bolbostemmae and Radix Angelicae Dahuricae is very effective when taken with a dose of 9 grams. If the patient is strong, the dosage can be increased to 15 grams. Usually after the first dosage, the illness may disappear. If not, a second dose is given."

Handbook of Holly Medicine reported: "The following formula, when decocted either in water or in wine, onion and ginger, is effective for pyogenic infection of the back of the hand:

Radix Glycyrrhizae 15g
Radix Glycyrrhizae (baked) 15g
Spina Gleditsiae 7.5g
Bulbus Bolbostemmae (baked with earth) 16.5g
Rhizoma Pinelliae 4.5g
Squama Manitis 7.5g
Rhizoma Anemarrhenae 7.5g "

RHIZOMA SMILACIS GLABRAE

Compendium of Materia Medica says: "The herb, slightly sweet in taste, flat in nature and nonpoisonous, is good for promoting the function of the spleen and the stomach and strengthening the bones and the muscles."

It is the dried root of *Smilax glabra* (*Liliaceae*). Li Shizhen wrote: "There are two types of smilax glabra, the white one is better than the red one when used as a herb."

ANTICANCER PHARMACOLOGICAL FUNCTIONS
1. Tests in vitro with JTC-26 showed that the hot water extract of the herb can completely inhibit JTC-26 with a concentration of $500\mu g/ml$, while bleomycinum ($5\mu g/ml$) has an inhibitory rate of 66%.
2. The herb also showed a certain inhibition on sarcoma cells.

EXPERIMENTAL FORMULAS
For meningoma:
Rhizoma Smilacis Glabrae 75g
Radix Polygoni Multiflori 25g
Ramulus Uncariae cum Uncis 25g
Semen Cassiae 20g
Flos Chrysanthemi 15g
Semen Persicae 15g
Rhizoma chuangxiong 10g
Radix Angelicae sinensis 50g
The herbs are taken in water decoction with a dose a day. (*Liaoning Journal of Traditional Chinese Medicine*)
For malignant lymphoma:
Ji Detang's Proved Recipes recommended decoction of the herb or porridge cooked with the slices or the powder of the herb. It also said that the herb contraindicates iron and fermentative food.
For thyroid cancer:
Rhizoma Smilacis Glabrae 15g
Radix Fagopyri 9g
Rhizoma Dioscoreae Bulbiferae 9g
Herba Solani Lyrati 15g
Radix Cayratiae 12g
Herba Taraxaci 12g
Radix Glycyrrhizae 6g

Flos Lonicerae 6g

The herbs are taken in water decoction, reported by *Zhejiang Journal of Folk Medicine*.

For papilloma of the bladder:

New Medical Bulletin reported in its third volume, 1978 that 60 grams of Fresh Rhizoma Smilacis Glabrae and 30 grams of Fructus Trachycarpi are decocted into a paste and are finally made into tablets, each 0.3 gram. The tablets are taken three times a day, each time 5 tablets.

For craniopharyngioma:

Journal of Liaoning Traditional Chinese Medicine reported in its third volume, 1978, the administration of the decoction of the following herbs:

Rhizoma Smilacis Glabrae 75g
Scorpio 10g
Rhizoma Dioscoreae Bulbiferae 10g
Flos Chrysanthemi 10g
Radix Polygoni Multiflori 25g
Sargassum 25g
Magnetitum 25g
Semen Plantaginis Asiaticae 25g
Concha Haliotidis 30g
Herba Scutellariae Barbatae 40g
Squama Manitis 10g
Rhizoma Chuanxiong 10g
Rhizoma Gastrodiae 10g
Rhizoma Arisaematis 5g

HISTORICAL COMMENTS

Comprehension of Materia Medica commended: "Rhizoma Smilacis Glabrae, which enters the collaterals to remove pathogenic dampness and heat, is used to relieve poisoning caused by hydrargyrum and calomelas through promotion of excretion. Hence, it is commonly used to treat syphilitic skin lesions, joint pain and sore throat and all malignant diseases.

Essential Properties of Medicinal Herbs said: "When applied, the decoction of Rhizoma Smilacis Glabrae is very effective for malignant carbuncles."

Essentials of Materia Medica recorded: "In its thin form, Rhizoma Smilacis Glabrae can get deep into the tissue, while in its thick form, it nourish the body. Taken in decoction as a tea, it is particularly effective for carbuncles."

THE AUTHOR'S NOTE

It was reported that the First Teaching Hospital of Beijing Medical University cured a patient with cancer of the urine bladder with the following formula and a special tea made out of Bufo and Herba Oldenlandiae Diffusae:

Rhizoma Smilacis Glabrae 30g
Medulla Junci 30g
Herba Solani Lyrati 30g
Herba Solani Nigri 30g
Herba Duchesneae 15g
Spora Lygodii 15g

FRUCTUS ZIZIPHI JUJUBAE

Luo Guoyang of the Qing Dynasty commended: "Fructus Ziziphi Jujubae reinforces the Middle-*jiao* with its sweet taste and replenishes *qi* with its mild nature. The acquired *qi* would be supplemented with it and a long term administration could help to build up the body."

It is the dried ripe fruit of Chinese date, *Ziziphus jujuba (Rhamnaceae)*. It has many varieties, but the red ones are used as a herb. Recently, it has been reported in Japan that the herb contains a lot of substance call cAMP, hence it is thought that the herb can promote immunity.

ANTICANCER PHARMACOLOGICAL FUNCTIONS
1. Tests in vitro proved that the hot water extract of the herb has an inhibition on the growth of JTC-26 with a rate of 90%, and it has also been found that the herb has a slight inhibition on the normal cells.

2. The intensity of its inhibition is closely related to its dose. Intense inhibition occurs to rats only when its concentration reaches $500\mu g/ml$. No inhibition takes place when the concentration is less than $100\mu g/ml$.

EXPERIMENTAL FORMULAS
For cardiac cancer:

Zhi Zhi Prescriptions reported that: "Get a date and have its core removed, then insert the body of a mylabris (without its head and wings) into the date and have it roasted. The body of the mylabris is removed away before eating the processed date on an empty stomach."

For spitting blood in lung cancer:

Equal portions of Fructus Ziziphi Jujubae (burned) and Galla Chinensis (processed with tea through fermentation) are ground into powder and taken 10 grams each time with rice porridge.

HISTORICAL COMMENTS
Ri Hua Zhi Materia Medica commended: "Fructus Ziziphi Jujubae removes hypochondriac lump."

Annotation on Shen Nong's Herbs said: "The herb, being sweet in taste, removes poison of any substance and is used to harmonize drugs used in a prescription."

Dutch Drug Mirror commended: "The sweetness of the drug functions to nourish the body, relieves poisoning and are indicative for cough, celostomia, sore throat, spitting blood due to long illnesses, infection of the blood, inflammation of the urinary tract and stranguria."

Luo's Mirror of Medicine recorded: "The drug is very sweet so it is contraindicative for abdominal distension, malnutrition in children, diseases due to phlegm heat and toothache."

THE AUTHOR'S NOTE
The author often prescribes the following formula for stomach cancer and has found it effective:

    Herba Agrimoniae 40g

    Fructus Ziziphi Jujubae 30g

The two herbs are decocted into a thick broth to be taken every 4 hours. A therapeutic course lasts for 40 days and the formula is found very effective for pain caused by stomach cancer. In 1981 *Journal of Medicinal Plants* reported that dates exported from China is rich in cAMP with a dried concentration of 100 to $500\mu g$ per gram. A Japanese scholar pointed out at the 15th Symposium on Chinese Medicinal Herbs that: "Cancer cells, containing low cAMP, may change to normal cells when cAMP is effused into them during culture." Undoubtedly, it is of benefit to increase the use of Fructus Ziziphi Jujubae in anticancer prescriptions.

BULBUS ALLII

Wang Ang in the Qing Dynasty commended that: "Bulbus Alii, bitter in taste and mild in nature, promotes the function of the spleen, subsides swelling and removes blood stasis and lumps."

It is the bulb of garlic, *Allium sativum* (*Liliaceae*), which grows over China and has a strong offensive odor.

ANTICANCER PHARMACOLOGICAL FUNCTIONS

1. Experimental tests on animals show that intraperitoneal injection of the infusion of the herb has certain therapeutical effect on Ehrlich's ascites cancer in rats.

2. The crude extract of the herb combats mitochysis of ascites cancer cells in rats.

3. Female rats fed with fresh garlic are immune to breast cancer.

4. It is also found that the herb has a certain inhibition on reticulosarcoma-180, parenchymal liver cancer and cervical cancer-14.

5. The inhibitory rate of the herb on JTC-26 is found to be 70-90%.

6. Clinical experiments showed that 64.8% of the patients had an increase in the transformation of lymphocytes.

EXPERIMENTAL FORMULAS

For cancer of the long:

Oral administration of 10 to 30ml of garlic juice, twice a day.

For leukemia:

The sublingual vein of the patients is cut and then rubbed with fresh garlic. This method is also good for lung cancer.

For other types of cancers:

Oral administration of garlic, peppermint oil and beer yeast is combined with intravenous injection of Vitamin F, K, E and chlorophyll.

A long term administration of garlic volatile oil can prevent the occurrence of cancer, reported by *Bulletin of Traditional Chinese Medicine* in Volume 6, 1974.

For various malignant tumors:

Collection of Tumor Data reported administration of garlic in the following ways:

1>. Intramuscular injection of 5ml of garlic distillation mixed with 2% novocaine each time, three times a day.

2>. Intramuscular injection of 1ml of garlic emulsion mixed with 2ml of 2% novocaine, twice a day.

3>. Intravenous drip of 25ml of garlicin mixed with 500ml of 10% glucose each time, once daily. A therapeutic course lasts for 2 weeks.

For carcinomatous thoracico-abdominal edema:

Diagnosis, Prevention and Treatment of Cancers reported the application of the mixed paste of Radix Kansui (9 grams), Fructus Amomi (9 grams) and fresh garlic, on the umbilicus.

HISTORICAL COMMENTS

Compendium of Medicinal Herbs recorded: "Garlic helps to digest grain and meat, cures furuncle and carbuncle. Its juice is indicative for vomiting blood and cardiac pain; its decoction for convulsion; combined with *Jiyu Pills* for diseases of the diaphragm; together with Concha Ostreae Ills for edema; with Minium Ills for dysentery and enteritis; and with Olibanum Ills for abdominal pain. When put into the anus, it cures obstruction and constipation."

"For cardiac pain due to inverted flow of the blood, 2ml of fresh Bulbus Allii is taken orally."

New Edition of Proved Prescriptions reports that: "When Hua Tuo met a patient with dysphagia and he told him to drink two or three bowls of vinegar in which Bulbus Allii had been immersed and to eat Bulbus Allii as much as possible."

THE AUTHOR'S NOTE

According to a Japanese bulletin (No. 53-27775 and No. 37-12000), Bulbus Allii is steamed for a short period of time to kill the activity of its enzyme, which is extracted later with methanol. The extracted enzyme is processed to get rid of its foul smell so as to obtain a substance for aesthetical purpose, resisting fatty liver and protecting vitamin C and B. It is thought that the substance is also effective for curing cancer. Since it has lost its irritating taste, the plant can be widely used as food. Recently, two Japanese scholars have developed a kind of tumor cells which contain the extract of Bulbus Allii. The cells, when injected into mice before the injection of millions of tumor cells, caused no tumor in the experimental animals. This is to say that the vaccine has an effective rate of 100% against tumor. In April 1958, *Questions Regarding Oncology* (English edition) reported that two Russian doctors treated 194 patients with white patch of lip cancer and 184 were completely cured. The effective rate was found to 95%.

RADIX ET RHIZOMA RHEI

Huang Gongxiu in the Qing Dynasty said that: "The drug, extremely bitter in taste and cold in nature, is characterized by properties of descending and dispersing."

The drug is obtained from the radix of *Rheum officinale Baill.* of the *Rheum* family and the *Polygonacene* genus, mainly produced in Hunan and Sichuan provinces in China. Drugs of the same family, such as *Rheum palmatum L.*, *Rheum tanguticum Maxim et Balf.*, and *Rheum wittrockii Lundstr.*, are used as the substitutes of the drug.

ANTICANCER PHARMACOLOGICAL FUNCTIONS

1. Intracutaneous injection of the unrefined extract of the drug causes damage to sarcoma-27 of mice.

2. Emodin evidently inhibits cellular respiration of ascites cancer, oxidization and deoxidization of certain kinds of amino acids and the products produced during glycometabolism.

3. Emodin evidently inhibits mice melanoma with an effective rate of 76%.

4. Rhein inhibits ascites cancer with an effective rate of 15% and mice sarcoma-180 with an effective rate of 21%.

5. Anthraquinone contained in the drug resists the activity of cancer.

6. The hot water extract of the drug inhibits mice sarcoma-180 with an effective rate of 48.8%.

EXPERIMENTAL FORMULAS

For uterine cancer:

Radix et Rhizoma Rhei 30g
Rhizoma Paridis 90g
Radix Paeoniae Lactiflorae 30g
Radix Angelicae Sinensis 30g
Radix Astragali 30g

The above herbs are ground into powder and rolled with honey into pills of 6 grams each. 2 of the pills are taken daily. (*Handbook of Medicinal Herbs in Northeast China*)

For rectocancer:

Radix et Rhizoma Rhei 3g
Fructus Bruceae 15g
Venenum Bofonis 0.015g

The herbs are ground into powder and taken once a day. (*Journal of Hunan Medicine*, Vol. 5, 1977)

For uteroma:

        Radix et Rhizoma Rhei 180g

        Radix Scutellariae 150g

        Radix Glycyrrhizae 210g

        Semen Persicae 360g

        Semen Pruni armeniacae 360g

        Radix Rehmanniae 600g

        Lacca Sinica Exsiccata 60g

        Tabanus 70

        Natrii Sulfas 300g

        Hirudo 70

The herbs are ground into powder, rolled with honey into pills for oral administration 9 grams each time, 3 times a day. (*Modern Prescriptions for Gynecology*)

For acute granulocytic leukemia:

        Radix et Rhizoma Rhei 9g

        Cortex Moutan 3g

        Radix Scrophulariae 9g

        Radix Rehmanniae 9g

        Folium Isatidis 9g

        Pulvis Glycyrrhizae Praeparatus 4.5g

        Periostracum Cicadae 4.5g

        Radix Trichosanthis 6g

The prescription is taken one dosage a day in decoction. (*Medical Research Correspondence*, Vol. 7-8, 1973)

For uterocancer at the primary stage:

        Radix et Rhizoma Rhei 2g

        Natrii Sulfas 3g

        Cortex Moutan 4g

        Semen Persicae 4g

        Semen Benincasae 4g

        Rhizoma Atractylodis Lanceae 4g

        Semen Coicis 8g

        Radix Glycyrrhizae 1g

The prescription is taken in decoction. (*Elucidation on Clinical Application*)

For ovarian cancer:

        Radix et Rhizoma Rhei 6g

        Cortex Phellodendri 3g

        Folium et Ramulus Biotae 6g

        Herba Lycopi 3g

        Herba Menthae 1.5g

The herbs are ground, decocted into a paste, mixed with some wine and applied to the abdomen before the patient is going to bed each night and removed the next morning. (*Prevention and Treatment of Common Tumors*)

HISTORICAL COMMENTS

In *Atlas of Materia Medica*, Li Shicai said that: "The drug is very violent in action, and therefore it is called a 'general commander'."

It is reported in *Confucian Medicine* that: "The drug bears a bitter taste and a fragrant odor, therefore it is used both as a tonic and a purgative. In fact, it is usually used as a purgative to treat dyspepsia or hyperhydrochloria."

It is said in *Materia Medica* that: "The drug is effective in curing hematostasis, amenia, cold-heat syndrome, abdominal mass, dyspepsia, constipation, damp-heat accumulation in the lower part of the body and disorder of the viscera." In the book, is recorded a prescription for curing uterine cancer: 30g of the drug is decocted in wine for oral taking. Another prescription recorded in the book is for breast tumor: 30g of the drug and 30g of Radix Glycyrrhizae are ground and decocted in wine into a paste for application to the lesion with a handkerchief and also for oral administration one spoonful a time.

It is reported in *Guide to Materia Medica* that: "The drug is forbidden for patients with deficiency of the stomach and the blood, when the disease develops to the *qi* phase. The functions of the drug are different when steeped in wine, steamed in wine, processed and unprocessed. The unprocessed drug is especially violent in action, therefore, Radix Scutellariae must be added as guiding element."

THE AUTHOR'S NOTE

In Zhongshan Hospital affiliated to Shanghai First Medical University, 14 cases of acute leukemia were treated with the drug and Semen Strychni as the main ingredients accompanied with Compound Cytarabine. The result was that 1 case of acute granulocytic leukemia was alleviated, 4 partially alleviated, 1 case of acute lymphatic leukemia and 2 cases of acute monocytic leukemia partially alleviated. The total alleviated rate was 57.1%. Orally administration of the crude drug powder has been proved to be very effective in stopping bleeding of the upper digestive tract, and the effective rate is reported to be 97.25%. It was reported in *Journal of Zhejiang Traditional Chinese Medicine* (Vol. 3, 1980) that a case of violent bleeding caused by an operation on colocancer, was cured with 9 grams of the drug powder blended with 140ml of salt water for enema, after the failure of transfusion of 1000ml of blood in three times and other therapies.

RADIX ET FOLIUM DOLICHI

It is defined in *Medicinal Herbs in Yunnan* that: "The drug is hot in taste, warm and toxic in nature, stopping hemorrhage to invigorate muscles, and subsiding inflammation to ease pain."

The drug is the leave or the root of *Dolichos falcatus klein* of the *Leguminosae* family, and its root contains triterpenoidal saponins and alkaloids. The drug is produced in Yunnan and Guangdong provinces.

ANTICANCER PHARMACOLOGICAL FUNCTIONS

1. The extract of the root of the drug evidently inhibits cellular respiration of the tissue of many transplanted tumors in mice.

2. The drug selectively damages cancer cells, with its effective element being saponins glucoside.

EXPERIMENTAL FORMULAS

For cervical cancer:

When pounded and applied to the lesion, the root of the drug is effective in reducing the size of the tumor, subsiding inflammation and stopping hemorrhage. (*Traditional Chinese Medicine Pharmacological Correspondence*, Vol. 2, 1977)

For bloody defecation caused by rectocancer:

3 to 9 grams of the calcined drug is decocted and taken three times a day orally. (*Medicinal Herbs in the Wen Mountains*)

HISTORICAL COMMENTS

Dictionary of Chinese Materia Medica says that: "The drug eases pain, subsides inflammation, stops hemorrhage, cures pain caused by wind-wetness, trauma, fracture, bleeding caused by exogenous factors, rhinorrhagia, blood-vomiting and bloody defecation, when 3 to 9 grams of the drug (15-30g when fresh) is decocted or steeped in wine for oral taking, or ground into powder for application to the lesion."

Medicinal Herbs in the Wen Mountains says that: "The drug promotes blood circulation to eliminate stasis and stops pain by subsiding inflammation and hemorrhage caused by trauma, when the pounded fresh leaves or the powder is applied to the lesion."

Selected Medicinal Herbs in Yunnan says that: "Pain due to wind-wetness and trauma can be treated with 6 grams of the drug steeped in wine for taking several times or 15-30g of the drug decocted and taken twice a day."

RADIX SOPHORAE SUBPROSTRATAE

Wang Ang in the Qing Dynasty said that: "The drug is bitter in taste and cold in nature, clearing away heat accumulated in the heart to protect the lung energy."

The drug is the dried root or rhizoma of *Sophora subprostrata* of the *Leguminosae* family, and mainly produced in Guangxi, Jiangxi and Guizhou. *Menispermum dauricum DC.* of the *Menispermaceae* family shares the same name with the drug in Chinese, but it does not resist cancer.

ANTICANCER PHARMACOLOGICAL FUNCTIONS

1. Animal experiment shows that the effect exerted by the drug on cancer is similar to that of immunity.

2. The hot water extract of the drug evidently inhibits cervical cancer.

3. Matrine and oxymatrine in the drug can prolong the life of mice with sarcoma-180, and trifolirhizin also bears this function.

4. Experiments with the drug on mice suffering from sarcoma and ascites hepatoma-180 showed that it cures the disease with an effective rate of 60%, and is effective in prolonging the survival of the dying rats and in resisting tumor. Oncological antigen has been found in the serum of the cured rats, and it is inheritable.

5. Methylene blue tube test with 2 grams of the crude drug per milliliter showed that the drug inhibits the cells of leukemia.

6. It is reported that the drug can stimulate the reticuloendothelial system.

7. The drug evidently inhibits transplanted cervical cancer-14, when the extract of the drug is administrate to mice orally with a dose of 60g/kg a day, for totally 16 to 21 days.

8. The efficiency of oxymatrine in chemotherapy is 7 or 8 times higher than that of Mitomycin C.

EXPERIMENTAL FORMULAS

For all kinds of cancer:

The paste or the liquid made from the drug are administered with a proper dosage. (*Medical Reference*, Vol. 2, 1972)

For laryngeal cancer:

        Radix Sophorae subprostratae 15g

        Radix Scrophulariae 15g

        Folium Isatidis 15g

        Radix Fagopyri 30g

The prescription is taken one dosage a day in decoction. (*Handbook of Practical Anticancer Drugs*)

For esophageal cancer:

        Radix Sophorae subprostratae 10g

        Flos Inulae 10g

        Haematitum 10g

        Semen Raphani 15g

        Radix Curcumae 10g

        Fructus Trichosanthis 20g

        Semen Canavaliae gladiatae 15g

        Rhizoma Paridis 20g

        Pericarpium Citri Reticulatae 10g

(*Traditional Chinese Medicine Oncology*)

For trophoblastic tumor:

The injection made from the drug is given intramuscularly. (*Journal of New Traditional Chinese Medicine*, Vol. 5, 1978)

HISTORICAL COMMENTS

It is reported in *Materia Medica* that: "The drug removes toxic materials in many drugs, stops pain, subsides inflammation and stops cough, cures pharyngitis when sucked, eliminates abdominal distension when ground and taken orally, relieves female abdominal distention due to the stagnation of blood when taken with wine, and treats baldness, snake bite, dog bite or spider bite when squeezed to get a juice for application to the lesion. For esophageal cancer and pharyngeal cancer, the drug is ground with vinegar for sucking."

It is said in *Elucidation on Materia Medica* that: "The drug is sweet-bitter in taste, cold and non-toxic in nature. It neutralizes toxicity with its sweet taste and eliminates heat with its cold nature. Toxic drugs are usually hot and sweet, and is removed spontaneously when combined with drugs that are cold, sweet and bitter." "The drug also cures breast cancer."

THE AUTHOR'S NOTE

It was defined in ancient times that: "The vines of the herb are evergreen and similar to those of a bean." It is certain that the herb belongs to the bean family, not the *Menispermaceae* family. The herb is a broad-spectrum anticancer drug, resisting different kinds of tumors. However it cannot be administered for a long time because of its bitter taste and cold nature. It was reported by the Ci County Anticancer Bureau, Hebei Province, that the effect of the drug on cancer tissues is different from that of the cellular toxicity and the anti-metabolism of the chemotherapeutic agents. The drug works through stimulating the anticancer immune mechanism of the patient and reinforcing his resistance against the growth of tumor. A patient suffering from severe headache caused by angioma in the left eye was treated with the drug together with Radix Amebiae, Radix Glycyrrhizae and Radix Semiaquilegiae. After taking 20 doses, the patient was relieved from headache and the eyesight was greatly improved.

It was reported in *Medical Abstract* (Vol. 4, 1960) that the drug produced in Japan was evidently effective in treating malignant tumor with no side-effect and danger to reduce the leukocytes. Animal experiments showed that the drug is safe for clinical use. A renowned Japanese doctor often prescribed the drug to treat cancer and has achieved certain curative effect. 17 cases of leukemia were treated with the drug in a hospital affiliated to Jiangxi Medical College and it was found significantly effective in 3 cases, and effective in 8 cases with different improvement of their condition. 30 cases of cervical cancer and laryngeal cancer were treated with the drug and the effect was evident. (*Hunan Medical Journal*, Vol. 5, 1977). In *Medical Essays* compiled by Wu Shangda in the Qing Dynasty, is recorded a prescription containing the drug for anal cancer:

Fructus Arctii
Radix Scutellariae
Cormus Iphigeniae
Scorpio
Flos Carthami
Radix Paeoniae Lactiflorae
Rhizoma Pinelliae
Semen Pruni Armeniacae
Radix Trichosanthis
Radix Kansui
Radix Euphorbiae Pekinensis
Periostracum Cicadae
Periostracum Serpentis
Radix et Rhizoma Rhei
Radix Sophorae Flavescentis

All the above herbs are effective against cancer and the prescription should be popularized and inherited.

LIGNUM ET RADIX ACRONYCHIAE

It is defined in *Handbook of Commonly Used Medicinal Herbs* that: "The drug is sweet in taste and mild in nature, invigorating *qi* to activate blood circulation."

The drug is the fruit, leaf, wood or root of a plant of *Acronychia pedunculata (L.) Miq.* of the *Rutaceae* family, containing ß-sitosterol in the wood, bauerenol and acronycine in the bark and volatile oil in the leaf, and being mainly produced in Guangdong, Guangxi, Yunnan, Guizhou and Taiwan.

ANTICANCER PHARMACOLOGICAL FUNCTIONS

1. Acronycine is significantly effective in treating reticulocytic leukemia-615. Oral administration of 40mg/kg will ensure mice with over 60 days of survival and with a curative effect of 100%.

2. The drug is effective in treating reticulohistiocytoma.

3. The drug inhibits mice liver cancer with an average effective rate of 52.5%.

4. The drug, administrated orally, inhibits mice cervical cancer-14 with an effective rate of 57.1%.

5. The drug inhibits the activity of animal myeloid leukemia-1499, plasma cell myeloma and adenocancer-755.

6. No change of body weight was seen in the mice in the above experiments, and after oral administration of the drug, no reactions of the digestive tract and no falling of their hair were observed in the animals.

7. Its anticancer mechanism lies in its inhibition of the carcinocytic synthesis of nuclear acid, but the drug shows no influence on normal nuclear acid of the animals.

EXPERIMENTAL FORMULAS

For stomach cancer, Hodgkin's disease, fibrosarcoma of bone, fibrosarcoma and liposarcoma:

Acronycine is taken orally 50mg a time and 2 to 3 times a day. 4 weeks make up a course of treatment. This drug is especially effective for Hodgkin's disease, the tumor of which will be reduced one or two weeks after the drug taken. (*Chinese Herbal and Medical Correspondence*, Vol. 11, 1977)

For various cancer:

15-30g of the bark of the root or tree is decocted or ground for oral administration. (*Dictionary of Chinese Materia Medica*)

HISTORICAL COMMENTS

Nomenclature of Medicinal Plants in Guangxi says that: "The twig and the leaf of the plant indicate for furuncle, sore and swelling; and the fruit promotes the circulation of *qi* to expel phlegm."

Handbook of Commonly Used Medicinal Herbs says that: "The twig and the leaf cure cough and trauma; the fruit cures dyspepsia; the internal wood or the root promotes the circulation of *qi* to invigorate the blood, activates the spleen and stops cough. The drug also cures lumbago, pain of the leg due to wind-wetness, pain due to trauma and gastralgia due to the stagnation of *qi*."

THE AUTHOR'S NOTE

Science of Medicinal Herbs (Vol. 8, 1966) reported that Acronycine extracted from a plant of the same family resists tumor and out of 17 oncological experiments, it showed significant curative effect in 12 experiments with cancers such as myelocytic leukemia C-1498, which are not sensitive to chemotherapy. A traditional herb with the same name in Chinese is not the drug, but *Dalbergia Sisso Roxb*.

FOLIUM PRUNI DAVIDIANAE

It is defined in *Collection of Comments on Materia Medica* that: "The drug is bitter in taste and mild in nature, curing amenorrhea and abdominal mass."

The drug is the leaf of *Prunus davidiana* (*Carr.*) *Franch* of the *Rosaceae* family, containing glucoside, naringenin, lycopene and cynogenic glycosides. *Prunus persica* (*L.*) *batsch* of the same family shares the same function.

ANTICANCER PHARMACOLOGICAL FUNCTIONS

1. The average inhibiting rate of the drug on mice sarcoma-180 is 41%.

2. Decoction of the drug reduces the enlarged spleen of mice with acute reticulocytic leukemia-615.

3. The powder or the 5% paste of the drug is effective in treating vaginal trichomoniasis. The paste shows a curative effect of 100%. It is thought that some insecticides are against the activity of cancer, because carcinocytic membrane is similar to the body membrane of insects in structure.

EXPERIMENTAL FORMULAS

For cervical cancer:

The leaf is pounded, wrapped and inserted into the vagina 3 to 4 times a day. (*Mengxi Prescriptions for Vaginal Sore*).

For nasal cancer:

The fresh internal part of the drug is pounded and applied to the nose frequently. (*Simple Prescriptions*)

HISTORICAL COMMENTS

Ri Hua Zhi Materia Medica says that: "The drug cures vomiting and high fever alternated with chill sensation."

Materia Medica says that: "The drug cures exogenous febrile disease, anhidrosis due to arthralgia caused by wind factors, headache, difficult urination and defecation and the abdominal pain due to cholera."

Collection of Folk Prescriptions in Guizhou says that: "The drug cures wind-wet syndrome when decocted for washing the body, and external application of the drug subsides inflammation."

Dictionary of Chinese Materia Medica says that: "Sores can be cured with 25kg of the drug steeped in 50kg of water, boiled for an hour, filtrated, boiled again into a paste and applied to the lesion 1 to 2 times a day."

RADIX CODONOPSIS LANCEOLATAE

It is defined in *Newly Compiled Materia Medica in Zhenan* that: "The drug is sweet in taste and mild in nature, clearing away heat in the lung, nourishing *yin* and removing toxic materials through expelling pus."

The drug is the root of *Codonopsis lanceolata Benth. et Hook.* of the *Campanulaceae* family, containing saponins, saccharides, protein and vitamin B, and is produced in most regions of China.

ANTICANCER PHARMACOLOGICAL FUNCTIONS
The drug inhibits the activity of transplanted sarcoma-180 of mice.

EXPERIMENTAL FORMULAS
For lung cancer:

> Radix Codonopsis Lanceolatae 30g
> Herba Houttuyniae 30g
> Herba Oldenlandiae Diffusae 30g
> Radix Codonopsis Pilosulae 12g
> Rhizoma Atractylodis Macrocephalae 12g
> Nidus Vespae 12g
> Poria 15g
> Polyporus 15g
> Semen Coicis 15g

The prescription is taken one dosage a day in decoction. (*Journal of Shanghai Traditional Chinese Medicine*, Vol. 3, 1979)

For thyroid cancer:

> Radix Codonopsis Lanceolatae 30g
> Spica Prunellae 9g
> Sargassum 9g
> Thallus Laminariae seu Eckloniae 9g
> Spina Gleditsiae 9g
> Squama Manitis 9g
> Cortex Moutan 6g
> Cormus Iphigeniae 6g
> Semen Sinapis 2.4g

The prescription is taken in decoction. (*Handbook of Tumor Prevention and Treatment with Chinese Medicinal Herbs*)

HISTORICAL COMMENTS
Records of Famous Doctors says that: "The drug cures dizziness, promotes *qi* and muscles."

Supplementation to Materia Medica says that: "The drug cures scrofula when the juice is administered with wine and the residue applied to the lesion."

Newly Compiled Materia Medica in Zhenan says that: "The drug is inferior to Radix Codonopsis pilosulae in reinforcing *qi*, but is superior in promoting moisture; inferior to Radix Adenophorae in nourishing the stomach to invigorate *yin*, but superior in promoting *yin* and lactation and removing toxic materials."

THE AUTHOR'S NOTE
Experiments on the comparison between the drug and Radix Codonopsis Pilosulae showed that both of them are capable of increasing erythrocytes and hemochrome, decreasing leukocytes and reinforcing the activity of the animals. But mice swimming experiment showed that the drug was superior to Radix Codonopsis Pilosulae. In treating patients with tumor characterized by deficiency of *qi* and blood, the author often uses large doses of the drug and Fructus Ziziphi Jupjubae and the effect is excellent.

CORMUS IPHIGENIAE

Miao Xiyong in the Ming Dynasty said that: "The drug is hot in taste and cold in nature, clearing away heat and subsiding inflammation."

The drug is obtained from Iphigenia indica *Kunth.* of the *Liliaceae* family, and is mainly produced in Yunnan and Tibet. The main element of the drug is colchicine.

ANTICANCER PHARMACOLOGICAL FUNCTIONS
1. Colchicine inhibits cellular mitochysis.
2. The external culture liquid when condensed to $0.1\mu g/ml$ affects mitochysis and resists cancer.
3. Demecolcine has a special function against cancer.
4. The drug inhibits carcinocytes in the blood to reduce the chances of metastasis of cancer through blood.
5. The drug inhibits sarcoma-180, cancer-256, solid liver cancer and lymphosarcoma, and also resists radiation.

EXPERIMENTAL FORMULAS
For thyroid cancer:
        Cormus Iphigeniae 4.5g
        Spica Prunellae 9g
        Sargassum 9g
        Thallus Laminariae seu Eckloniae 9g
        Lapis Pumicis 9g
        Rhizoma Pinelliae 9g
        Bulbus Fritillariae Thunbergii 9g
        Radix Angelicae Sinensis 9g
        Rhizoma Cyperi 9g
        Rhizoma Dioscoreae Bulbiferae 15g
        Pericarpium Citri Reticulatae 4.5g
The prescription is taken one dosage a day in decoction. (*Journal of New Traditional Chinese Medicine*, Vol. 2, 1980)
For various cancer accompanied with pain:
        Cormus Iphigeniae 30g
        Radix Notoginseng 30g
        Rhizoma Paridis 30g

Rhizoma Corydalis 30g
Rhizoma Dioscoreae Bulbiferae 30g
Radix Aconiti 30g
Borneol 9g

The prescription is ground into powder and taken 3g a time and three times a day. (*Diagnosis and Treatment of Tumor*)

For unulcerous breast cancer:
Cormus Iphigeniae 30g
Bulbus Bolbostemmae 15g
Galla Chinensis 15g
Radix Angelicae Pubescentis 15g
Rhizoma Cyperi 15g
Rhizoma Arisaematis 15g
Rhizoma Pinelliae 15g

The prescription is ground into powder to be blended with vinegar into a paste for application to the lesion. The treatment is renewed once a day. (*Journal of Jiangsu Traditional Chinese Medicine*, Vol. 1, 1958)

For skin cancer and breast cancer:
The fresh drug is pounded, mixed with millet vinegar and applied to the lesion. Chinese Injection-81 made from Colchicine is very effective in treating cancer. (*Tianjin Medical Journal*, Vol. 2, 1973)

For breast cancer:
Cormus Iphigeniae 9g
Sargassum 30g
Herba Taraxaci 30g

The prescription is taken one dosage a day in decoction. (*Handbook of Practical Anticancer Drugs*)

For esophageal cancer and stomach cancer:
120g of the drug is washed, decocted in water, then mixed with 120g of white honey to make a paste for oral administration 9-15g a time and twice a day. (*Collection of Experienced Prescriptions of Traditional Chinese Medicine*)

HISTORICAL COMMENTS

Guide to Materia Medica says that: "The drug is especially effective in clearing away pathogenic heat to disperse stasis, curing furuncles, sores, inflammation, scrofula, snake and dog bite."

True Materia Medica says that: "The drug can be used externally and internally to treat furuncle, carbuncle, urticaria, malignant sore, snake bite and scrofula. But the drug cannot be taken in large dose because of its cold nature."

THE AUTHOR'S NOTE

Colchicine is neutral and dissolvable in water, different from any other kinds of alkaloid substances. 90 cases of breast cancer were treated in Tianjin People's Hospital with a colchicine preparation, and 66.6% of the patients survived for over 5 year. In addition, colchicine may cause vomiting, poor appetite, abdominal distention and constipation. Sometimes it even causes intestine disorder and numbness of the four extremities. The drug may also result in leukopenia and reduction of the platelets, but seldom results in serious osteomyelitis which will disappear spontaneously after the cessation of the drug. The drug can still cause phlebitis and necrosis of the local tissues if the liquid of the drug leaks out of the vein. The drug is forbidden for patients with week physique, poor liver function and cardiovascular diseases.

FRUCTUS CRATAEGI

It is defined in *Daily Materia Medica* that: "The drug is sweet-sour in taste and non-toxic in nature, removing hemostasis and the *qi* stagnation."

The drug is the fruit of *Crataegus pinnatifida Bge.*, *C. cuneata Sieb. et Zucc.* of the *Rosaceae* family. Citric acid of the latter contains malic acid, crataegolic acid, tannins, saponins and vitamin C. The fruit of *Crataegus pinnatifida Bge.* contains amygdalin.

ANTICANCER PHARMACOLOGICAL FUNCTIONS

1. The decoction of sliced *Crataegus pinnatifida Bge.* can prolong the life of animals with transplanted tumor.

2. The drug resists bacteriophage, this indicating that it inhibits the activity of cancer.

3. The drug evidently inhibits the cells of mice ascites cancer.

4. The decoction of the drug's fruit inhibits JTC-26 with an effective rate of 50-70% in the external experiments.

EXPERIMENTAL FORMULAS

For osteocancer:

      Fructus Crataegi 30g
      Radix Astragali 30g
      Poria 30g
      Semen Coicis 30g
      Herba Oldenlandiae Diffusae 30g
      Radix Angelicae Sinensis 10g
      Radix Trichosanthis 10g
      Rhizoma Cibotii 12g
      Radix Dipsaci 12g
      Rhizoma Dioscoreae Bulbiferae 12g
      Fructus Mume 10g
      Rhizoma Dioscoreae 15g

The prescription is taken one dosage a day in decoction. (*Journal of Hubei Traditional Chinese Medicine*, Vol. 6, 1980)

For reinforcement after the operation of stomach cancer:

      Fructus Crataegi 12g
      Poria 12g
      Massa Medicata Fermentata 12g
      Radix Codonopsis Pilosulae 12g
      Radix Astragali 15g
      Rhizoma Paridis 15g
      Rhizoma Atractylodis Macrocephalae 10g
      Radix Paeoniae Lactiflorae 10g
      Radix Paeoniae Alba 10g
      Fructus Hordei Germinatus 10g
      Fructus Oryzae Germinatus 10g
      Fructus Aurantii Immaturus 10g
      Pericarpium Citri Reticulatae 10g
      Radix Actinidiae Chinensis 60g

The prescription is taken one dosage a day in decoction. (*Journal of Hubei Traditional Chinese Medicine*, Vol. 1, 1979)

For stomach cancer:

> Calcined Fructus Crataegi 500g
>
> Fructus Mume 500g
>
> Roasted Rhizoma Dioscoreae 2000g
>
> Poria 250g

The herbs are ground into powder, mixed up with honey to make pills of 6g each. Three pills are taken daily after each meal. (*Journal of Shaanxi Traditional Chinese Medicine*)

For ovarian cancer:

> Fructus Crataegi 30g
>
> Herba Leonuri 15g
>
> Radix Angelicae Sinensis 9g
>
> Rhizoma Corydalis 9g
>
> Radix Arnebiae 9g
>
> Rhizoma Chuanxiong 6g

The prescription is taken one dosage a day in decoction. (*Introduction to Oncology*)

For chorioepithelial cancer:

> Fructus Crataegi 18g
>
> Radix Angelicae Sinensis 9g
>
> Herba Lycopi 9g
>
> Zujia 9g
>
> Poria 12g
>
> Radix Salviae Miltiorrhizae 15g
>
> Nidus Vespae 6g

The prescription is taken one dosage a day in decoction and 5 days will make one course of treatment. (*Anticancer Preparation in Traditional Chinese Medicine*)

HISTORICAL COMMENTS

Materia Medica says that: "The drug promotes digestion, digests accumulated meat and cures phlegm-distention and hemostasis."

Records of Integrated Western and Chinese Medicine says that: "The drug accompanied with drugs of sweet taste removes hemostasis without damaging the new blood, expels the stagnation of *qi* without damaging the vital energy. The nature of the drug is especially mild."

History of Herbs Reinforcing Each Other says that: "The fruit helps cooking old chickens when several of it added."

PROSPIROBOLUS

Li Shizhen in the Ming Dynasty said that: "The drug is hot in taste, warm and toxic in nature, curing malaria."

The drug is obtained from *Prospirobolus joannsi* of the *Prospirobolus* genus and the *Strongylosomidae* family. Its secretion contains cyanic acid and quinoid substances, and resists cancer.

ANTICANCER PHARMACOLOGICAL FUNCTIONS

1. Paste made with the drug is proved to be effective in inhibiting mice sarcoma-180.

2. The curative effect of the drug (33.3%) is similar to that of Bleomycin (36.4%) in treating experimental squamous carcinoma of mice.

3. The content abstracted with dimethyladenine inhibits mice spermatocytes, this indicating that it resists the activity of cancer.

EXPERIMENTAL FORMULAS

For dermatocancer:

    Prospirobolus 18g

    Semen Ricini 6g

    Old Lime 3g

    Powder of tobacco 3g

    Radix Boehmeriae 18g

The paste made from the prescription is applied to the lesion once a day or once the other day. (*Sichuan Traditional Chinese Medicine Correspondence*, Vol. 1. 1974)

HISTORICAL COMMENTS

Materia Medica says that: "The drug, seldom used in ancient times, mainly cures abdominal cancer, stagnation, polyp, malignant sore, tinea capitis, heat accumulated in the abdomen, abdominal distention and malaria." "The drug is only for external use because of its toxicity."

THE AUTHOR'S NOTE

It is reported in *Traditional Chinese Medicine Research Reference* that 64 cases of dermatocancer were treated with a paste made with the drug from 1972-1976 in Sichuan Antibiotic Industry Academy. The total effect was 38.6%

SEMEN STRYCHNI

It is defined in *Dictionary of Chinese Materia Medica* that: "The drug is bitter in taste, cold and toxic in nature, clearing away heat accumulated in blood and subsiding swelling to stop pain."

The drug is the fruit of *Strychnos nux-vomica L.* of the *Loganiaceae* family, mainly produced in Yunnan. *S. wallichiana Steud. ex DC.* of the same family, produced in India, Sikkim and Hainan Island in China, is used as the substitute for the drug.

ANTICANCER PHARMACOLOGICAL FUNCTIONS

1. The drug inhibits mice sarcoma-180.

2. The drug inhibits the activity of the cells of leukemia.

EXPERIMENTAL FORMULAS

For acute leukemia:

    Semen Strychni 1.5g

    Radix Glycyrrhizae 4g

    Rhizoma Paridis 12g

    Radix Sophorae Subprostratae 9g

    Rhizoma Belamcandae 6g

    Radix Rubiae 9g

    Radix Angelicae Sinensis 6g

    Radix Codonopsis Pilosulae 6g

    Radix Astragali 30g

    Herba Pteridis Multifidae 16g

    Calculus Bovis 0.6g

The prescription is taken in decoction one dosage a day. (*Research and Prevention of Tumor*, Vol. 2, 1976)

For dermatocancer:

Semen Strychni

Radix Arnebiae

Scolopendra

Rhizoma Polygoni Vivipari

Equal portions of the above herbs are made into a paste and applied to the lesion three times a day.

For uterine cancer:

Semen Strychni

Semen Persicae

Lacca Sinica Exsiccata

Agkistrodon

Pericarpium Zanthoxyli Bungeani

Radix et Rhizoma Rhei

Scolopendra

Scorpio

Equal portion of the above herbs and two portions of Radix et Rhizoma Rhei are ground and made into pills with honey. 3 pills are taken a day. Patients with weak physique should take the pills with great caution. (*Journal of Jiangsu Traditional Chinese Medicine*, Vol. 7, 1960)

For nasopharyngeal cancer, cancer on the digestive tract and breast cancer:

Semen Strychni 9g

Radix Glycyrrhizae 2.5g

Rhizoma Chuanxiong 6g

Realgar 3g

Squama Manitis 9g

Radix Angelicae Sinensis 9g

Cornu Rhinoceri 6g

Scorpio 6g

Scolopendra 6g

Semen Strychni is roasted yellow in oil, ground into powder with other ingredients and rolled with honey into pills of 1.5g each. The pills are taken one a time and twice a day. (*Diagnosis and Treatment of Tumor*)

For anal cancer:

The drug is ground into powder, blended with vinegar and applied to the lesion. (*Handbook of Practical Anti-cancer Drugs*)

For brain cancer:

Semen Strychni 120g

Scorpio 30g

Herba Ephedrae 15g

Rhizoma Gastrodiae 15g

Radix Glycyrrhizae 15g

Radix Aucklandiae 15g

Pericarpium Citri Reticulatae 15g

Rhizoma seu Radix Notopterygii 15g

Cortex Eucommiae 15g

Olibanum 15g

Myrrha 15g

Radix Morindae Officinalis 15g

The prescription is ground into powder, blended with old vinegar and flour and made into pills of mung bean size. The pills are taken 0.3-0.5g after each meal with boiled water and three times a day.

There should be one day interval after each six days of administration. The dose can not be increased. (*National Collection of Prescriptions of Famous Doctors in Traditional Chinese Medicine*)

For cancer on the digestive tract:

30 grams of Semen Strychni is steeped in water and then, peeled, dried, cut into slices, roasted yellow in sesame oil, ground into powder with 9 grams of Radix Glycyrrhizae and made into pills with rice flour coating of the size of Semen Firmianae. The pills are taken 0.3-0.6g a time and 2 to 3 times a day with boiled water. (*National Collection of Prescriptions of Famous Doctors in Traditional Chinese Medicine*)

HISTORICAL COMMENTS

It is recorded in *Tang Yao's Experienced Prescriptions* that: "To cure pharyngitis, one of the drug and 0.9 gram of Radix Auckandiae are ground with water and then mixed with 9 grams of Fel Ursi and 1.5 gram of Chalcanthitum for application to the throat."

It is said in *Selected Prescriptions of Yang Qi's Recipes* that: "Radix Aucklandiae and Radix Sophorae Subprostratae, when ground and blown into the throat, is effective for pharyngitis."

It is reported in *Materia Medica* that: "The drug cures exogenous febrile disease, pharyngitis and abdominal mass when sucked."

It is said in *Origin of Materia Medica* that: "The drug is violently toxic for birds, dogs and human beings."

It is suggested in *Elucidation on Materia Medica* that: "The drug is forbidden for patients with deficiency of qi, blood, spleen and stomach."

THE AUTHOR'S NOTE

54 cases of esophageal cancer were treated with the drug in the Second Hospital in Luda City and it was found effective in 45 cases, not effective in 5 and 3 patients became worse after the administration and 1 died. The total effect rate was 83.3%.

The drug is highly toxic, therefore it must be used with great caution. Emergent measures for its poisoning: 1) 1:2000 $KMnO_4$ for gastric lavage; 2) Ether for mild anesthesia or barbital for intravenous injection if convulsion occurs; 3) Morphine is forbidden; 4) The patient is moved to a darkroom to prevent convulsion.

The toxic element is strychnine, 5-10mg of which will result in poisoning and 30mg will cause death. Therefore, the drug must be processed before using. The procession pattern is: boiled first, steeped in water, stripped off the peel, cut into slices, and roasted yellow in sesame oil.

SEMEN IRIDIS

It is defined in *Canon of Materia Medica* that: "The drug is sweet in taste and mild in nature, clearing away heat accumulated under the skin and in the stomach."

The drug is obtained from the seed of *Iris lactae Pall. var. chinensis Koidz* of the *Iridaceae* family, and ranked as the top medicine in *Shennong's Pharmacopoeia*.

ANTICANCER PHARMACOLOGICAL FUNCTIONS

1. Pallason A extracted from the drug inhibits acute leukemia and solid tumor.

2. Its anticancer mechanism lies in its inhibition of ^3H-TdR's penetration, affecting the synthesis of DNA in cancer cells.

3. Immune experiment indicates that the drug can reinforce non- specific immunological macrophagic function, promoting cell immunity.

4. The drug inhibits the cells of mice cervical cancer-14, ascites cancer, lymphosarcoma, solid and ascites liver cancer.

EXPERIMENTAL FORMULAS

For cervical cancer:

        Semen Iridis 6g

        Fructus Ailanthi 6g

        Herba Equiseti Hiemalis 9g

        Herba Indigoferae 15g

        Herba Houttuyniae 15g

        Caulis Sargentodoxae 15g

        Os Sepiae 24g

        Rhizoma Smilacis Glabrae 24g

        Radix Damnacanthi 30g

        Radix Loropetali 30g

The prescription is taken in decoction one dosage a day. (*Introduction to Oncology*)

HISTORICAL COMMENTS

Tang Materia Medica says that: "The drug cures incised wound and furuncle."

Ri Hua Zhi Materia Medica says that: "The drug cures upsetness caused by menopathy."

Medical Compilation says that: "The drug eliminates hemostasis and disperses mass."

Explanation on Materia Medica says that: "The drug is special for eliminating stagnation. For cold-deficiency syndrome, the drug is forbidden."

FRUCTUS TRITICI LEVIS

It is defined in *Chinese Medical Dictionary* that: "The drug is hot in taste, cold and non-toxic in nature, curing skin verrucosis and nevus, and decayed muscles."

The drug is obtained from wheat stalk of the *Gramineae* family, produced in the regions North of the Yellow River, containing cellulose and polysaccharides.

ANTICANCER PHARMACOLOGICAL FUNCTIONS

1. Polysaccharides inhibits mice sarcoma-180 with an effective rate of 85-100%, when used with a dose of 100-200mg/kg.

2. Polysaccharides can stimulate the reticuloendothelial system, increase the immune reaction of the host against the specific antigen of the cancer cells.

3. Bacteriophagic screening test shows that the drug resists bacteriophage, indicating that it is against the activity of cancer.

4. Celiac injection of polysaccharides extracted from wheat bran for ten days inhibits white mice sarcoma-180 (250 mg/kg) with an effective rate of 61.9%.

5. The extract from the leaves and the roots can selectively inhibit sudden variation of carcinogenic material in Ames experiment.

6. Phytohemagglutinin extracted from the malt can directly agglutinize cells of lymphoma and ascites cancer, this indicating that is can kill cancer cells.

EXPERIMENTAL FORMULAS

For thyroid tumor:

Wheat flour and fresh Folium Artemisiae Argyi are made into steamed cake for oral taking daily. (*Anticancer Consultation*)

For yellowish skull cancer:

Fructus Tritici Levis 30g
Radix Codonopsis Pilosulae 10g
Radix Paeoniae Alba 10g
Rhizoma Atractylodis Macrocephalae 10g
Poria 10g
Radix Angelicae Sinensis 10g
Fragmenta Cornus Cervi 10g
Rhizoma Deynariae 10g
Fructus Psoraleae 10g
Herba Taxilli 15g
Fructus Ligustri Lucidi 15g
Radix Glycyrrhizae 6g

The prescription is taken one dosage a day in decoction. (*Journal of Shanghai Traditional Chinese Medicine*, Vol. 5, 1980)

For acute mononuclear cellular leukemia:

Fructus Tritici Levis 30g
Fructus Corni 30g
Concha Ostreae 30g
Radix Rehmanniae 30g
Radix Adenophorae 30g
Radix Codonopsis pilosulae 30g
Radix Ginseng 12g
Rhizoma Dioscoreae 15g
Radix Paeoniae Alba 9g
Radix Glycyrrhizae 9g
Radix Ophiopogonis 9g
Fossilia Ossis Mastodi 9g
Semen Ziziphi Spinosae 9g
Fructus Schisandrae 3g
Fructus Ziziphi Inermis 10

The prescription is taken one dosage a day in decoction. (*Medical Research Correspondence*, Vol. 7-9, 1973)

HISTORICAL COMMENTS

Ri Hua Zhi Materia Medica says that: "The young wheat can eliminate restlessness, clear away extreme heat, cure pestilence and calm the small intestine."

Supplementation to Materia Medica says that: "The drug cures jaundice and drunkenness."

THE AUTHOR'S NOTE

To treat patients suffering from cancer with the deficient of heat, the author often, a part from the normal prescription, prescribes a handful of the young wheat for the patients to take as tea for clearing away heat and nourishing the vital energy. It is reported in *American and International News* that colocancer can be effectively prevented by taking 15 grams of wheat bran each day. It was also reported in *Traditional Chinese Medicine Research Information* (Vol. 6, 1978) that the drug was widely used in Japan to prevent and treat tumor.

HERBA CEPHALANOPLORIS

It is defined in *Dictionary of Chinese Materia Medica* that: "The drug is sweet in taste, warm and non-toxic in nature, nourishing the essence and invigorating the blood."

The drug is obtained from *Cephalanoplos segetum* (*Bge.*) *Kitam.* of the *Compositae* family, produced in most regions of China and used clinically with Herba seu Radix Cirsii Japonici. The extract of Cnicus bene dictus of the same family is used externally to treat dermatocancer in some foreign countries.

ANTICANCER PHARMACOLOGICAL FUNCTIONS
The drug inhibits ascites cancer.

EXPERIMENTAL FORMULAS
For uterine cancer:

        Herba Cephalanoploris 18g
        Herba seu Radix Cirsii Japonici 18g
        Herba Menthae 9g

The prescription is taken in decoction. (*Handbook of Medicinal Herbs in Northeast China*)
For cystocancer:

        Herba Cephalanoploris 30g
        Herba seu Radix Cirsii Japonici 30g
        Herba Scutellariae Barbatae 30g
        Pollen Typhae Carbonisatus 30g
        Semen Plantaginis Asiaticae 30g
        Rhizoma Dryopteris Crassirhizomae Carbonisatus 30g
        Flos Sophorae Immaturus Carbonisatus 30g
        Herba Oldenlandiae Diffusae 30g
        Rhizoma Anemarrhenae 12g
        Poria 12g
        Polyporus 12g
        Cortex Phellodendri 12g
        Radix Rehmanniae 12g

The prescription is taken in decoction one dosage a day. (*Practical Oncology*)
For various cancer:

15 grams of the whole herb is taken in decoction. (*Traditional Chinese Medicine Research Information*, Vol. 6, 1978)
For lymphosarcoma:

90 grams of the radix of the drug is decocted with thin pork. Both of the pork and the decoction are taken. The prescription is taken once a day. (*Journal of New Traditional Chinese Medicine*, Vol. 5, 1977)

        For malignant tumor of the bile duct:
        Herba Cephalanoploris 15g
        Spora Lygodii 12g
        Herba Artemisiae Capillaris 12g
        Radix Curcumae 12g
        Corium Stomachichum Galli 9g
        Radix Scutellariae 9g
        Radix Bupleuri 6g
        Radix Aucklandiae 9g

Radix Glycyrrhizae 6g

Herba Desmodii Styracifolii 30g

Radix Adinae 30g

The prescription is taken one dosage a day in decoction. (*Prevention and Treatment of Tumors*)

HISTORICAL COMMENTS

Tang Materia Medica says that: "Both Herba Cepholanoploris and Herba seu Radix Cirsii Japonici can eliminate hemostasis, but the former only focuses on treating blood disorder, while the latter subsides swelling."

Ri Hua Zhi Materia Medica says that: "The drug clears away heat, improves appetite and deficiency." The leaves of Herba seu Radix Cirsii Japonici eliminate abdominal hemostasis."

Prescriptions of Universal Relief says that: "Glossorrhagia can be cured by the drug when pounded with wine and taken orally."

CONCHA MERETRICIS

Chen Cunren said that: "The drug is salty in taste, mild and non-toxic in nature, curing ulcerous sore and hemorrhoids."

The drug is obtained from *Meretrix meretrix L.* of the *Veneridae* family. The shell is 3-10cm in length, large and thick, oval in the middle, protruding on the top, smooth on the surface and lustrous. The two shells are identical. The drug is produced in the areas near the sea.

ANTICANCER PHARMACOLOGICAL FUNCTIONS

1. The extract from the liver of Concha Meretricis can prolong the survival period of animals with Moloney leukemia.

2. The liquid extract from the tissue of Concha Meretricis with complex color inhibits mice sarcoma-180 with an effective rate of 30%, ascites cancer with an effective rate of 96-262.5%, ascites liver cancer and solid liver cancer with an effective rate of 40% or 50%.

3. Mercenene, a sort of sugar protein, extracted from edible Concha Meretricis, inhibits sarcoma-180 and ascites cancer-2, cures mice tumor induced by A_{12} and SV_{40} when injected into the tumor mass.

4. The water extract of the liver of Concha Meretricis evidently inhibits L_{1210} (cells of lymphatic leukemia).

EXPERIMENTAL FORMULAS

For thyroid cancer:

Sargassum

Concha Meretricis

Rapana

Os Sepiae

Thallus Laminariae seu Eckloniae

Equal portions of the above herbs are made into pills with honey. 2 of the pills are taken daily. (*Chinese Marine Medicinal Plants*)

For gastrocancer:

Concha Meretricis 15g

Concha Ostreae 15g

Sargassum 15g

Thallus Laminariae seu Eckloniae 15g

Thallus Porphyra 15g
The prescription is taken in decoction. (*Chinese Marine Medicinal Plants*)

HISTORICAL COMMENTS

It is reported in *Materia Medica* that: "The drug clears away pathogenic heat to promote drainage, eliminates phlegm and abdominal mass, cures bloody dysentery, abdominal blood stasis, perspiration seen in the exogenous febrile disease, convulsion and paralysis of limbs caused by apoplexy."

Supplementary Explanation on Materia Medica says that: "Menoxenia can be cured with meat of Concha meretricis."

RADIX TRICHOSANTHIS CUCUMEROIDIS

Yany Shitai in the Qing Dynasty said that: "The drug is bitter in taste and cold in nature, promoting blood circulation to expel hemostasis caused by heat accumulation."

The drug is obtained from a plant of the *Trichosanthes* genus and the *Cucurbitaceae* family, the root of which is for medical use. The drug is mainly produced in Jiangsu, Zhejiang, Hubei and Taiwan. In Jiangsu and Zhejiang, the peel of the fruit is used as Pericarpium Trichosanthis and the seed is used as Semen Trichosanthis.

ANTICANCER PHARMACOLOGICAL FUNCTIONS

1. Most of the plants of the *Cucurbitaceae* family contain cucurbitacin which has been proved to inhibit the respiration and anaerobic glycolysis of the cells of ascites cancer.
2. The drug inhibits cells ascites carcinoma, sarcoma-180 and JTC-26.

EXPERIMENTAL FORMULAS

For nasopharyngeal cancer:

10 grams of the drug is cut into slices, steeped in 25ml of 75% ethanol, added with 25ml of distilled water first and 50ml more three days later, and then filtrated out the residue with sterilized gauze and added with 20ml of glycerin. The preparation is dropped into the nose 3-6 times a day. This treatment may be accompanied with a prescription containing: 3 Scolopendra, 3 grams of Squama manitis, 3 grams of Eupolyphaga seu Steleophaga and 3 grams of Lumbricus, which are ground into powder, mixed with Radix Notoginseng Powder, millet wine and Xinyi Powder. The prescription is taken three times a day in decoction. (*Collection of Papers from a National Display of New Traditional Chinese Medicine Therapies*)

For gastrocancer cancer:

The drug and 6 grams of Gastrocalming Powder are decocted for oral taking. (*History of Sichuan Medicinal Herbs*)

For hematochezia due to enterocancer:

  Radix Trichosanthis Cucumeroidis 30g
  Radix Rehmanniae 60g
  Rhizoma Coptidis 15g

The prescription is made into honey-coated pills for oral administration 30 grams a time with millet porridge. (*Guiding Prescriptions*)

HISTORICAL COMMENTS

Canon of Compendium of Materia Medica says that: "The drug cures interior disorder and amenorrhea."

Records of Famous Doctors says that: "The drug clears away accumulated heat and subsides inflammation."

Compendium of Materia Medica says that: "The drug cures black complexion and facial sore."

Synopsis of Golden Chamber says that the drug cures leukorrhagia, menstrual disorder, and abdominal distension.

Introduction to Medicine says that: "The drug cures dysphagia."

Materia Medica for Daily Use says that: "The drug subsides swelling, cures jaundice, promotes lactation and menstruation."

THE AUTHOR'S NOTE

The drug used alone is effective in easing pain caused by cancer. 65 cases of pain due to trauma, operation and gastroenteric disorder were treated with pills made from the drug (0.5g-1g a time for adult) in Nongyai County, Fujian Province, 48 relieved and 11 improved, according to the report in *Collection of Papers from a National Display of New Traditional Chinese Medicine Therapies* in 1970. The effect was gained 5 to 30 minutes after the administration of the drug and continued for 0.5 to 72 hours.

CORIOLUS

It is defined in *Journal of New Traditional Chinese Medicine* that: "The drug is sweet in taste and slightly cold in nature, nourishing spleen to promote drainage and curing cancer."

The drug is the Sporphore or the Mycelium of *Coriolus* of the *Polyporaceae* family and it was found resisting cancer in 1979.

ANTICANCER PHARMACOLOGICAL FUNCTIONS

1. PS-K has been proved to resist cancer through reinforcing the specific immunofunctions of the tumor.

2. PS-K evidently increases delayed cutaneous hypersensitivity of mice with tumor.

3. The effect of PS-K against cancer agrees with the restoration of IgG generation.

4. The drug inhibits many tumors of experimental animals, such as cervical cancer-14, mice sarcoma-180, ascites cancer, adenocancer-755, lympholeukemic cell-7212 and lympholeukemic cell-388.

5. PS-K (200mg/kg) inhibits mice sarcoma-180 with an effective rate of 70.2-77.5% and reduces tumor size with an effective rate of 50-57%.

6. Intravenous injection of ATSO (1mg/kg) inhibits Swiss white mice sarcoma-180 with an effective rate of 99.3% and reduces tumor size with a 100% effective rate.

7. Coriolan obtained from the mycelia of the herb has a strong action against cancer, even stronger than ATSO and the coriolan obtained from Ganoderma and Polyporus. It inhibits mice sarcoma-180 with a 99.9% effective rate and reduces tumor mass with a 100% effective rate.

8. The effective rate of ATSO in resisting lung cancer is 77.2%, and that of Coriolan is 80.9%; and the effective rate of ATSO in inhibiting Shiono's carcinoma is 70.7% (for females) and 69.2% (for males), and that of Coriolan is 82.1% and 76.4% respectively.

9. Coriolan showed no evident effect on white mice without thoracic gland and hair when coriolan was administered with a dose of 100mg/kg, and the life span of only 20% of the mice were prolonged. It can be inferred that this sort of polysaccharides, like an interferon inducer, resists cancer through reinforcing the cellular immunity of the thoracic adenolymphocytes.

EXPERIMENTAL FORMULAS

For malignant tumor:

1>. 3 to 6 grams of PS-K is taken orally each day.

2>. Coriolus Polysaccharides Injection is administered intramuscularly 40 grams a time and twice a day. 4 weeks will be a course of treatment and between two courses there is a 2 week interval. Or 120-160mg of the injection mixed with 300ml of 10% glucose is administered intravenously each day. This treatment may be continued for 10 days and, after 1 or 2 weeks of interval, renewed for 10 more days. (*Journal of New Traditional Chinese Medicine*, Vol. 6, 1979)

THE AUTHOR'S NOTE
In Japan, gastrocancer is treated with chemotherapy accompanied with ATSO. The drug is easy to be cultivated with soybean sauce, sugar and onion as the basic substances.

RADIX ASPARAGI

Zhang Yuansu in the Yuan Dynasty said that: "The drug is bitter and sweet in taste, eliminating hemostasis and nourishing kidney."

The drug is the root of a plant of the *Asparagus* genus and the *Liliaceae* family, produced in the south and the central regions of China. *Asparagus spinosissimus Wang et S.C. Chen* produced in Tibet is used as a substitute of the drug.

ANTICANCER PHARMACOLOGICAL FUNCTIONS
1. The drug inhibits mice sarcoma-180 and leukemic cells.
2. The drug can prolong the surviving period of the antibody and reinforce the immunity of the body fluid.
3. Experiments in vivo showed that A. meioclados Levl. resists the activity of cancer.
4. The ethanol extract inhibits human tumor, causing changes in 51-100% of the cancer cells.

EXPERIMENTAL FORMULAS
For mammary cancer:
1>. The peeled fresh drug is boiled with millet wine for 30 minutes and then the millet wine is taken orally.
2>. The fresh drug is peeled and eaten in raw with millet wine.
3>. The fresh drug is squeezed to get juice to be mixed with 0.1% benzoic acid and taken 3 times a day (50 grams each) with millet wine. The dosage can be gradually increased to 150 grams a time if the effect is not significant. (*New Medical Information*, Vol. 4-5, 1972)

For Leukemia and breast cancer:
The drug is diacolated with 70% ethanol and the liquid is condensed into 1:4 before being mixed with some 95% ethanol to make a liquid with 70-80% ethanol. After the clear liquid is collected and the ethanol is removed, normal saline is added to dilute the liquid to such a solution with each milliliter containing 5 grams of the crude drug. The preparation is administered either intravenously or intramuscularly 2-4ml a day.

For malignant lymphoma:
> Radix Asparagi 30g
> Spica Prunellae 30g
> Flos Lonicerae 24g
> Radix Scrophulariae 24g
> Thallus Laminariae seu Eckloniae 12g
> Radix Ampelopsis 12g
> Rhizoma Belamcandae 12g
> Rhizoma Paridis 12g

The prescription is taken in decoction. (*Selected Prescriptions from an Oncological Symposium Held in Hunan*)

HISTORICAL COMMENTS

Approach to Medicine says that: "Swelling and carbuncles can be cured with 30-150g of the fresh drug when washed, ground, filtrated with wine and taken orally."

Prescriptions for Surgery says that: "Chronic stomatitis can be cured with an equal portion of Radix Asparagi, Radix Ophiopogonis and Radix Scrophulariae made into honey-coated pills and sucked with one pill a time."

Materia Medica of Pharmaceutical Properties says that: "The drug eliminates foul odor emitted from the body."

Pharmaceutical Properties says that: "The drug cures pyogenic lung cancer."

Prescriptions Worth a Thousand Gold says that: "The drug cures abdominal mass, pyogenic sore and carbuncles."

Newly Edited Materia Medica says that: "The drug is cold and slippery in nature, forbidden to be used for patients with splenogastropenia and diarrhea with undigested food."

THE AUTHOR'S NOTE

In Dongshan People's Hospital, Wu county, Jiangsu Province, 41 cases of malignant lymphatic cancer were treated with the drug and Herba Oldenlandiae Diffusae as the main ingredients, and 36.9% of the patients were clinically cured, 22.% proved significantly effective and 29.3% effective, with a total effective rate of 87.9%. 23 cases were treated with the drug and Herba Oldenlandiae alone, and the total effective rate was 87.9%, according to a report in *New Medicine* (Vol. 4, 1975). Compared with other anticancer drugs, these two drugs were quick in action, significant in efficacy, safe in use and effective for patients with resistance to other drugs. Therefore, these two drugs can be used alone or with other drugs to treat malignant lymphoma.

119 cases of various tumors were treated with the drug combined with Western medicine in Suzhou Hygiene Bureau, among which 48 were cured, 25 were proved significantly effective, 27 effective and the total effective rate was 84%. This indicates that the drug is effective in treating breast cancer, lymphoma and metastasized cancer according to a report in *Correspondence of Chinese Herbal Medicine* (Vol. 4, 1972).

RADIX TRICHOSANTHIS

Huang Gongxiu in the Qing Dynasty said that: "The drug is sour, slightly bitter and sweet in taste, slightly cold in nature, eliminating heat-phlegm accumulated above the diaphragm."

The drug is obtained from *Trichosanthis Ririlowii Maxim.* of the *Trichosanthes* genus and the *Cucurbitaceae* family.

ANTICANCER PHARMACOLOGICAL FUNCTIONS

1. The extract from the drug cures chorioepithelioma with a rate of 50% and malignant hydatidiform mole with a rate of 100%. It increases leukocytes, but has no side effect on the liver and the kidney.

2. The drug inhibits cervical cancer-14, sarcoma-180 and ascites cancer.

3. The drug inhibits JTC-26 with a 90% effective rate.

4. Its anticancer mechanism lies in: 1). Causing necrosis to trophocytes; And 2). Interfering the respiration and anaerobic glycolysis of the cancer cells. The effective element is glucoprotein.

EXPERIMENTAL FORMULAS

For malignant hydatidiform mole and chorioepithelioma:

The fresh drug is washed, sterilized with alcohol, squeezed into juice and put into refrigerator for deposition. The clear liquid is collected and frozen. The whole Fructus Gleditsiae Abnormalis is washed, sterilized with alcohol, calcined, ground into powder, filtrated with distilled water and frozen. The two frozen drugs are blended with a 9 to 1 ratio and filled into 0.275g-0.5g capsules for inserting into the vaginal fornix 5-7 days a time. Before the administration, the patient should urinate, defecate, wash the vagina with warm boiled water. The patient should lie on bed to rest after a capsule inserted. The dosage should begin from the minimum and the preparation has some side effect. (*Selected Medical Research Papers*)

For mammary cancer:

   Radix Trichosanthis 30g
   Concha Ostreae 30g
   Spica Prunellae 30g
   Sargassum 9g
   Thallus Laminariae seu Eckloniae 9g
   Nidus Vespae 9g
   Radix Scrophulariae 3g
   Bulbus Bolbostemmae 15g
   Scolopendra 2g

The prescription is taken one dosage a day in decoction. (*Diagnosis and Treatment of Tumor*)

For esophageal cancer:

   Radix Trichosanthis 18g
   Radix Codonopsis Pilosulae 15g
   Rhizoma Dioscoreae 15g
   Radix Asparagi 9g
   Radix Ophiopogonis 9g
   Semen Persicae 9g
   haematitum 30g

The prescription is taken one dosage a day in decoction. (*Selected Experienced Prescriptions in Shaanxi*)

For malignant hydatidiform mole:

When injected intramuscularly, the drug necroses the mole tissue, prevents and the womb from enlarging and evidently reduces the size of the enlarged womb. In some cases, the mole would come out spontaneously 3-6 days after the administration. (*Medical Research Correspondence*, Vol. 7, 1978)

For the side effect of chemotherapy:

   Radix Trichosanthis 30g
   Rhizoma Phragmitis 60g
   Radix Rehmanniae 15g
   Radix Scrophulariae 12g
   Radix Ophiopogonis 12g
   Herba Dendrobii 30g

The prescription is taken one dosage a day in decoction. (*Hunan Journal of Tumor Research and Treatment*, Vol. 1, 1980)

HISTORICAL COMMENTS

Ri Hua Zhi Materia Medica says that: "The drug smoothens small intestine, subsides swelling, cures breast abscess and expels pus to promote muscle development."

Classification and Prescriptions says that: "Breast abscess can be cured with 30 grams of the drug and 3 grams of Olibanum when ground into powder and taken 6 grams a time with wine."

Dietetic Prescriptions of Mengxi says that: "Primary carbuncles or swelling can be cured by the drug when decocted in millet wine, dried and ground. The powder is blended with millet wine, spread on paper and applied to the lesion." "Equal portion of the drug and Semen Phaseol Calcarati is ground, blended with vinegar and applied to the lesion."

RHIZOMA ARISAEMATIS

Mao Xiyong in the Ming Dynasty said that: "The drug is hot and bitter in taste, violent in action and toxic and warm in nature, dispersing pathogenic factors and eliminating stasis or stagnation."

The drug is obtained from *Arisaema erubescens (Wall.) Schott* of the *Arisaema* genus and the *Arisaema* family, mainly produced in Yunnan, Hunan, Northeast and Southeast of China. *A. heterophyllum Bl.*, *A. Amurense Maxim.*, *A. thunbergii Blume*, *A. ambiguum Engl.* and *A. fraternum Schott* of the same family are used as the substitutes of the drug.

ANTICANCER PHARMACOLOGICAL FUNCTIONS
1. D-mannitol extracted from the fresh drug inhibits the activity of cancer.
2. The extracted liquid from the fresh drug strongly inhibits Hela cell.
3. The drug eases experimental pain induced on mice.
4. Intramuscular injection of the extracted liquid from the drug into mice (0.1ml each) with experimental tumor evidently inhibits the tumor.

EXPERIMENTAL FORMULAS
For malignant tumor of the never system:
     Rhizoma Arisaematis 30g
     Rhizoma Pinelliae 30g
     Herba Xanthii 15g
     Semen Astragali Complanati 15g
     Rhizoma Zingiberis
The prescription is taken in decoction. (*Handbook of Practical Anticancer Drugs*)
For lung cancer:
     Rhizoma Arisaematis 30g
     Dinodon Pulveratum 30g
     Rhizoma Bletillae 30g
     Pericarpium Citri Reticulatae 30g
     Fructus Trichosanthis 30g
     Radix Glehniae 60g
     Radix Quinquefolium 15g
     Carapax Trionycis 45g
     Olibanum 20g
     Myrrha 20g
     Cinnabaris 12g
The herbs are ground into powder and taken 1 gram a time and three times a day. (*Guide for Clinical Treatment of Tumor*)
For thyroid tumor:
One of the drug is ground with 5-7 drops of vinegar and applied to the lesion. (*Yan Zhili's Holly Prescriptions*)

For dermatoma:

The drug is blended with vinegar and applied to the lesion. (*Simple Prescriptions*)

For cervical cancer:

1>. The drug (15 to 45 grams) is decocted and taken as tea for 3 months.

2>. Local administration:

1). Medicinal Bag: 9 grams of the radix of the drug is washed (not steeped in water), added with 0.5ml of 75% ethanol, pounded into a paste, wrapped with gauze and inserted into the vagina on the lesion and changed once a day.

2). Suppository or claviformation: A suppository, containing 50g of the crude drug, is inserted to the os of the uterus; A claviformation, containing 10g of the crude drug, is inserted into the os of the uterus.

3). The extracted liquid from the drug is used for pelvic ionic dialysis.

(*Selected National Medical Research Papers*, Vol. 2, 1972)

For nasopharyngeal cancer:

Rhizoma Arisaematis 50-150g

Herba Selaginellae 100g

Fructus Trichosanthis 15g

Herba Xanthii 15g

Radix Glehniae 15-50g

The prescription is taken one dosage a day in decoction. (*Practical Oncology*)

HISTORICAL COMMENTS

Pharmaceutical Properties of Materia Medica says that: "The drug cures abdominal mass and enteritis."

Materia Medica says that: "The drug cures convulsive diseases, face-distortion, laryngitis, stomatitis, glossitis and tuberculosis."

Elucidation on Materia Medica says that: "The drug eliminates stasis and stagnation, subsides swelling, calms the thorax and disperses blood to induce abortion."

THE AUTHOR'S NOTE

It is recorded in *Holy Prescriptions* that the paste made from the drug cures dermatoma: one of the drug is washed, ground, blended into a paste with some vinegar, spread on a piece of paper, applied to the tumor that has been punctured with a small needle. The plaster is administered 3-5 times a day.

FRUCTUS ET FOLIUM SOLANI INDICI

It is defined in *Zhennan Materia Medica* that: "The drug is bitter in taste and cold in nature, curing sinusitis."

The drug is obtained from *Solanum indicum L.* of the *Solanaceae* family, produced in Yunnan, Guangdong, Sichuan and Taiwan, the fruit of which contains 0.1% Solanine and the leaf 0.02%. *Solanum nigrum L.* of the same family is also of clinical anticancer effective.

ANTICANCER PHARMACOLOGICAL FUNCTIONS

1. The powder of the leaves causes damage to tumor, enabling the decayed tumor tissue to come off.

2. The drug has a curative effect on some tumors.

3. The extract from Atropa belladome of the same family inhibits experimental tumor; *Solanum nigrum L.* inhibits stomach cancer cells in animals; *Solanum lyratum Thunb.* evidently inhibits mice sarcoma-180 and cancer-256.

EXPERIMENTAL FORMULAS
For ulcerous breast cancer:

The fresh leaves are dried, ground, sterilized by autoclave and then sprinkled on the ulcerous lesion and covered with sterilized gauze. The treatment is given once or twice a day. Before sprinkling a new powder, the ulcerous lesion must be washed with normal saline. The powder cannot be sprinkled on the fresh muscle or the normal skin membrane lest dermatitis or eczema may occur. (*Dictionary of Chinese Materia Medica*)

HISTORICAL COMMENTS
Fujian Medical Herbs says that: "Ulcer can be cured with the powder of the leaves of the drug."

Record of Lingnan Herbal Medicine says that: "To treat retained food or water in the stomach, the drug is washed, dried, calcined yellow, ground into powder, blended with sugar and mixed with 8 to 15 grams of boiling water before oral administration on an empty stomach.

Handbook of Common Chinese Medicinal Herbs reports: "The drug functions to remove stasis and relieve swelling, inflammation and pain, and is indicative for pharyngitis, tonsillitis, lymphatic tuberculosis and gastralgia. To cure gastralgia, 9 to 15 grams of the drug is taken in decoction."

HERBA HYDROCOTYLI SIBTHORPIOIDITIS

It was reported in *Essential Properties of Medicinal Herbs* that: "The herb, bitter in taste and cold in nature, is used to cure tinea capitis, fetid ear and infections above the nasal region."

Herba Hydrocotyli Sibthorpioiditis is the dried whole plant of *Hydrocotyle Sibthorpioides Lam.* of the family *Umbelliferae*, which is found growing in East China, Central China and other places. It is also known as Herba Centipedae and contains flavonoid glycosides.

ANTICANCER PHARMACOLOGICAL FUNCTIONS
1. Fluorescent microscopy in vitro showed that the herb has an antileukocytic action with an rate of 84.8%.

2. Bacteriophagic tests indicated that the herb had an antiphagic action. It is hence inferred that the drug has an active antineoplastic effect.

EXPERIMENTAL FORMULAS
For cancer of the liver:

      Herba Hydrocotyli Sibthorpioiditis 60g
      Herba Scutellariae Barbatae 30g
      Herba Lobeliae Chinensis 30g
      Herba Oldenlandiae Chrysotrichae 30g
      Semen Coicis 30g

The formula is taken one dose daily in decoction and it can be prepared into injections for use.
For nasal bleeding due to cancer of the nasal cavity:

Fresh Herba Hydrocotyli Sibthorpioiditis is put into the nostrils after being pounded to pieces. (*Prevention and Treatment of Tumors in Traditional Chinese Medicine*)

For urinary bleeding and pain caused by cancer of the urinary bladder:

Herba Hydrocotyli Sibthorpioiditis and Herba Polygoni Aviculare (120 grams each) are pounded to pieces to get its juice for oral administration with white sugar.

For squamous epithelial carcinoma:

Certain amount of the drug is decocted to make a plaster for applying to the lesion. (*New Collection of Materia Medica of Zhenan*)

For cancer of the stomach:

> Herba Hydrocotyli Sibthorpioiditis 60g
> Herba Scutellariae Barbatae 30g
> Herba Lobeliae Chinensis 30g
> Herba Oldenlandiae Chrysotrichae 30g
> Semen Coicis 30g
> Radix Hostae Plantagineae 1.5g

The decoction of the herbs is taken once daily and 2-4 months make a therapeutic course. (*Anticancer Herbal Preparations*)

HISTORICAL COMMENTS

It was stated in *Compendium of Medicinal Herbs* that: "The herb can help relieve nasal obstruction, clear the nine senses, and spit out phlegm due to pathogenic wind." "It functions to remove toxic materials, improve vision and dissipate skin swellings."

Found in *Supplement to Compendium of Medicinal Herbs* was that: "To heal nebula, the herb is crushed and filled into the nostrils."

In *Imperial Collection of Poems*, there was a poem about Herba Hydrocotyli Sibthorpioiditis: "If nebula follows conjunctivitis, Herba Centipedae is put in the nostrils and replaced frequently, consequently eyesight will be restored in three days."

In *Dietetic Materia Medica* it was declared that: "The herb cures hemorrhoid."

THE AUTHOR'S NOTE

Biyun San, an ancient formula, which consists of Herba Hydrocotyli Sibthorpioiditis for detoxication as a principal drug and Indigo Naturalis for removing heat and Rhizoma Chuanxiong for sending up and expelling wind as auxiliary drugs, was used for the treatment of nebula and nasal polyp. In addition, Herba Hydrocotyli Sibthorpioiditis sometimes causes leukopenia during administration, but it will disappear automatically after the withdrawal of the herb.

RADIX ET HERBA SEMIAQUILEGIAE

It was claimed in *Materia Medica of Southern Yunnan* that: "The herb is cold in nature and bitter, acrid in taste, and cures breast cancer as hard as rock."

Radix et Herba Semiaquilegiae is the dried tuberous root or the whole plant of Semiaquilegiae, *Semiaquilegiae adoxoides* (*DC.*) *Mak.* of the family *Ranunculaceae*, which is primarily distributed in Jiangsu and Zhejiang Province and contains mainly alkaloids.

ANTICANCER PHARMACOLOGICAL FUNCTIONS

The herb was found to have an inhibitive action on sarcoma-180 of rats.

EXPERIMENTAL FORMULAS

For cancers of the nasopharynx and esophagus:

Radix et Herba Semiaquilegiae (0.5kg) is pulverized and immersed in 5kg of sorghum or cereal wine for 7 days. Then, the wine is taken three times a day with a dose of 50ml each time. Salmiacum preparations can also be given at the same time. (*Selected Data from a National Exhibition on New Medical and Medicinal Techniques*)

For cancer of the urinary bladder:

Radix et Herba Semiaquilegiae 15g

Folium Pyrrosiae 15g

Herba Lysimachiae 30g

Rhizoma Smilacis Glabrae 30g

A decoction of the herbs is taken once daily.

For cancer of the lung:

Radix et Herba Semiaquilegiae 15g

Herba Bulbophylli 15g

Rhizoma Fagopyri Cymosi 30g

Herba Lepidogrammitis 30g

A decoction of the herbs is taken once daily. (*Practical Anticancer Handbook*)

For cancer of the breast:

Radix et Herba Semiaquilegiae 4.5g

Bulbus Fritillariae Cirrhosae 9g

Concha Ostreae 12g

Radix Glycyrrhizae 3g

The decoction of the herbs is taken once daily. (*Folk Medicinal Herbs of Zhejiang Province*)

For malignant lymphoma:

Radix et Herba Semiaquilegiae 15g

Rhizoma Dioscoreae Bulbiferae 15g

Radix Kadsurae 15g

Rhizoma Paridis 15g

Rhizoma Arisaematis (first boiled for 2 hours) 30g

The decoction of the herbs is taken once daily. (*Diagnosis, Treatment and Prevention of Tumors*)

HISTORICAL COMMENTS

Compendium of Medicinal Herbs points out that: "The herb can help discharge urinary stone. To treat tiger and snake bite, squeeze out the juice of the herb and drink it; When applied to the surface of the wound, the drug may serve as a detoxicant and analgesic."

In *Origin of Materia Medica* it was commented that: "The herb is mainly used to cure internal injuries due to phlegm fire. In addition, it cures scrofula and malignant boils, and becomes more powerful particularly after being immersed in wine."

THE AUTHOR'S NOTE

Recorded in *Mirror of Ancient and Modern Medicine* was *Tiankui Wan* (Radix et Herba Semiaquilegiae Pill), which is mainly indicated for scrofula and is used by doctors who try to treat thyroid cancer and lymphoma. The Pill consists the following herbs:

Radix et Herba Semiaquilegiae 45g

Sargassum 30g

Thallus Eckloniae 30g

Thallus Laminariae 30g

Bulbus Fritillariae Cirrhosae 30g

Radix Platycodi 30g

Os Sepiae 15g

All the above herbs are put together and ground into fine powder to be blended with wine to make pills of the size of Semen Firmianae. 70 pills are taken each time with warm wine after meal.

FRUCTUS FICI

In *Rest and Diet Recipes*, it was recorded that: "The herb is sweet, cold, acts to reduce heat and loosens the bowel."

Fructus Fici is the dried succulent receptacle, root and leaf of *Ficus carica L.* of the family *Moraceae*, which contains antineoplastic agents in the dried and immature fruit and its juice. In addition to its medicinal functions, Fructus Fici is edible because it is sweet in taste.

ANTICANCER PHARMACOLOGICAL FUNCTIONS

1. The juice of the whole plant, when injected into guinea pigs, has an inhibitive effect on the transplanted sarcoma.

2. The dregs of the water extract of the dried fruit precipitated with acetone has an active action against Ehrlich's sarcoma.

3. The juice extracted from its immature fruit inhibits transplanted sarcoma in rats, spontaneous mastocarcinoma of mice and causes necrosis of the tumor. It may as well delay the growth of transplanted adenocarcinoma, myeloid leukemia and make the tumor degenerate.

EXPERIMENTAL FORMULAS

For cancers of the stomach and the bowel:

Five pieces of the fresh Fructus Fici are eaten or a decoction of 20 grams of the dried fruit is taken after meals every day. (*Research Data on Medicinal Herbs*, Vol.6, 1978)

For esophageal cancer:

Fresh Fructus Fici (500g) is stewed with lean meat (100g) for half an hour and both the broth and the meat are taken altogether. (*Herbal Handbook*)

For cancer of the urinary bladder:

Fructus Fici (30g) and Caulis Aristolochiae Manshuriensis (15g) are decocted for oral administration daily. (*Prevention and Treatment of Tumors in Traditional Chinese Medicine*)

HISTORICAL COMMENTS

In *Materia Medica of Yunnan Province*, it was pointed out that: "Mixed with cereal oil, the herb may be applied to all sorts of anonymous pyrogenic infections such as cellulitis, carbuncle, scabies, impetigos, breast mass and ulcerated smallpox."

In *Flower Mirror*, it was described that: "There are seven advantageous aspects concerning the herb: First, it is sweets harmless and suitable for people old and young; Second, it looks and tastes like persimmon when dried under the sun; Third, maturing fruit collected in early autumn will be sufficient for use for three montls; Fourth, it is one of the most productive and fastest growing trees, which, once planted, bears fruit at ihe same year and may become a big tree the next year, but peach and plum trees are quite different, they grow 3-4 years to bear fruit; Fifth, the leaves of the plant is the best herb for hemorrhoid; Sixth, the immature fruit can be collected and boiled with sugar; Seventh, the plant can grow anywhere it is planted."

In *Compendium of Medicinal Herbs* it was commented that: "The herb cures sore and painful throat and pharynx, and different types of hemorrhoid."

It was indicated in *Jiangsu Flora* that: "The white juice of the fresh fruit cures verruca when applied externally."

THE AUTHOR'S NOTE

According to a report in *Medical Reference Data* (Vol. 2, 1972), the extract of Fructus Fici was used in some foreign countries to treat 5 cases of advanced gastric cancer and it seemed effective. After

30-50 days of intravenous administration with a dose of 10-40ml three times a day, the tumor finally disappeared. The drug has a broad scope of antineoplastic actions and has no toxic side effects. Besides, it is sweet and edible as fresh fruit and should be included in the list of anticancer diet for cancer patients. In West Germany, juice of the fruit has been applied to cure verruca since the ancient time, while in Japan, the herb has been processed into injections for the treatment of pharyngolaryngeal cancer, adenocarcinoma, cervical cancer and cancer of the urinary bladder.

The ficoin in the juice of Fructus Fici is an anthelmintic which is effective both for roundworms and whipworms. The antineoplastic activity of traditional anthelmintics used in various countries has been carefully studied in Japan since 1970s and certain achievements have been made.

CORTEX ACANTHOPANACIS

In *Canon of Materia Medica* it was indicated that: "The herb is acrid and warm, and is used to supplement *qi* and cure the lame."

Cortex Acanthopanacis is the dried root or bark of *Acanthopanax gracilistylus W. W. Smith* of the family *Araliaceae*. *Acanthopanax henryi (Oliv.) Harms.*, *Acanthopanax giraldii Harms.*, *Acanthopanax leucorrhizus Harms.*, *Acanthopanax sessiflorus Seem.*, *Acanthopanax verticillatus Hoo.* are all pharmacologically used as Cortex Acanthopanacis. The root contains large quantities of glucosides and saccharides, and also possesses substances which react to sterol and triterpenordal saponins.

ANTICANCER PHARMACOLOGICAL FUNCTIONS
1. The alcohol extract of Cortex Acanthopanacis has an inhibitory rate of 40.2-68.0% against solid Ehrlich's ascites carcinoma and sarcoma-180 in rats.

2. Cortex Acanthopanacis strengthens human body defensive function against pathogens and promotes resistance against harmful stimulants (chemical, physical and biological) from the natural environment. It has been proved that oral administration of Cortex Acanthopanacis can help human body produce large quantities of antibodies which are of significant importance for the immunity to cancers and for the increase of leukocytes.

3. The alcohol extract of *Acanthopanax henryi (Oliv.) Harms.* of the family *Araliaceae* may inhibit metastatic diffusion of Walker's cancer in rats.

4. In Japan, tests in vitro with Cortex Acanthopanacis revealed that the hot water extract of the drug had an inhibitory rate of over 90% on JTC-26.

EXPERIMENTAL FORMULAS
For cancer of the stomach:

The extract of Cortex Acanthopanacis is processed into pills containing 1.5 gram of the crude drug each and 3 pills are taken each time, 3 times daily. The drug also prevents and treats bone marrow arrest due to chemotherapy. (*Shanghai Journal of Medicinal Herbs*, Vol.1, 1980)

To prepare the extract, certain amount of the crude powder of the root and the stem of the herb is immersed in two-fold of 70% alcohol under room temperature for 24 hours, and then more 70% alcohol is added for continuously extracting in a steam jar for 10-12 hours. The liquid will concentrate to adhesive plaster after alcohol is recovered. Five grams of the plaster corresponds to 100 grams of the raw material.

For cancer of the digestive canal:

10-15ml of the mixture of Pericarpium Juglandis and Cortex Acanthopanacis is taken three times a day.

To prepare the mixture, fresh fruit of walnut is immersed in 60% alcohol for 20 days, during which stirring is given once or twice daily. The extract is then filtered with 80% of the alcohol removed.

Water is added to keep the concentration of the crude herb to 60%. Then 20% of the extract of Cortex Acanthopanacis is added to make the mixture. (*Heilongjiang Research Journal of Traditional Chinese Medicine, 1975*)

For the prevention and treatment of leukopenia due to chemotherapy and radiotherapy:

Fresh Cortex Acanthopanacis (15 to 30 grams) is steamed in a cooking steamer for oral administration. (*Anticancer Herbal Preparations*)

Fresh fruit of walnut and the root of Cortex Acanthopanacis are immersed in white wine for two months and the immersion is widely used to treat tumors of the digestive system.

HISTORICAL COMMENTS

It was expounded in *Records of Famous Physicians* that: "The drug cures impotence, infection of the scrotum, dribbling urination in males, pruritus vulvae, pain along the spinal column, pain and numbness of the feet in females. It improves and replenishes the vital essence, consolidates muscles and bone, and strengthens the will power. Prolonged administration will make a person's body light and prevent him from aging."

In *Prescriptions Worth a Thousand Gold* it is reported that: "To cure five kinds of strain and seven kinds of impairment, the leaves, the root and the stem of Cortex Acanthopanacis are collected and taken orally with wine one gram each time, three times a day."

THE AUTHOR'S NOTE

An outstanding feature of Cortex Acanthopanacis is its regulation of the balance of body functions, known as adaptagen action or balance effect. It is similar to lentinan that has been recently studied in Japan. Adaptagen action, as is called, is to keep a person's body in a state of non-specifically increased resistance (SNIR). According to a report in *New Scientists* (Vol. 8, 1980) of England, in the 1980th Olympic Games, Soviet athletes administered a unique record-promoting drug, Cortex Acanthopanacis, also known as Siberian Ginseng. Cortex Acanthopanacis was administered by astronauts during their stopover in Salute-6 and Union 32 space station. They took 4ml of the extract of Cortex Acanthopanacis every morning. Animals, that were frozen, heated, enclosed, radiated, exposed to altered atmospheric pressure and oxygen content or induced to develop cancer and other diseases by poisonous drugs or chemicals, were found to survive much longer if they had been given Cortex Acanthopanacis. As an example, the survival period of the group of rats who were given Cortex Acanthopanacis was prolonged twice the original after having received 3000 rad of τ-ray.

FLOS ET FOLIUM HIBISCI MUTABILIS

It was written in *Illustrated Materia Medica* that: "The Herb is acrid, neutral and is applied topically for pyrogenic infections."

Flos et Folium Hibisci Mutabilis is the dried flower, leaves or root of *Hibiscus Mutabilis L.* of the Family *Malvaceae*. Its leaves contain flavonoid glycosides, amino acid and tannic substances while its flower contains hyperoside, rutin, etc.. Flos et Folium Hibisci Mutabilis has three different colors during a day, yellowish in the morning, pink at noon and deep reddish in the evening. In the morning the flower does not contain anthocyanin, but at noon and in the evening it does. The concentration of anthocyanin in the evening is three times of that at noon.

ANTICANCER PHARMACOLOGICAL FUNCTIONS

Drug sensitivity tests showed that the herb was sensitive to stomach cancer cells.

EXPERIMENTAL FORMULAS

For lung cancer:

        Folium Hibisci Mutabilis 30g

        Folium Cordylini Fruticosae 30g

        Herba Euphorbiae Lunulatae 15g

A decoction of the herbs is taken once daily. (*Handbook of Practical Anticancer Drugs*)

For mammary cancer:

An adhesive plaster made by blending Folium Hibisci Mutabilis powder with 25% vaseline is applied to the affected surface of the tumor once or twice daily. (*Anticancer Herbal Preparations*)

For cancer of the digestive system:

Folium Hibisci Mutabilis is dried in the oven and then ground to powder to be applied to the tumor mass; For esophageal cancer, 3 grams of the powder is taken each time, twice a day. (*Handbook of Practical Anticancer Drugs*)

HISTORICAL COMMENTS

It is stated in *Compendium of Materia Medica* that: "The leaf clears the lung, cools the blood and serves as an antipyretic and detoxicant. It cures all sizes of carbuncle, cellulitis, pyrogenic infections and malignant boils through relieving swelling, evacuating pus and relieving pains."

In *Records of Lingnan Herbs* it is reported that: "The herb, decocted in good wine, cures acute mastitis completely."

Described in *Medicinal Herbs of Chongqing* is that: "The following herbs, when stewed together with pig's heart and lung and a little sugar or salt, cure consumptive diseases and cough: Folium Hibisci Mutabilis 60-120g

        Herba Pyrolae 30g

        Yellow Sugar 30g

It is mentioned in *Yujiu's Annotation on Medicinal Herbs* that: "The leaf of the herb clears away pathogenic wind, reduces heat, cools blood and relieves swelling."

FRUCTUS CHAENOMELIS

Wang Shixiong of the Qing Dynasty remarked that: "The herb is sour and neutral to regulate *qi*, harmonize the functions of the stomach, nourish the liver, relieve flatulence, relax muscles, calm pathogenic wind and remove dampness."

Fructus Chaenomelis is the dried fruit of *Chaenomeles lagenaria (Loisel.) Koidz.* of the family *Rosaceae*, which is mainly produced in Southwest China. *Chaenomeles lagenaria (Loisel.) Koidz. var. wilsonii Rehd.* and *Chaenomeles lagenaria (Loisel.) Koidz. var. cathayensis Rehd.*, both have the same pharmacological functions as Fructus Chaenomelis. The major component of the herb is carpaine.

ANTICANCER PHARMACOLOGICAL FUNCTIONS

1. Carpaine of the herb has a remarkable effect against the activation of lymphocytic leukemia-1210.

2. Carpaine has an intermediate action against lymphocytic leukemia-388 and cancer cells of nasopharyngeal carcinoma.

3. The water decoction and alcohol extract of Fructus Chaenomelis apparently have inhibitive effects on Ehrlich's ascites carcinoma in rats.

4. Malic acid and potassium malate in Fructus Chaenomelis highly inhibit ascites carcinoma in rats.

5. Experiments in vitro showed that the water decoction of Fructus Chaenomelis has an inhibitory rate of 70-90% on JTC-26.

EXPERIMENTAL FORMULAS

For various types of cancer, an injection of Fructus Chaenomelis is administered intramuscularly with a dose of 50mg twice a day. (*Bulletin of Medicinal Herbs*, Vol 6, 1976)

For prolonged pains of abdominal tumors:

Fructus Chaenomelis 30g

Folium Mori 15g

Fructus Ziziphi Inermis 3 piece

A decoction of the herbs is taken frequently. (*Dietetic Materia Medica*)

HISTORICAL COMMENTS

It was described in *Collection of Holy Prescriptions* that: "The drug cures flatulence and pain caused by the attack of *qi* on the abdominal and costal regions due to the deficiency and coldness of the kidney. Thirty fresh Fructus Chaenomelis are peeled with its core removed, then filled with 500 grams of the powder of Flos Chrysanthemi and salt, finally steamed and pounded to plaster to be mixed with 1000 grams of Folium Artemisiae Argyi for making into pills of the size of Semen Firmianae. Thirty pills are taken each time, twice a day."

In *Supplement to Compendium of Medicinal Herbs* was written that: "To cure cardiac attack due to foot *qi*, an immature Fructus Chaenomelis, with its seeds removed, is decocted and taken. Fructus Chaenomelis strengthens muscles and bones, keeps cold wind flowing downward, relieves nausea, cures heart and diaphragm syndrome and promotes digestion."

Noted in *Lei's Treatise on Preparation of Drugs* was that: "The drug regulates *ying* and *wei* and supports the essence derived from food."

THE AUTHOR'S NOTE

It was found in Changhai Hospital in Shanghai that 2.5% Fructus Chaenomelis crystal has a higher inhibition rate on Ehrlich's ascites carcinoma in rats. Further experiments revealed that the antineoplastic substances were not the tartaric acid, citric acid and ascorbic acid it contained.

CAULIS ARISTOLOCHIAE MANSHURIENSIS

In *Shen Nong's Classic Herbs* it was recorded that: "The herb, acrid in taste and neutral in nature, acts to clear the nine orifices and promote blood circulation and joint movement."

Caulis Aristolochiae Manshuriensis is the dried xylem stalk of *Akebia trifoliata (Thunb.) Koidz. var australis Rehd.*, *Akebia trifoliata (Thunb.) Koidz.* and *Akebia quinata (Thunb.) Decne.* of the family *Aristolochiaceae*, which contains akebin that can be hydrolyzed into hederagenin, oleanolic acid, glucose and rhamnose. Both its fruit and seed are anticancer drugs.

ANTICANCER PHARMACOLOGICAL FUNCTIONS

1. The dried powder, obtained from the hot water extract of Caulis Aristolochiae Manshuriensis through distillation, when administered to JTC-26 in vitro with a dose of 500μg/ml, was found to have an inhibiting rate of over 90% while the fruit 50-70% under the same dose.

2. Experiments in vivo showed that the alcohol extract of Caulis Aristolochiae Manshuriensis had an inhibition rate of 4.4% on ascitic sarcoma-180 of rats while the hot water extract 21.5%.

EXPERIMENTAL FORMULAS

For pancreatic cancer, tumor of the common bile duct, cancer of oral cavity and lymphosarcoma:

Xiao Zheng Pian (a pill composed of Semen Plantaginis Asiaticae (0.027g), Mylabris (0.015g) and Talcum (0.03g) is taken by mouth twice a day, each time 1 to 2 pills. (*New Traditional Chinese Medicine*, Vol. 3, 1980)

For blood in urine due to cancer of the urinary bladder:

        Caulis Aristolochiae Manshuriensis 3g
        Radix Achyranthis Bilentatae 3g
        Radix Rehmanniae 3g
        Radix Asparagi 3g
        Radix Ophiopogonis 3g
        Fructus Schisandrae 3g
        Cortex Phellodendri 3g
        Radix Glycyrrhizae 3g

The above herbs are taken in decoction. (*Annotation on Shen Nong's Herbs*)

HISTORICAL COMMENTS

It was stated in *Essentials of Materia Medica* that: "Caulis Aristolochiae Manshuriensis is indicated for strong fire-syndrome while Rhizoma Alismatis for a minor one. Though both function to relieve water retention, they are used differently."

Written in *Ocean Materia Medica* was that: "The drug is primarily used to cure fistula and sore throat and is preferably to be taken in decoction. The powder can be kept in month for resolving as an emergent therapy."

In *Ri Hua Zi Materia Medica* it is commented that: "The herb relieves upsetness of mind through calming the heart, quenches thirst and alleviate fever. It cures amnesia, improves visual and auditory acuity, treats nasal obstruction, clears intestine and purges away water. The herb dissolves agglomerated blood clot, evacuates pus, relieves pain, and cures furuncle and breast cancer."

FLOS AND RADIX BOMBAI

In *Chinese Medical Dictionary* it is described that: "The herb, sweet, warm and nonpoisonous, is mainly indicative for metrorrhagia and incised wound."

Flos and Radix Bombai is the dried flower, bark and root of *Bombax Malabarica L.* of the family *Bombacaceae*. Belonging to deciduous arbors, it grows up to 25 meters, much higher than its neighboring trees. Covered with deep grey bark, both its young trunks and old branches have short and strong conical thorns, which becomes thicker at the base. The branches are whorled and flat, growing upward in layers with palmate compound leaves (5 to 7 pieces). The leaves begin to grow in early spring with fascicle flowers borne at the end of the branches, the corolla appearing to be red or orange red. The large capsule, xyloid, elliptic and as long as 15 cm, becomes divided to 5 pieces when being ripe. There are white filiform hairs in the petal, where many black and smooth seeds are stored. Flos and Radix Bombai is mainly distributed in the provinces of Southern China.

ANTICANCER PHARMACOLOGICAL FUNCTIONS

Screening tests in vivo showed that the herb had an inhibitive effect on tumor.

EXPERIMENTAL FORMULAS

For cancer of the stomach, Flos and Radix Bombai (1150 grams) and lean pork (150 grams) are boiled in 5kg of water for 7-8 hours to the volume of one bowl and taken once daily. Usually the pain may become alleviated after a week's administration, but the prescription should Le continued till the patient is fully recovered. (*Diagnosis and Treatment Based on Differentiation of Symptoms and Signs*)

HISTORICAL COMMENTS

It was recorded in *Compendium of Medicinal Herbs* that: "When burnt to ashes, the drug mainly cures metrorrhagia and incised wound." "The oil of Flos and Radix Bombai, being acrid, hot and slightly poisonous, is mainly used to cure pyrogenic infection, scabies, tinea and the injury of the eyes by fire."

In *National Herbal Collection*, it was reported: "The root of the herb, slightly bitter and cool, is used to dissipate hard mass and relieve pain, while the bark, also slightly bitter and cool, is effective for expelling pathogenic wind, removing dampness, promoting blood circulation and removing swelling."

THE AUTHOR'S NOTE

Southern China Tumor Hospital adopted the method of stewing lean pork with the bark of the plant to treat gastric and esophageal cancer and achieved an overall effective rate of 64%. One of their patients with esophageal cancer who could not eat any food at all, was able to eat 100 grams of food after two months' administration. The tumor size was reduced from 8cm to 3cm in diameter. And the same treatment was given to three other patients with esophageal cancer and it was also found to have certain effect.

HERBA CATHARANTHI

It was recorded in *Dictionary of Chinese Medicinal Herbs* that: "The herb, slightly bitter and cool, functions to cure malignant tumors."

Herba Catharanthi is the dried whole plant of *Catharanthus roseus. (L.) G. Don* of the family *Apocynaceae*.

Among the 70 types of alkaloids separated from the plant, 6 have anticancer actions. They are vinblastine, vincristine, leurosine, leurosidine, isoleusosine and lochneridine. 5 have antiviral actions and 6 have actions to reduce high blood pressure. The content of alkaloids is 0.37-1.16% in leaf, 0.46% in stem, 0.7-2.4% in root, 0.14-0.84% in flower, 1.14% in bark and 0.18% in seed.

It was reported that the herb is mainly used for lymphocytic reticulosarcoma (Hodgkin's Disease), chorioepithelioma, acute leukemia (especially of children). The toxicity of vincristine is primarily involved with nerves and muscles. The toxin may accumulate to cause degeneration of nerve cells. Vinblastine mainly arrests bone marrow and granulocytes. The clinical manifestations of the toxicity are anorexia, nausea, alopecia, and in many people, general asthenia. In addition, toxic reactions of the central and the peripheral nervous system are mental depression, abnormal sensation, subsided tendon reflex, headache and hyperspasmia.

ANTICANCER PHARMACOLOGICAL FUNCTIONS

1. Vincristine has an apparent inhibitive action on Ehrlich's ascites carcinoma of rats.

2. Vinblastine has a remarkable inhibition on transplanted chronic lymphocytic leukemia-1534.

3. Vinblastine inhibits cell mitosis and causes metakinesis, as a result that the cell's ability to synthesize ribonucleic acid is lost. In the telophase of the cell cycle, vinblastine reduces the solubility and increases the synthesis of RNA so as to affect the synthesis of protein.

4. With total cellular volumetric method, the alcohol and the hot water extract of vinblastine was found to inhibit sarcoma-180 of rats, with rates of 100% and 95.7% respectively.

EXPERIMENTAL FORMULAS

For acute lymphocytic leukemia:

1>. A decoction of Herba Catharanthi (15 grams) is taken.

2>. Vincristine sulfate, dissolved in 10ml of normal saline with a dose of 0.025-0.05 mg/kg of body weight, is administered intravenously once a week. Side effects, including baldness, abdominal pain, nausea, constipation, sourness and pain of muscles, finger numbness and fever, may occur but will disappear upon the cessation of the drug. (*Treatment and Prevention of Tumors*)

HISTORICAL COMMENTS

It was recorded in *Handbook of Common Medicinal Herbs* that: "The drug, slightly bitter and cold, is used as a sedative and tranquilizer, to calm the mind and the liver, to reduce blood pressure and to cure hypertension."

In *Records of Medicinal Plants in Guangxi*, it was commented that: "The plant cures leukemia, pulmonary cancer, chorioepithelioma and lymphatic tumor."

It was stated in *Dictionary of Chinese Medicinal Herbs* that: "6 to 15 grams of the herb is decocted and taken daily."

THE AUTHOR'S NOTE

When administered in injection, the drug often causes injury to the peripheral nerves with reactions such as numbness of the extremities, muscular tremor and reduced tendon reflex. These reactions, particularly, the numbness of the fingers and the toes, are slow to get over. After 1 to 3 weeks of administration, leukocytopenia and thrombocytopenia may occur. The drug is contraindicative for patients who have apparent arrest of bone marrow due to chemotherapy or radiotherapy.

FRUCTUS CROTONIS

It was reported in *Essentials of Materia Medica* that: "The drug ia acrid, hot and extremely poisonous. Its toxicity is more severe when immature but becomes less severe when ripe."

Fructus Crotonis is the dried seed of *Croton tiglium L.* of the family *Euphorbiaceae*, which is distributed in most places of China. Its root, leaf, bark and the croton oil of kernel are also of medical use. The seed contains 34-57% of croton oil, in addition to crotin, crotonoside and ß-sitosterol.

ANTICANCER PHARMACOLOGICAL FUNCTIONS

1. Tumor-inhibiting experiments in vivo with rats proved that the extract of Fructus Crotonis had a remarkable inhibitive effect on solid and ascitic sarcoma-180, solid and ascitic cervical carcinoma-14, solid liver carcinoma and Ehrlich's ascites carcinoma. The inhibition rate is over 30% (P < 0.05).

2. Trypan-blue staining method showed that the extract of Fructus Crotonis or Fructus Crotonis injection had an action to kill cells of Ehrlich's ascites carcinoma and ascitic liver carcinoma in tube.

3. The hot water extract of Fructus Crotonis has an inhibitory rate of 50-70% on JTC-26.

EXPERIMENTAL FORMULAS

For cervical cancer:

Fructus Crotonis, peeled and coated with yellow wax is taken 5 to 6 granules once daily and ten doses make a therapeutic course. (*Shanghai Journal of Medicinal Herbs*, Vol. 9, 1984)

For ulceration of tumor:

Fructus Crotonis is peeled, baked, powdered and finally made into plaster for application to the ulcer. (*Proved Recipes for Carbuncle and Cellulitis*)

For cancer of the nasopharynx, the rectum and the urinary bladder:

           Fructus Crotonis 7 granules
           Arsenium 15g
           Fructus Ziziphi Jujubae 7 pieces
           Chinese Onion Tassels 3.5Kg

Crush Fructus Crotonis (peeled) and Arsenium into fine powder, and pound Fructus Ziziphi Jujubae and Chinese Onion Tassels into paste after steaming. Then put the powder and the paste together and wrap it up in a piece of cloth to be held in hands for 12 hours each time, every other day. The hands should be washed afterwards. (*Diagnosis, Treatment and Prevention of Tumors*)

HISTORICAL COMMENTS

It was described in *Materia Medica in Decoction* that: "To cure acute diseases of the digestive tract, the herb is taken raw with its peel, kernel, skin and oil removed. To cure chronic diseases such as food retention and abdominal mass, the herb is burnt black and pulverized into powder before administration. It is widely known that the drug clears the bowel and cures diarrhea."

It was reported in *Essentials of Materia Medica* that: "Acute paralysis of the throat may cause death if delayed. *Jiedu Wan*, made of Realgar (30 grams), Radix Curcumae (3 grams) and peeled Fructus Crotonis (14 granules), is very effective for this illness, when 1.5 gram of it is taken each time. Realgar clears away accumulated *qi*, Radix Curcumae dissipates extravasated blood and Fructus Crotonis moves away thick saliva. The pill is very devastating and should be used with care."

THE AUTHOR'S NOTE

Despite its antineoplastic action, Fructus Crotonis is limited in usage because of its toxicity. Experiments with rats showed that exposure of rat's skin to croton oil for a long period of time will cause papilloma and carcinoma. It is thought that croton oil is not carcinogenic but the crotyl dihydroxybenzene alcoholate in the oil is. Thereupon, when used as an antineoplastic drug, it is better to have the oil removed before use.

FRUCTUS POLYGONI ORIENTALIS

In *Materia Medica of Southern Yunnan*, it was reported that: "The herb, bitter in taste and cold and neutral in nature, is used to eliminate blood stasis, cure abdominal mass in children and other chronic and uterine mass."

Fructus Polygoni Orientalis is the dried fruit of *Polygonum orientale L.* of the family *Polygonaceae*, and is an annual plant growing as high as 3 meters.

ANTICANCER PHARMACOLOGICAL FUNCTIONS

1. Experiments in vitro revealed that the herb had an inhibitive action on tumor cells.
2. Experiments in vivo showed that administration of the decoction, tincture, or petroleum ether extract of Fructus Polygoni Orientalis to guinea pigs by oral perfusion for 10 days in succession proved that it has certain unsteady inhibition on the solid and ascitic Ehrlich's ascites carcinoma and sarcoma-180.

EXPERIMENTAL FORMULAS

For cancer of the thyroid:

30 grams of fresh Fructus Polygoni Orientalis is decocted and taken daily, while a proper amount of it is pulverized into a paste for external application. (*Diagnosis and Treatment Based on Differentiation of Symptoms and Signs*)

For malignant lymphoma:

A certain amount of Fructus Polygoni Orientalis (half baked and half unprocessed) are ground into fine powder and taken with wine, each time 6 grams, three times a day. (*Amplified Materia Medica*)

For tumors of the abdominal cavity:

Fructus Polygoni Orientalis 6g

Radix et Rhizoma Rhei 3g
Natrii Sulfas 3g
Fructus Gardeniae 3g
Calcaria 3g

The herbs are mixed with wine yeast (about the size of an egg) and smashed to paste to be spread on a piece of cloth for application to the mass. The plaster will be removed after three days and the skin looks deep black because of the application. (*Complete Medical Records*)

HISTORICAL COMMENTS
In *Amplified Materia Medica* it was stated that: "The drug cures scrofula."

It was cited in *Chinese Pharmacopeia* that: "The drug quenches thirst, relieves fever, improves vision and promotes the flow of *qi*."

In *Proved Recipes of Li Fu Tang* it was commented that: "The drug cures abdominal mass. One bowl of the flower or the fruit of Fructus Polygoni Orientalis is stewed to paste to be applied to the mass or to be mixed with wine for oral administration. Greasy food is forbidden while taking the drug."

THE AUTHOR'S NOTE
The eighth volume of New Edition of *Proved Prescriptions* written by Bao Xiang, a noted physician in the Qing Dynasty, cited an eliminating tumor mass plaster, called *Xiao Pi Gao*, which can be used as a trial therapy for cancer of the liver and the stomach and other abdominal tumors. The formula of the plaster is:
Lithargyrum 180g
Resina Ferulae 150g
Rhizoma Notopterygii 30g
Fructus Polygoni Orientalis 30g
Squama Manitis 9g
Moschus 3g

The herbs are normally decocted to make paste. 3 grams of Moschus is added at the end of the decoction. The paste is spread on a piece of cloth to be applied on the mass. The plaster should be the same size of the mass, no large and no small. Meanwhile, Fructus Polygoni Orientalis (9g) is pounded to powder, immersed in 1kg of heated wine and drunk frequently till the mass disappears."

HIRUDO

Huang Gongxiu of the Qing Dynasty pointed out: "Hirudo lives in gloomy and damp places and is proficient in sucking human blood. It is salty and bitter in taste, neutral and poisonous in nature, and is used medically to clear water passage, reduce blood stasis and induce abortion."

Hirudo is the dried body of an annelida animal, *Whitmania pigra Whitman* of the family *Hirudinidae*, commonly known as leach. The body of Hirudo is long, flat and greenish black, with linear yellow strips on the back. It has five pairs of eyes on both sides of its head and a mouth underneath the head. The biggest worm is 6-10cm in length and 1cm in width. It lives in pond and paddy field and is skillful in sucking blood of the vertebrates with the sucking disk in its mouth. In the middle of its anterior disk, there are three serrated palate plates. As its mouth is trident, the lambdoid wound in the skin of its victim can be observed after being bitten. Its body stretches and contracts smoothly, looking like a small ball when it contracts and being in undulant form when it is swimming in water. Out of water, it moves with its sucking disk. Hirudo is found mainly in Central China and South China.

ANTICANCER PHARMACOLOGICAL FUNCTIONS

1. Injection prepared with Hirudo inhibits the division of spermatogonium.

2. It has been proved with eosin method in vitro that the injection has an inhibitive effect on tumor cells.

3. Experiments in vivo showed the drug has an inhibitive action on liver cancer of mice.

EXPERIMENTAL FORMULAS

For adenocarcinoma of the uterine body:

        Hirudo 15g

        Radix Astragali 30g

        Radix Angelicae Sinensis 6g

        Rhizoma Scirpi 9g

        Rhizoma Zedoariae 9g

        Squama Manitis 12g

        Semen Persicae 18g

        Corium Stomachichum Galli 9g

All the above herbs are put together and ground into fine powder for oral administration twice a day, each time 3 grams. (*Diagnosis, Treatment and Prevention of Tumors*)

For cancer of the skin:

        Hirudo 30g

        Rhizoma et Radix Rhei 5g

        Indigo Naturalis 3g

The above drugs are ground into fine powder to be decocted with sesame oil (60g) and yellow wax (9g) to make a plaster for external application. (*Prevention and Treatment of Common Tumors in Qinghai*)

For cancer of the large intestine:

Powdered Hirudo is taken with water or wine, 1 gram each time. (*Progress in Research on tumor Prevention and Treatment Inside and Outside of China*, 1978)

For tumor of the oviduct and the ovary:

Dried Hirudo is ground into fine powder for oral administration daily with millet wine in the morning and in the evening, 3 grams each time. (*New Traditional Chinese Medicine*, Vol. 5, 1975)

For hysteromyoma:

1>.   Hirudo 30g

        Radix Astragali 45g

        Rhizoma Scirpi 15g

        Rhizoma Zedoariae 15g

        Radix Angelicae Sinensis 18g

        Rhizoma Anemarrhenae 18g

        Semen Persicae 18g

All the above drugs are ground into fine powder and mixed with honey for rolling into pills of the size of Semen Firmianae. 6 grams are taken in the morning and in the evening. It is not administered during the period of menstruation. (*Journal of Traditional Chinese Medicine*, Vol. 8, 1963)

2>.   Hirudo 30

        Tabanus 30

        Semen Persicae 20

        Rhizoma et Radix Rhei 9g

The above herbs are decocted and the broth is divided into two portions for taking in the morning and in the evening. (*Collection of Herbal Prescriptions in Modern Gynecology*)

Historical Comments

In *Records of Combined Traditional Chinese and Western Medicine*, it was stated that: "Hirudo removes blood stasis without causing any damage to the fresh blood."

It was reported in *Supplement to Compendium of Medicinal Herbs* that: "The drug cures carbuncle and poisonous swelling."

Practical Materia Medica commented that: "The drug is effective for menopause, uterine mass and abdominal mass."

It was claimed in *Essential Prescriptions Worth a Thousand Gold* that: "To cure metrostaxis, Hirudo is baked and crushed into powder for oral administration with wine, 3 grams each time, twice a day, until the extravasated blood disappears."

It was recorded in *Collection of Prescriptions for Saving Lives* that: "The drug cures postpartum faintness and blood stasis accumulated in the chest, the abdomen and the hypochondrium. 3 grams of each of Hirudo, Tabanus (with its wings and feet removed), Myrrh and Maschus is baked, powdered and taken together with *Si Wu Tang*. The pain will be relieved once the retained blood is removed. *Si Wu Tang* should be continued."

It was expounded in *Prescriptions for Rescuing the Sick* that: "To cure trauma, injury, blood stasis and flatulence in the chest and the abdomen, constipation and anuresis, and critical symptoms of the dying, the following formula is recommended:

      Hirudo 15g
      Calix 15g
      Radix et Rhizoma Rhei 60g
      Semen Pharbitidis 60g

The above drugs are powdered and taken 6 grams each time with warm wine, till the extravasated blood is completely removed.

HYDRARGYRUM

Huang Gongxiu of the Qing Dynasty remarked: "Hydrargyrum is acrid in taste and extremely cold and poisonous in nature. It is heavy and can flow smoothly."

Being a metal element abstracted from mineral mines, Hydrargyrum is a silver-colored and lustrous liquid under room temperature, but it coagulates into octahedral crystals under a temperature 40°C below zero, slightly evaporates under ordinary temperature and completely evaporates in high temperature. Produced mainly in Kunming or Yunnan Province, Hydrargyrum, being soluble in strong nitric acid solution, has a specific gravity of 1.35 and its boiling point is 360°C. Before administration, Hydrargyrum is often smelted with other mineral drugs to make a mixtures called *Sanxian Dan*, *Hongsheng Dan*, *Baijiang Dan* and *Wuhu Dan*.

ANTICANCER PHARMACOLOGICAL FUNCTIONS

1. *Wuhu Dan* has a destructive action on cancer cells of the skin, with a protoplasmic toxicity of Hg^{++} to cells.

2. *Hongsheng Dan* has an inhibitive action on tumors of guinea pig.

EXPERIMENTAL FORMULAS

For esophageal cancer:

Hydrargyrum and Sulfur (3 grams each) are pulverized and taken with millet wine or ginger soup with a dose of 1.5 to 3 grams each time, twice daily. (*Manual of Medicinal Herbs*)

For various types of sarcoma:

      Hydrargyrum 3g
      Gambir 3g

Borax 3g

Borneol 0.4g

Moschus 9g

Sanguis Draconis 9g

Cortex Phellodendri 1.5g

The herbs are ground into powder and applied to the affected Lesion. (*Secret Prescriptions Inherited from a Divine Doctor——Hua Tuo*)

For cancer of the skin and the breast:

Hydrargyrum 180g

Alumen 180g

Melanteritum 180g

Natrii Sulfas 180g

The drugs are melted to make white crystals for external application. (*Hunan Journal of Medicine and Drugs*, Vol.1, 1976)

For cervical cancer:

Ten portions of the white crystals of the above formula and one equal portion of pulverized Venenum Bufonis are mixed with starch or boiled rice as an excipient to make prismatic drug-nails of the size of a cotton swab about 1.5-2cm in length for use after it becoming dry. After the cervix is exposed with a speculum and disinfected, a drug-nail is implanted 0.8-1cm deep in the base or in the body of the tumor. If the implantation is difficult, poke a hole in the selected part of the tumor with a sharp knife and then insert the nail. Note that the drug-nail is fully inserted into the tissue of the tumor and make sure that it would not come out or off. Check that no segments of the drug are left in the vagina, then rinse the vagina at the end of the operation. The drug-nail will be dissolved and absorbed several days after the implantation, and the therapy is repeated till the full exfoliation of the tumor tissues. (*Data of National Medical and Health Researches*, Vol. 9, 1972)

For malignant hydatidiform mole metastasized to the lung:

The powder of *Hongsheng Dan*, composed of Hydrargyrum, Natrii Sulfas, Alumen, Melanteritum, Realgar and Cinnabaris, is packed into capsules for oral administration once a week with a dose of 0.4-1.0 gram. (*On Drugs and Prescriptions*)

For various types of cancer:

Lingyao (major component: Hydrargyrum) 3g

Jindan (major component: Cerussa) 3g

Yincui (major component: Silver) 3g

The above drugs are crushed into powder to be rolled with flour paste into pills of the size of soy bean, weighing 0.3 gram each and coated with Malachitum. A pill is taken once daily in the evening till the symptoms fully disappear. If toxic reactions appear, the drug should be stopped. (*On Drugs and Prescriptions*)

HISTORICAL COMMENTS

It was reported in *Holy Prescriptions* that: "When taken together with rice flour, the drug has a quick effect to promote the lactation of milk of the primipara and cure sore throat with the feeling of a bean in the pharynx."

It was commented in *Collection of Holy Prescriptions* that: "The following formula is administered for patients with stomach cancer:

Folium Pini Thunbergis 4.5g

Hydrargyrum 4.5g

Sulfur 15g

Cortex Cinnamomi 3g

The above drugs are put together and crushed into powder for oral administration. Each time, 1.8 grams of the powder is taken after being mixed with a broth containing half rice porridge and half ginger juice.   In *Li Lou's Prescriptions for Odd Symptoms and Signs* it was said that: "The drug cures malignant boil with putrid flesh. A 14-year-old girl had a painful and purple tumor in one of her wrist with the size of a soybean. Half of the tumor grows deep in the flesh and she did not respond to a variety of drugs. She was given 120 grams of Hydrargyrum and two pieces of soft paper, with which she rubbed the drug on the tumor. Three days after application, the tumor mass exfoliated spontaneously."

Recorded in *Handbook of Prescriptions for Emergencies* was that: "The following formula is effective for all sorts of malignant boils:

> Hydrargyrum 250g
> Rhizoma Coptidis 250g
> Cerussa 250g

All the above drugs are crushed into powder for external application."

Prescriptions worth a Thousand Gold says that: "Application with Hydrargyrum for several times will cure leukoderma immediately."

THE AUTHOR'S NOTE
In Dandong Hospital of Traditional Chinese Medicine, Anticancer Drug No.1 and Anticancer Drug No.2, prepared with Hydrargyrum and other minerals, were used to treat 48 advanced cancer patients, and they reported that the effective rate was 39.5%. As being very poisonous, Hydrargyrum must be used with great care."

HERBA ET RADIX GEI

In *Dutch Drugs Mirror* it was commented that: "Being acrid, warm, fragrant and astringent, the herb smells like Flos Syzyqii Aromatici and is effective for scrofula and other pyrogenic infections."

Herba et Radix Gei is the whole plant or tuberous root of *Geum aleppicum Jacq*. of the family *Rosaceae*, which is found growing mainly in Zhejiang, Anhui and Yunnan Province. *Adina pilulifera (Lam.) Franch.* and *Adina rubella (Sieb. et Zucc.) Hance* of the family *Rubiaceae* are also called "Herba et Radix Gei" and has been recognized to have an antineoplastic activity, inhibiting cells of cervical cancer, sarcoma-SAK and Walker's cancer-256 in rats. Herba et Radix Gei, recorded in *Compendium of Medicinal Herbs* belongs to the family Rosaceae, not to the family Rubiaceae. In clinical reports, the two kinds of herbs are often confused. But as for the anticancer effects, the two are quite similar and can substitute each other.

ANTICANCER PHARMACOLOGICAL FUNCTIONS
1. Experiments in vivo with total cellular volumetric method revealed that the inhibition rate of the hot water extract of Herba et Radix Gei on sarcoma-180 in rats was 54%.
2. Tests in vitro showed that the water decoction of Herba et Radix Gei had an inhibition rate of over 90% on JTC-26.

EXPERIMENTAL FORMULAS
For cancers of the liver and the stomach:
A decoction of Herba et Radix Gei (120g) and Herba Pteridis Multifidae (30g) is taken daily. (*Essential Points of Tumors*)
For lymphoma:
Pills of Herba et Radix Gei (1.5-3g) prepared with honey are taken all the year; or Herba et Radix Gei (30g) is immersed in white wine (400ml) for some time and a tea spoonful of the wine is taken

each time, 3 to 4 times a day; or 45 grams of Herba et Radix Gei is decocted in 500ml of water to get 250ml of broth for oral administration with a tea spoonful each time every half an hour. (*Dutch Drugs Mirror*)

For cancer of the digestive canal:

        Radix Gei 30g

        Herba Solani Glabrae 30g

        Herba Salviae Chinensis 30g

        Radix Aucklandiae 9g

The recipe is taken in decoction daily. (*Practical Anticancer Handbook*)

HISTORICAL COMMENTS

It was described in *Dutch Drugs Mirror* that: "Herba et Radix Gei, an effective herb for invigorating the mind, contains a sort of oil and bitter salt, which warm up and reinforce the nerve, the heart and the stomach and act to some extent as a diaphoretic and diuretic. With its action to relieve spasm, the herb is used effectively for the treatment of various syndromes due to relaxation and weakness of the fibers. In addition, the drug drives away pathogenic wind, cures pain caused by hernia and always takes effect when used to cure putrefactive fever and intermittent fever. Moreover, it is indicative for prolonged diarrhea, deficiency syndrome caused by dysentery with bloody stool, metrorrhagia, metrostaxis, leukorrhea and vomiting blood. Those with excessive loss of blood are advised to take it."

In *Compendium of Medicinal Herbs* it was stated that: "The drug is acrid, warm, nonpoisonous and is mainly used for the treatment of furuncle and other types of pyrogenic infections."

In *Dictionary of Chinese Materia Medica* it is explained that: "The drug restores *qi* and tonifies the kidney, with indications for dizziness, lassitude of the extremities, spermatorrhea, impotence, cold due to exterior deficiency, cough, hematemesis, abdominal pain due to the cold of insufficiency type, irregular menstruation, furuncle and fracture."

In *Records of Herbs in Hunan* it was recorded that: "The drug warms the middle-*jiao*, promotes circulation of *qi* and alleviates pains."

HERBA PTERIDIS MULTIFIDAE

In *Properties of Categorized Medicinal Herbs* it was reported that: "The drug, being cool and nonpoisonous in nature, is used to remove toxic heat, resolve swelling and clear away the fire."

Herba Pteridis Multifidae is the dried whole plant of *Pteris multifida Poir*. of the family *Pteridaceae*, which is extensively distributed from South Korea to the subtropical areas of Asia."

ANTICANCER PHARMACOLOGICAL FUNCTIONS

1. It has been proved that the herb inhibits sarcoma-180, sarcoma-37 and Walker's cancer-256 in rats.

2. Radix Pteridis Multifidae showed an inhibition rate of 30-50% on Yoshida's sarcoma of rats.

EXPERIMENTAL FORMULAS

For chorioepithelioma and malignant hydatidiform mole:

        Herba Pteridis Multifidae 60g

        Radix Gei 60g

        Hielianthus annucis 1

A decoction of the herbs is taken once daily in succession for six months. (*Zhejiang Bulletin of Science and Technology*, Vol. 2, 1972)

For cancer of the large intestine:

Herba Pteridis Multifidae 30g
Rhizoma Smilacis Chinensis 30g
Bolus Rubra 30g
Limonitum cum Terra 30g
The decoction of the herbs is taken daily. (*Manual of Practical Anticancer Drugs*)
For lung cancer:
Herba Pteridis Multifidae 30g
Herba Scutellariae Barbatae 30g
Ramus Araliae Chinensis 30g
Fructus Pratiae 30g
The above herbs are decocted for oral administration daily. (*Prevention and Treatment of Commonly-Seen Tumors*)
For cervical cancer:
Herba Pteridis Multifidae 30g
Herba Selaginellae 30g
The herbs are decocted for oral administration daily. (*Anticancer Herbal Preparations*)
For cancer of the breast:
Herba Pteridis Multifidae 15g
Radix Codonopsis Lanceolatae 15g
Caulis Trachelospermi 15g
Herba Isodi 30g
Flos Damnacanthi 30g
Corium Erinacei 9g
Flos Sophorae 9g
Spica Prunellae 9g
Excrementum Vespertilionis 9g
Radix Clematidis 6g
Fructus Trichosanthis 12g
The herbs are decocted for oral administration daily. (*Essential Points of Tumors*)

HISTORICAL COMMENTS

In *Collection of Herbs* it was asserted that: "It is a holy drug for retropharyngeal abscess."

It was commented in *Essential Properties of Medicinal Herbs* that: "To stop bleeding and promote the growth of new flesh, juice squeezed out of the herb is mixed with wine for oral administration and the dregs left are for application to the wound. Ground to powder and stored in a container, the drug cures pains caused by the disorder of *qi*."

In *Materia Medica of Lu Chan Yan* it was reported that: "Being cold in nature, the drug can not be administered for a long time to patients who are old."

It cautioned in *Materia Medica of Eastern Fujian* that: "The herb should not be prescribed for pregnant women and patients with cold or recurrent dysentery."

FOLIUM ET SEMEN CYCIS REVOLUTAE

In *Folk Medicinal Herbs of Fujian* it was reported that: "The herb, being sweet, slightly warm and a little poisonous, is used to promote blood circulation, eliminate blood stasis, dispel the wind and remove toxic materials."

Folium et Semen Cycis Revolutae is the dried leaf, flower and seed of *Cycas revoluta Thunb.* of the family *Cycadaceae*, which contains compounds such as biflavone, long-chain hydrocarbon, ethanol and large amount of wax in the leaf; xylose, glucose and galactose in the stalk; cycasin A, B, C, laminaribiose, fats, trigonelline, choline, malic acid, tartaric acid and zeaxanthine in the seed.

ANTICANCER PHARMACOLOGICAL FUNCTIONS
1. Animal experiments showed anticancer effects of cycasins on a variety of tumors.
2. Cycasin was found to be sensitive to the cancer cells of the stomach in drug sensitivity tests.
3. The inhibitive rate of the hot water extract of Folium Cycis Revolutae on JTC-26 is estimated to be 50-70%.

EXPERIMENTAL FORMULAS
For cancer of the breast:
        Folium Cycis Revolutae 15g
        Cormus Iphigeniae 15g
        Herba Pteridis Multifidae 9g
        Herba Siphonostegiae 9g
        Nidus Vespae 9g
        Xylotrupes 9g
        Lignum Suberalatum Evonymi 9g
        Herba Solani Lyrati 30g
        Radix Ranunculi Ternati 30g
        Periostracum Serpentis 3g
The above formula is decocted in water and taken daily. (*Practical Oncology*, Vol.2)
For cancer of the stomach:
        Folium Cycis Revolutae 30g
        Semen Coicis 30g
        Herba Lobeliae Chinensis 30g
        Herba Solani Lyrati 30g
The above formula is decocted in water for oral administration once daily. (*Exhibited Prescriptions of Medicinal Herbs of Wuhan*)
For skin cancer:
        Folium Cycis Revolutae 500g
        Herba Oldenlandiae Diffusae 500g
        Herba Lobeliae Chinensis 500g
        Flos Lonicerae 500g
        Fructus Meliae Toosendan 500g
The above herbs are pounded to crude powder and decocted three times in water with ratios of 1:4, 1:3, 1:2 respectively. The three decoctions are mixed and condensed to 1/5 of the original volume, and then the sediment is deposited with alcohol twice. The broth is processed with activated charcoal, filtered, bottled and sterilized. The injection is given twice a day, each time 2-4ml. In addition, this preparation is also effective for cancers of the breast, lip and penis. (*Selection of Data on Medicine and Health from National Scientific and Technologic Research Programs*)
For cervical cancer:
        Folium Cycis Revolutae 120g
        Fructus Ziziphi Inermis 12
The above two herbs are taken in decoction daily. (*Clinical References of Traditional Chinese Medicine*)
For cancer of the liver:
        Folium Cycis Revolutae (green) 9g
        Folium Cycis Revolutae (red) 9g

Herba Oldenlandiae Diffusae 60g
Herba Scutellariae Barbatae 60g
Rhizoma Phragmitis 30g
The above formula is taken in decoction daily. (*New Traditional Chinese Medicine*)

HISTORICAL COMMENTS

In *Supplement to the Compendium of Medicinal Herbs* it was mentioned that: "The drug calms the liver and cures all kinds of pains caused by the liver *qi*."

It was stated in *Guiding Recipes* that: "Three pieces of Folium Cycis Revolutae are decocted in a bowl of water and taken orally for the treatment of dystocia."

In *Principal Toxic Plants in South China* it was described that: "The seeds and the crown of the plant is poisonous, causing symptoms such as dizziness and vomiting. To relieve it, gastrolavage is conducted with 1/1000-1500 potassium permanganate or 0.5-4% tannin. Emetic reaction may be provoked with a finger or a chicken feather by stimulating the pharyngeal region so that the toxic materials in the stomach may be vomited out."

HERBA ET RADIX RANUNCULI JAPONICI

In *Supplement to the Compendium of Medicinal Herbs* it was reported that: "The herb is acrid, warm and poisonous, being primarily used for the treatment of malignant boil, carbuncle, swelling and pain."

Herba et Radix Ranunculi Japonici is the dried whole plant of *Ranunculus japonicus Thunb.* of the family *Ranunculaceae*, which is found largely growing in Northeast China and South China and contains a principal chemical substance as protoanemonin. In different areas, *Ranunculus Sieboldii Miq.*, *Ranunculus Smirnovii Ovez.* and *Ranunculus Cantoniensis DC.* of the same family are pharmacologically used as Herba et Radix Ranunculi Japonici.

ANTICANCER PHARMACOLOGICAL FUNCTIONS

1. It has been proved in animal and clinical experiments that the volatile oil of Herba et Radix Ranunculi Japonici inhibits tumor and causes acute necrosis of tumor cells.

2. So far as its anticancer action concerned, the fresh ripe herb has the best effect, and its root is more often selected for medical use than its seedling. The herb, having been preserved for a long time or becoming stale, has the worst effect.

3. The inhibitive effect of Herba et Radix Ranunculi Japonici on animal tumors is possibly through its inhibition on phosphofructokinase.

EXPERIMENTAL FORMULAS

For squamous carcinoma, undifferentiated carcinoma and melanotic carcinoma of the lung:

The volatile oil obtained from Herba et Radix Ranunculi Japonici through distillation is diluted in 5% glucose and given intravenously. (*Research Reference of Traditional Chinese Medicine*, Vol. 2, 1974)

For cancer of the breast, the cervix and the skin:

1>. The volatile oil distilled from the root of the herb is mixed with three equal portions of the whole herb decoction for oral administration with a dose small at the beginning and gradually increased later.

2>. The volatile oil distilled from the root of the plant is mixed with two equal portions of the powder of the whole herb and processed into a solid plaster with lard for external application.

3>. Fresh Herba et Radix Ranunculi Japonici is dried in low temperature, pulverized into powder and then mixed with ox oil to make an ointment for external use. (*Bulletin of Medicinal Herbs*, Vol. 6, 1979)

HISTORICAL COMMENTS

It was expounded in *Compendium of Medicinal Herbs* that: "Crushed and applied, the leaves and the seeds of the herb, acrid, warm and poisonous, is used for the treatment of malignant boil and carbuncle, with swelling and pain, but without ulceration. Care must be given not to cause flesh decay. If a person catches malaria, a handful of the plant is crushed to pieces and applied to the arm."

In *Supplement to Compendium of Medicinal Herbs* it was stated that: "Herba et Radix Ranunculi Japonici and Rhizoma Zingiberis are ground to powder and applied to the abdomen to dispel cold wind."

In *New Materia Medica* it was pointed out that: "Externally used, Herba et Radix Ranunculi Japonici stimulates the skin and is indicative for scrofula, arthritis, tuberculosis of the joint and the bone, bronchial gasp and all kinds of unulcerated boil and carbuncle."

THE AUTHOR'S NOTE

According to a report of Xuzhou Medical College, a preparation made of the crude extract of Herba et Radix Ranunculi Japonici was used to treat 33 cases of lung cancer with remarkable effect in 7 cases and general effect in 6 cases. Protoanemonin derived from Herba et Radix Ranunculi Japonici was also used in a control group of 17 cases of lung cancer and 5 cases showed remarkable effect and 2 showed general effect. Protoanemonin seems to have a better effect.

The herb is usually prescribed for external use, as protoanemonin is irritating and may cause gastroenteritis if the mucous membrane of the digestive tract is stimulated. The administration of a large dose of protoanemonin caused complications such as nephritis and symptoms of the nervous system in animals. According to a report in *Research Data of Medicinal Herbs* (6,1978), Radix Anemone Cernua Thunb of the same family was used in Japan for the treatment of various types of cancer, through decocting 2-5 grams of its root in 200ml of water for oral administration in three portions.

RADIX ACONITI

It was described in *Changsha's Annotation of Medicinal Herbs* that: "The herb is warm-dry and of downward nature, and is able to dispel pathogenic factors between the interior and the exterior."

Radix Aconiti is the dried tuberous root of *Aconitum carmichaeli Debx.* or *Aconitum kusnezoffii Reichb.* of the family *Ranunculaceae*, with aconitine as its main component.

ANTICANCER PHARMACOLOGICAL FUNCTIONS

1. An injection prepared with the extract of Radix Aconiti (both Radix Aconiti and *Radix Aconiti Kusnezoffii*) was found to have an inhibition rate of 47.77-47.38% on the sold liver cancer of rats ($p < 0.01$).

2. With a dose of $200\mu g/ml$, the extract of Radix Aconiti inhibits live and proliferative cancer cells of the stomach.

3. It has been proved that the drug inhibits sarcoma-180 of rats and this action raises with the increase of the dosage.

4. Studies in vitro indicated that the herb is able to inhibit mitosis of cancer cells of the stomach in human beings.

EXPERIMENTAL FORMULAS

For various types of tumors:

Radix Aconiti 30g
Rhizoma Dioscoreae Bulbiferae 30g
Radix Notoginseng 30g
Rhizoma Paridis 30g
Rhizoma Corydalis 30g
Rhizoma Phragmitis 30g
Cormus Iphigeniae 30g
Borneol 6g

The herbs are crushed to powder for oral administration with hot water three times daily, each time 3 grams. The formula is very effective for tumors with severe pain. (*Diagnosis, Treatment and Prevention of Tumors*)

For malignant lymphoma:

1>. Equal portions of Radix Aconiti praeparata and Cortex Phellodendri are ground into powder, mixed with rice vinegar and applied to the tumor mass daily. (*Golden Mirror of Medicine*)

2>. *Xiao Jin Dan* is taken with a half cup of warm millet wine, one bolus in the morning and one in the evening. *Xiao Jin Dan* is prepared with the following herbs:

Radix Aconiti kusnezoffii 45g
Resina Liquidambaris 45g
Faeces Trogopterorl 45g
Lumbricus 45g
Semen Momordicae 45g
Olibanum 27.5g
Myrrh 27.5g
Radix Angelicae Sinensis 27.5g
Moschus 9g
Black Charcoal 3.6g

All the above herbs are pulverized and blended with glutinous rice flour (36g) to make approximately 250 boluses or pills. (*Oncology of Traditional Chinese Medicine*)

HISTORICAL COMMENTS

It was described in *Secrets of Therapeutics* that: "The herb has six functions: The first one is to remove cold; The second to relieve epigastric mass; The third to warm and nourish the viscera; The fourth to heal the diverse wind symptoms; The fifth to alleviate the stagnation of *qi*; And the sixth to cure abdominal pain due to cold."

It was commented in *Collection of Ancient and Modern Proved Recipes* that: "The herb cures carbuncle and pyrogenic infections. For the treatment of polyp, 5 pieces of Radix Aconiti are immersed in 120ml of bitter wine for 3 days and the liquid is used to wash the polyp three to four times very day."

THE AUTHOR'S NOTE

In the First Peoples' Hospital in Jinan, the extract of Radix Aconiti (or the hydrolysate of Radix Aconiti) was used clinically to treat 271 cases of advanced alimentary cancers such as liver cancer and stomach cancer, with a dose of 1.6mg/ml for intramuscular injection twice daily. It prolonged the survival period and alleviated symptoms in most patients, with a pain-relieving effect of 100%. It has also been verified in Dongzhimen Hospital affiliated to Beijing College of Traditional Chinese Medicine that the drug is effective for esophagus cancer, colon cancer and rectum cancer.

FRUCTUS MUME

Li Shizhen of the Ming Dynasty commented: "The herb, warm in nature, acid in taste and nonpoisonous, is indicative for regurgitation and dysphagia, with function to astringe the lung and the bowel."

Fructus Mume is the dried fruit of *Prunus Mume (Sieb.) Sieb. et Zucc.* of the family *Rosaceae*, which is distributed largely in Gansu and Shaanxi Province and contains such chemical elements as malic acid, citric acid, tartaric acid, succinic acid, ß-sitosterol, inositol and triterpenoids in its immature fruit; cyanogenetic glycosides and fatty oil in its seed; and volatile oil (mainly benzoic acid and benzaldehyde) in its flower.

ANTICANCER PHARMACOLOGICAL FUNCTIONS

1. It has been verified, through experiments in vitro with plate culture method of cells of ascites carcinoma, that the herb inhibits the activation of cancer cells.

2. Bacteriophagic method has proved that sarcocarp of Fructus Mume has an anticancer function.

3. Tests in vivo indicates that the herb has an inhibitive action on sarcoma-180 of rats.

4. The herb was found able to reinforce the phagocytic function of leukocytes and reticular cells and promote immunological function of the body.

5. Screening tests with bean sprout method have revealed that the herb has an antineoplastic effect.

6. The hot water extract of the herb has exhibited an inhibition rate of over 90% on JTC-26.

EXPERIMENTAL FORMULAS

For cancer of the stomach and the esophagus:

100 grams of Herba Scutellariae Barbatae is decocted in 1500ml of water to 750ml of broth, and then mixed with 50ml of the decoction of Fructus Mume. The mixed broth is filtered three times and taken after meal, three times a day, each time 50ml. (*Diagnosis, Treatment and Prevention of Tumors*)

For malignant reticulosis:

2.5mg of prednisone is taken once daily with the decoction of the following herbs:

> Fructus Mume 18g
> Radix Semiaquilegiae 9g
> Semen Coicis 60g
> Rhizoma Dioscoreae Bulbiferae 6g
> Radix Glycyrrhizae 6g
> Herba Oldenlandiae Diffusae 9g

(*Determination of Treatment Based on Differentiation of Symptoms and Signs*)

For cancer of the penis and the cervix uteri:

27 pieces of Fructus Mume is decocted with 1000ml of brine in a casserole or enamel cup on small fire for about 20 minutes upon its boiling. The boiled drug is then put aside for 24 hours before being filtered for use. The dosage for adults is 3ml each time, six times a day, that is, the drug is taken immediately before and after each meal. Brown sugar, white wine, or anything sour or pungent should be abstained during the period of administration. Recently, the drug is available in bolus, injection and plaster and is used extensively for a variety of tumors. The drug can also be used for external application or rubbing on tumors of the body surface. (*National Collection of Medicinal Herbs*)

For various types of cancer:

It is suggested that the jam made of sarcocarp of fresh Fructus Mume be taken in small dose every day for a long period of time. (*Data of Medicinal Herbs*, Vol. 6, 1978)

HISTORICAL COMMENTS

In *Classic Herbs* it was pointed out that: "The herb cures melanotic nervus and rotten flesh."

It was described in *Li Lou's Prescriptions for Odd Symptoms and Signs* that: "For the treatment of pyrogenic infection of the finger, especially when complicated with severe pain, sarcocarp of Fructus Mume and jellyfish are pounded for external application to the lesion."

It was reported in *Holy Prescriptions* that: "To cure exogenous febrile diseases and diseases related to insect-bite in the lower part of the body, 90 grams of Fructus Mume is parched into powder and mixed with honey for making into pills of the size of Semen Firmianae. 20-30 pills are taken with a decoction of Cortex Granati before meal."

In *Handbook of Prescriptions for Emergencies* it was mentioned that: "For abdominal distention and pain and for those who are short of breath and dying, 27 pieces of Fructus Mume are decocted in 200ml of water for oral administration."

It was commented in *Gong's Classic Prescriptions* that: "The herb is used to cure globus hystericus. Half green and half ripe Fructus Mume are soaked in brine for a night and then dried in the sunshine. The process is repeated until the fruit is completely dehydrated. Then 2 Fructus Mume are placed and tied between 3 old coins (with holes in the middle) with thread, to be packed in a enamel jar and buried in earth for a hundred days. The longer the preservation, the better the effect. The preserved fruit is kept in mouth for resolving and it can cure globus hystericus quickly and effectively."

In light of modern science, a Japanese journal, *Glory of Families* (6, 1974) reported various effects of Fructus Mume, which was regarded as a very ideal life-prolonging substance. One section of the report was particularly devoted to the preparation of various Fructus Mume diets, many of which are thought to be effective for the prevention and treatment of tumors. Here are some of the dietary recipes:

1>. Cuttlefish with Fructus Mume: Fructus Mume is denucleated, cut to pieces and blended with cooking wine, sugar and broad-bean sauce. The cuttlefish is sliced and steamed done. Then spread the mixture on the steamed slices and wrap them in Radix Arnebiae seu Lithospermi before eating. It is really tasty.

2>. Fish Soup with Fructus Mume: When cooking soup with coilia extenes, sardine or Mylophrygodon aethops, adding one or two Fructus Mume will not only make the taste of the soup better, but also increase its tonic properties.

3>. Pickled Fructus Mume: Folium Menthae is washed clean, placed in a bamboo basket for drop dry, scattered with salt and placed in a jar, with a sour soup prepared from Fructus Mume poured in. A heavy piece of stone is put on the top of the leaves to keep it from floating up. The leaves are edible in a week's time.

4>. Fructus Mume beverage: Various tasty and health-promoting beverages can be made from Fructus Mume, the simplest of which is prepared by mixing up 1/3 vinegar made from Fructus Mume, 1/3 honey and 1/3 water in a cup. In hot summer, a small piece of ice or several drops of lemon juice can be added.

RHIZOMA CIMICIFUGAE FOETIDAE

It was reported in *Origin of Medicine* that: "The herb, warm in nature and acrid in taste, serves as a medicinal guide of other drugs to tonify the spleen and the stomach."

Rhizoma Cimicifugae Foetidae is the dried rhizome of *Cimicifuga foetida L.*, *Cimicifuga dahurica (Turcz.) Maxim.* or *Cimicifuga heracleifolia Kom.* of the family *Ranunculaceae*, which is found growing in Jiangsu, Hubei, Qinghai and other places and contains such chemical elements as cimicifugine, salicylic acid, caffeic acid, ferulic acid, tannin and fatty acid.

ANTICANCER PHARMACOLOGICAL FUNCTIONS

When 20ml of the hot water extract of the herb, with a concentration of $500\mu g/ml$, is added to the culture medium of JTC-26, it was found to have an inhibiting rate over 90% on tumor cells and a slight inhibition on the normal cells.

EXPERIMENTAL FORMULAS
For laryngeal carcinoma:
> Rhizoma Cimicifugae Foetidae 30g
> Zixue San 30g
> Cornu Rhinoceri 30g
> Cornu Saigae Tataricae 30g
> Gypsum Fibrosum 30g
> Calcitum 30g
> Radix Scrophylariae 60g
> Radix Glycyrrhizae 24g
> Lignum Aquilariae Resinatum 15g
> Radix Aucklandiae 15g

These herbs are ground to powder for oral administration 3 grams each time, twice a day. The prescription is very effective for laryngeal carcinoma at early stages without ulceration. (*Diagnosis, Treatment and Prevention of Tumors*)
> For cancer of breast:
> Rhizoma Cimicifugae Foetidae 2g
> Radix Astragali 2g
> Radix Angelicae Sinensis 3g
> Radix Paeoniae Alba 3g
> Rhizoma Chuanxiong 3g
> Radix Arnebiae 3g
> Rhizoma et Radix Rhei 15g
> Flos Lonicerae 15g
> Concha Ostreae 4g
> Radix Glycyrrhizae 1g

The decoction of the herbs is taken daily. (*Explanation to Clinical Prescriptions of Traditional Chinese Medicine*)

For cancer of the tongue:

Rhizoma Cimicifugae Foetidae is infused in 50% alcohol to make a liquid extract. Herba Solani Lyrate and Radix Semiagnilegiae (30 grams each) are pounded into fine powder to be mixed with the liquid for oral administration, 3 to 5 grams each time, with certain amount of potassium iodide and water. In abroad, the liquid extract of the whole plant is used for the treatment of axillary carcinoma metastasized from tongue cancer and breast cancer after operation and it is found very effective. (*Bulletin of Medicinal Herbs*, Vol. 6, 1974)

HISTORICAL COMMENTS
It was described in *Handbook of Prescriptions for Emergencies* that: "Rhizoma Cimicifugae Foetidae is pulverized and blended with vinegar to be applied externally for the treatment of various types of pyrogenic infections."

It was reported in *Materia Medica in Decoction* that: "The herb cures the root decay of the teeth with fetid smell."

In *Properties of Medicinal Herbs* it was pointed out that: "For the treatment of carbuncle and eruptive diseases, the herb is decocted and applied to the sores with silk floss."

THE AUTHOR'S NOTE

Rhizoma Cimicifugae Foetidae is known as "a holy herb for patients of skin diseases", extraordinarily effective for various pyrogenic infections, eruptive diseases and miliaria. When these signs are seen in tumor patients, the dose of Rhizoma Cimicifugae Foetidae should be increased.

RADIX RUMEI CRISPI   *Sheep Sorrel*

It was reported in *Simple Herbal Prescriptions* that: "The herb is bitter in taste and administered to promote blood circulation and replenish vital essence and strength."

Radix Rumei Crispi is the dried root of *Rumex crispus L.* of the family *Polygonaceae*, which is mainly distributed over Northeast and Northwest China and contains elements such as emodin and rhapontin.

ANTICANCER PHARMACOLOGICAL FUNCTIONS

6 days after the implantation of sarcoma-37 to the muscles of a mouse's thigh, the alcohol extract of Radix Rumei Crispi was injected subcutaneously. Then the tumor tissues were removed for examination after 6-48 hours and it was found that the drug caused damage to the tissues. It has been proved that the acid extract of the herb is more efficient.

EXPERIMENTAL FORMULAS

For acute leukemia:

1>. A dose of 30-60 grams of Radix Rumei Crispi is taken in decoction daily. (*Handbook of Internal Medicine*)

2>. The following herbs are taken in decoction once daily:

        Radix Rumei Crispi 60g

        Radix Arnebiae 60g

        Herba Galii Aprinis 60g

        Cortex Moutan 9g

(*Practical Manual of Anticancer Drugs*)

HISTORICAL COMMENTS

It was indicated in *Materia Medica of Eastern Fujian* that: "The herb, used as an antipyretic, anthelmintic, and an agent to remove pus and toxic materials, is indicative for tinea capitis, nail-like boils and furuncle."

In *Handbook of Herbal Treatment in Highland Regions* it was recorded that: "It relieves fever, cools down blood, loosens and relaxes the bowels, with indications for acute hepatitis, amenorrhea, abdominal distention and anonymous pyrogenic infections.

It was suggested in *Medicinal Herbs of Chungking* that: "Fresh Radix Rumei Crispi is stewed with lean pork for oral administration."

It was said in *Medicinal Herbs of Jilin* that: "A decoction of Radix Rumei Crispi (150g) and Periostracum Cicadae (3) is taken twice daily."

In *Herbal Records of Sichuan* it was warned that: "The herb is contraindicative for diarrhea due to hypofunction of the spleen."

THE AUTHOR'S NOTE

In the United States, the extract of the root of Rume hymenosepulus of the same family as Radix Rumei Crispi was used for the treatment of skin cancer, with a bandage completely soaked in the extract, wrapped around the lesion, and changed frequently.

FRUCTUS ET RADIX ARCTII

Miao Xiyong, a physician in the Ming Dynasty, pointed out: "The herb, being acrid to resolve mass and bitter to remove heat, is effective for removing stasis of *qi* in the viscera."

Fructus et Radix Arctii is the dried root, seed and whole plant of *Arctium lappa L.* of the family *Compositae*, which is widely distributed all over China and contains arctiin, fatty oil, sterol, vitamin A-like substances and vitamin B in the fruit; volatile oil and vitamin B in the leaf and 5% inulin, mucilage, tannic substance and proteins in the root.

ANTICANCER PHARMACOLOGICAL FUNCTIONS

A culture solution was prepared with JTC-26 ($1x10^5$/ml), 90% of Eris' solution and 10% of embryo serum of calf. Then the hot water extract of Fructus et Radix Arctii was added and the concentration was adjusted to 500μg/ml, with each plate containing 20ml of the mixed solution. The medium was kept under 27°C for 134 hours and the result showed that the drug inhibits the proliferation of cancer cells of JTC-26 with a rate of 90%. This suggests that the herb has a strong antineoplastic activity.

EXPERIMENTAL FORMULAS

For cancerous edema:

Fructus et Radix Arctii (60g) is fried and pulverized for oral administration 6 grams three times daily. (*Holy Prescriptions*)

For cancer of throat:

Fructus et Radix Arctii and Semen Iridis (1.8 grams each) are ground to powder to be taken with warm water before meal. In addition, Fructus et Radix Arctii (90g) and salt (60g) are pounded into powder and fried hot before application around the laryngeal protuberance. (*Universal Prescriptions*)

For various types of cancer:

In some foreign countries, Herba Arctii, Radix Rumei Obtusifolii (or Radix Rumei Crispi) and Rhizoma Smilacis Chinae are prescribed for oral administration, and it is very effective. (*Bulletin of Medicinal Herbs*, Vol.6, 1974)

For malignant lymphoma:

Radix Arctii 15g
Radix Trichosanthis 15g
Radix Bupleuri 9g
Bulbus Bolbostemmae 12g
Radix Sophorae Subprostratae 30g
Rhizoma Smilacis Glabrae 30g
Nidus Vespae 30g
Radix Isatidis 30g
Radix Scrophulariae 30g
Herba Bideni Bipinatae 30g
Herba Euphorbiae Humifusae 30g
Fructus Forsythiae 30g

The decoction of these herbs is taken daily. (*Shaanxi Traditional Chinese Medicine*, Vol. 1, 1980)

For cervical cancer:

Equal portions of Radix Arctii and Fructus Broussonetiae are pulverized for oral administration with a dose of 6 grams each time, twice daily. (*Proved Recipes of Experienced Doctors of Traditional Chinese Medicine*, 1983)

For various types of cancer:

7 Fructus Arctii is decocted in 1000ml of water and the decoction is divided into 3 portions to be taken in the morning, afternoon and evening. (*Research Data of Medicinal Herbs*, Vol. 6, 1978)

For rectal cancer:

Radix Arctii 70g

Radix Angelicae Sinensis 7g

Semen Phaseoli 7g

Rhizoma et Radix Rhei 7g

Herba Taraxaci 7g

All the herbs are ground to powder to be taken with warm water twice a day, each time 6 grams. (*Proved Recipes of Experienced Doctors of Traditional Chinese Medicine*, 1983)

HISTORICAL COMMENTS

It was reported in *Prescriptions for Longevity* that: "To cure swelling due to heat pathogens in the throat, Radix Arctii (15g) is decocted in 200ml of water to a volume of 40ml for oral administration three times."

In *Universal Prescriptions* it was stated that: "Radix Arctii is pounded and its juice is swallowed slowly for the treatment of pharyngeal swelling of children."

It was described in *Prescriptions Worth a Thousand Gold* that: "For the treatment of chronic malignant boil, ulcerous mass and stubborn anal fistula (similar to skin cancer), Radix Arctii is pounded and blended with lard (obtained in December or January) to seal the wound every day."

It was recorded in *Universal Prescriptions* that: "To cure absence of menstruation, mass and severe distention in the abdomen, Radix Arctii (1000g) is steamed 3 times, put in a silk bag and then immersed in 1000ml of wine for 5 days. A small cup of the wine is taken before each meal every day." The author thinks this prescription can be given to patients with hysteromyoma as a trial.

CALCULUS BOVIS

Huang Gongxiu of the Qing Dynasty remarked: "The drug, bitter in taste and cool in nature, is effective to expel pathogenic heat in the Heart Channel, clear the orifices and eliminate phlegm."

Calculus Bovis is the gallstone of *Bos taurus domesticus Gmelin* of the family *Bovidae*. Currently in use is the artificial ox gallstone or Calculus Bovis Factiticus.

Calculus Bovis is a light, yellowish, round mass as large as an egg or as small as a bean, which is composed of many thin layers that are overlapping and, when pierced with a hot needle, may peel off. When split, a white spot is seen in the middle. It still gives yellow color when dissolved in water or rubbed on chalk. It is soluble in saliva and smells fragrant. It is mainly produced in the Northwest, Southwest and Northeast China and contains cholic acid, cholesterol, ergosterol, fatty acid, lecithin, bilirubin and other elements such as calcium, iron and copper. Calculus Bovis Factiticus is similar in composition to Calculus Bovis.

ANTICANCER PHARMACOLOGICAL FUNCTIONS

1. The suspension of Calculus Bovis Factiticus, when fed to hybrid mice with implanted sarcoma-180 with a dose of 408.9-437.6 mg/kg of body weight, was found to have an inhibitive rate of 60.9% whereas the inhibitive rate of camptothecine, in the control group was only 40.8%.

2. The inhibitive rate of Calculus Bovis Factiticus on sarcoma-37 was found to be 54.3% and 72.2% respectively in two different groups.

3. The inhibitive rate of the herb on solid Ehrlich's ascites carcinoma is 18.9%, suggesting that the drug has certain inhibition on cell division of ascites carcinoma, but does not inhibit its growth completely.

4. Calculus Bovis Factiticus is low in toxicity and capable of promoting the proliferation of erythrocytes in rats, and hence is an antisarcoma agent that works "to strengthen the body resistance and restore the normal function of the body".

5. A non-dialyzable substance obtained from the bile of oxen has been verified to have an inhibitive effect on the growth of Walker's cancer-256 and cause extensive necrosis of tumor with a proper dosage given through intraperitoneal administration. Calculus Bovis Factiticus has been found to have the same effects.

EXPERIMENTAL FORMULAS

For esophageal cancer:

1>.   Calculus Bovis Factiticus 6g
       Salmiacum 3g
       Radix Isatidis 30g
       Herba Euphorbiae Iunulatae 30g
       Rhizoma Arisaematis 9g
       Radix Clematidis 60g

This formula is pounded to powder for oral administration with a dose of 1.5 grams each time, four times a day. (*Anhui Information for Science and Technology*, Vol. 5, 1976)

2>.   Calculus Bovis 1.5g
       Alumen 1.5g
       Alumen (baked) 1.5g
       Realgar 1.5g
       Succinum 1.5g
       Olibanum 1.5g
       Myrrha 1.5g
       Margarita 1.5g
       Hydrargyrum Chloratum Compositum 1.5g
       Rhizoma Arisaematis 300g
       Concha Arcae 45g
       Arsenicum 1.5g
       Moschus 1.5g

The powder of the above herbs are blended with bile of Mylopharyngodon aethops and made into pills as large as Semen Sinapis for oral medication, or mixed with *Shenwenwei Gao* for application to the acupoint of *Chungwan* (*Ren* 12). (*Discourses on External Therapy*)

For cancer of the liver:

       Calculus Bovis Factiticus 30g
       Fructus Akebiae 30g
       Rhizoma Smilacis Chinae 90g
       Rhizoma Pinelliae 15g
       Rhizoma Arisaematis 15g
       Radix Astragali 30g
       Radix Medicata Fermentata 30g

(*Jilin Traditional Chinese Medicine and Drugs*, Vol. 1, 1984)

For cancer of the breast:

The decoction of Calculus Bovis (0.9g) and Spica Prunellae (60-90g) is taken orally. (*Data of Medicine and Drugs*, Vol. 4, 1974)

For leukemia:

Niuhuang Jiedu Pian (Calculus Bovis Detoxicating Pill) is taken 4 pills each time, three times a day. (*Manual of Practical Anticancer Drugs*)

HISTORICAL COMMENTS

In *Universal Prescriptions* it was stated that: "To treat epilepsy induced by terror and the disturbance of the mind, Calculus Bovis (as large as a bean) is crushed into powder, mixed with honey and fed to the patient."

In *Wang's Prescriptions for Smallpox and Measles* it was reported that: "To cure collapsed smallpox, 2 pieces of Calculus Bovis and 0.3 gram of Cinnabaris are ground to powder, dipped in honey and mixed with rouge for external application once daily."

Recorded in *Chinese Pharmacopeia* is that: "As an oral medicine, it cures furuncle, carbuncle, cellulitis and many other kinds of infections, while as an external medicine, it drastically functions as an analgesic and detoxicant."

THE AUTHOR'S NOTE

It was reported in Anhui Province that the preparations of Calculus Bovis Factiticus has a curative effect of 88.7% for intermediate and advanced esophageal cancer. In Chinese Academy of Medical Sciences, *Rengong Niuhuang San* (comprised of Borneol, pig's bile, Calculus Bovis and Cinnabaris) was administered to 6 cases of esophageal cancer. Among the 3 cases who took the drug for three months, one patient was greatly improved, the condition of one case became stable and one case died. (*Practice of New Medicine*, Vol. 3 and 4, 1975). Under the entry of Calculus Canis in the same category as Calculus Bovis in Li Shizhen's *Compendium of Materia Medica*, there was a formula for the treatment of dysphagia, which can also be prescribed for esophageal cancer. The formula is composed of pulverized Calculus Canis (0.3g), Radix Clematidis (60g) and salt (6g). The above drugs are pound into mass to be mixed with a cup of water for oral administration. Two of the preparation is taken daily. Upon complete recovery, tonic medicine is administered.

BULBUS FRITILLARIAE

In *Origin of Herbal Canon* it was recorded that: "Bulbus Fritillariae is sweet and most effective, while Bulbus Fritillariae thunbergii is slightly bitter and less effective."   Bulbus Fritillariae is the dried bulb of both *Bulbus Fritillariae Cirrhosae* and *Bulbus Fritillariae thunbergii* of the family *Liliaceae*. Bulbus Fritillariae Cirrhosae originates from *Fritillaria cirrhosa D. Don.*, *Fritillaria unibracteata Hsiao et K. C. Hsia* and *Fritillaria delavayi Franch.*, mainly growing in Sichuan and Yunnan Province. Bulbus Fritillariae Thunbergii is largely distributed over Zhejiang Province. In historical literatures before *Compendium of Materia Medica*, Bulbus Fritillariae had not been classified into Bulbus Fritillariae Cirrhosae and Bulbus Fritillariae Thunbergii. The name of Bulbus Fritillariae Thunbergii first appeared in *Mirror of Materia Medica* of the Qing Dynasty. The major components of both Bulbus Fritillariae Cirrhosae and Bulbus Fritillariae Thunbergii are alkaloids, and they have the same structures, functions and indications.

ANTICANCER PHARMACOLOGICAL FUNCTIONS

1. The inhibitive rate of the hot water extract of Bulbus Fritillariae on JTC-26 ranges from 70% to 90%.

2. Screening tests in vitro showed that both Bulbus Fritillariae Thunbergii and *Cardiocrinum cathayanum (Wils.) Mak.* have anticancer effect.

EXPERIMENTAL FORMULAS

For cervical cancer:

Bulbus Fritillariae Thunbergii (9-15g) is stewed together with a healthy male rabbit and the meat is divided into two portions taken in the morning and in the evening every day. If the patient's constitution is not bad, brown sugar can be added to the meat to achieve better therapeutical effect. (*New Medicine*, Vol. 2, 1976)

For cancer of the breast:

        Bulbus Fritillariae 10g
        Radix Ginseng 10g
        Rhizoma Cyperi 10g
        Poria 10g
        Pericarpium Citri Reticulatae 10g
        Radix Rehmanniae 10g
        Rhizoma Chuanxiong 10g
        Radix Angelicae Sinensis 10g
        Radix Paeoniae Alba 10g
        Rhizoma Atractylodis Macrocephalae 12g
        Radix Platycodi 6g
        Radix Glycyrrhizae 6g
        Rhizoma Zingiberis 3
        Fructus Ziziphi Inermis 2

This formula is taken in decoction. (*Oncology of Traditional Chinese Medicine*)

HISTORICAL COMMENTS

It was stated in *Descriptions of Materia Medica* that: "The herb cures furuncle, swelling and tumor mass with the functions to reinforce the viscera and protect the heart, as an astringent and detoxicant."

In *Interpretation of Drugs* it was described that: "With its downward and dispersing nature, the drug eliminates toxic materials, relieves stagnation and boosts blood circulation. It is therefore used for the treatment of consumptive diseases of the lung, pulmonary abscess, goiter, subcutaneous nodule, carbuncle, cellulitis and many other sorts of infections."

RADIX SALVIAE MILTIORRHIZAE

It was recorded in *Essentials of Materia Medica* that: "The herb is neutral in nature and used to invigorate the heart, promote blood generation and remove blood stasis."

Radix Salviae Miltiorrhizae is the dried root of *Salvia miltiorrhiza Bge.* of the family *Labiatae*, containing many elements such as tanshinone, tanshinol and vitamin E, essential to promote blood circulation and to remove blood stasis.

ANTICANCER PHARMACOLOGICAL FUNCTIONS

1. An obvious antineoplastic effect of Radix Salviae Miltiorrhizae on Ehrlich's ascites carcinoma of mice has been discovered.

2. The inhibitive rate of the hot water extract of Radix Salviae Miltiorrhizae on ascitic sarcoma-180 of mice was found to be 33.6%.

3. The antineoplastic mechanism of Radix Salviae Miltiorrhizae may lie in its inhibition on the respiration and glucolysis of cancer cells.

EXPERIMENTAL FORMULAS

For esophageal cancer:

Radix Salviae Miltiorrhizae 15g
Radix Adenophorae 15g
Sargassum 15g
Thallus Laminariae seu Eckloniae 15g
Bulbus Fritillariae Cirrhosae 10g
Radix Curcumae 10g
Folium Loti 12g
Fructus Amomi 6g
Haematitum 24g
Herba Oldenlandiae Diffusae 60g
Mel 60g

The herbs are decocted for oral administration daily. (*Medicine and Drugs in Jiangsu Province*, Volume of Traditional Chinese Medicine, 1979)

For cancer of the thymus gland:
Radix Salviae Miltiorrhizae 25g
Flos Carthami 25g
Rhizoma Atractylodis Macrocephalae 25g
Radix Astragali 25g
Radix Codonopsis Pilosulae 25g
Rhizoma Dioscoreae 25g
Rhizoma Pinelliae 15g
Radix Paeoniae Alba 15g
Rhizoma Zedoariae 15g
Radix Bupleuri 15g

The herbs can be increased and decreased according to the symptoms and are decocted for oral administration daily. (*New Traditional Chinese Medicine*, Vol. 11, 1983)

For cancer of the abdominal cavity:
Radix Salviae Miltiorrhizae 9g
Rhizoma Zedoariae 9g
Rhizoma Scirpi 9g
Spina Gleditsiae 3g

The herbs are decocted for oral administration. (*Selected Herbs of Shaanxi, Gansu, Ningxia and Qinghai Province*)

HISTORICAL COMMENTS

It was expounded in *Female Manners* that: "The decoction of Radix Salviae Miltiorrhizae has the same function as *Si Wu Tang* (Decoction of Four Ingredients)."

It was commented in *Ri Hua Zi Materia Medica* that: "The drug nourishes the mind, reinforces willpower, unblocks the *guan* pulse and cures goiter and pyogenic infections."

In *Origin of Herbal Canon* it was cautioned that: "Patients with loose bowels of the non-excess type should not take the drug."

THE AUTHOR'S NOTE

In Japan, Radix Salviae Miltiorrhizae is often added to *Qige* Powder for the treatment of cancer of the stomach. But, in another report, it was said that Radix Salviae Miltiorrhizae obviously accelerated metastasis and hematogenous diffusion of cancer cells on the one hand and enhanced the power of chemotherapy on the other. (*Bulletin of Pharmaceutics*, Vol. 7, 1980)

RADIX GLYCYRRHIZAE

Wu Yiluo of the Qing Dynasty reported: "The herb is sweet in taste and neutral in nature and is used as a drug for reinforcing or reducing the body functions, curing illnesses of the exterior or the interior, with ascending or descending properties."

Radix Glycyrrhizae is the dried tuberous root of *Glycyrrhiza* genus of the family *Leguminosae*, which grows in Northeast, Northwest and Northern China. The crude drug is used for purging pathogenic fire and when fried with honey, it warms the middle-*jiao*.

ANTICANCER PHARMACOLOGICAL FUNCTIONS

1. Glycyrrhetinic acid has an inhibitive action on implanted Oberling Guerin myeloma in rats.

2. The mixture of ammonium glycyrrhizinate, sodium glycyrrhetininate and the derivatives of glycyrrhetinic acid has an inhibitive effect on Ehrlich's ascites carcinoma and sarcoma of mice. When administered orally, the mixture still has the same effect.

3. Glycyrrhizin and liquiritin are found to induce morphological changes in cells of ascitic liver cancer and Ehrlich's ascites carcinoma in mice.

4. Glycyrrhizin inhibits the growth of subcutaneous Yoshida's sarcoma.

5. Glycyrrhizin is a prophylactic agent against cancer. The mice in the experimental group, fed with carcinogen 3-Me-DAB and injected with 1mg of glycyrrhizin intramuscularly every week, did not develop liver cancer and liver damage, and the structure of the liver cells in most of the mice remained normal by the time when the experiment came to an end. Whereas the mice of the control group presented a different picture. Severe liver damage appeared from the third month and among the 4 mice killed at the end of the 12th month, 3 developed liver cancer.

6. The hot water extract of Radix Glycyrrhizae has an inhibitive rate of 70-90% on cells of JTC-26, with slight involvement of normal cells.

EXPERIMENTAL FORMULAS

For chorioepithelioma:

> Radix Glycyrrhizae 15g
> Herba Scutellariae Barbatae 15g
> Herba Taraxaci 15g
> Herba Patriniae Scabiosaefoliae 15g
> Radix Sophorae Subprostratae 15g
> Radix Arnebiae 30g
> Semen Phaseoli 30g
> Colla Corii Asini 9g

These herbs are decocted for oral administration daily. (*Prevention and Treatment of Tumors*)

For cancerous ulcer of the vulva:

> Radix Glycyrrhizae 15g
> Galla Chinensis 15g
> Fructus Mume 15g
> Cortex Phellodendri 15g
> Alumen 15g

These herbs are ground to powder for external application. (*Concise Dermatology of Traditional Chinese Medicine*)

For obstruction due to esophageal cancer:

> Radix Glycyrrhizae 300g
> Salmiacum 30g
> Borax 150g

Galla Turcica 150g

Fructus Mume 9g

These herbs are pulverized, blended with honey and made into pills (each weighing 0.9g) for oral administration with a pill each time, three times a day. (*New Edition of Traditional Chinese Medicine*)

For tumor of the spinal column:

Radix Glycyrrhizae 6g

Radix Paeoniae Alba 6g

The two herbs are decocted to be taken with the powder of Radix Sophorae Subprostratae (2g). (*Explanation to Clinical Prescriptions of Traditional Chinese Medicine*)

For esophageal cancer:

Radix Glycyrrhizae 2g

Radix Ginseng 2g

Radix Ophiopogonis 5g

Rhizoma Pinelliae 5g

Fructus Oryzae 5g

Fructus Ziziphi Inermis 3

These herbs are decocted in 600ml of water to 300ml of broth, which is divided into four portions for oral administration three times during the day and one time at night. (*Explanation to Clinical Prescriptions of Traditional Chinese Medicine*)

For cancer of the stomach:

Radix Glycyrrhizae 2g

Rhizoma Zingiberis 4g

Fructus Ziziphi Inermis 4g

Radix Paeoniae Alba 6g

Saccharum Granorum 20g

The first four of the above herbs are decocted and filtered to remove the dregs. Then Saccharum Granorum is added and dissolved with further decoction for 5 minutes. The decoction is divided into three portions and taken in three times. (*Harbin Traditional Chinese Medicine*, Vol. 9, 1960)

For cancer of the tongue:

A thick decoction is made from Radix Glycyrrhizae for gargling while it is warm." (*Compendium of Medicinal Herbs*)

HISTORICAL COMMENTS

In *Practical Materia Medica*, Huang Gongxiu pointed out: "The drug is a tonic when used in mediating recipes, an antipyretic in cooling recipes, an agent to dispel pathogenic factors in the muscles in diaphoretic recipes, an agent to restore the vital-*qi* in radical recipes and an agent to nourish the blood and expel toxic materials in relaxing recipes."

In *New Materia Medica*, Wu Yiluo expounded: "Radix Polygalae, Radix Euphorbiae Pekinensis, Flos Genkwa, Radix Kansui and Sargassum are not compatible with Radix Glycyrrhizae. But there are cases in which these herbs are used in combination with Radix Glycyrrhizae: Hu Qia added Radix Glycyrrhizae to *Shizao Tang* for the treatment of accumulation of phlegm in hypochondrium; Dong Yuan used the drug in combination with Sargassum to cure tuberculosis; Dan Xi employed Flos Genkwa together with Radix Glycyrrhizae for treating tuberculosis. Those who do not have excellent command of the drugs can not comprehend this."

In *Selected Compilation of Materia Medica* it was reported that: "When extremely hot and extremely cold drugs are prescribed, Radix Glycyrrhizae must be added to mediate the intensity; When cold drugs and hot drugs are used in combination, Radix Glycyrrhizae also should be included to harmonize the properties."

THE AUTHOR'S NOTE

Radix Glycyrrhizae has fairly good analgesic effect. Hot plate experiment with rats has confirmed a remarkable analgesic action of FM-100 (one of the effective ingredients of Radix Glycyrrhizae). Therefore, it may play a supplementary role in the relief of cancerous pain. Though Radix Glycyrrhizae has low toxicity, a long period of administration will develop edema and hypertension, which may disappear upon the withdrawal of the drug. This suggests that the drug should be used with care for cancer patients complicated with nephric diseases and hypertension. During his management of patients with lung cancer, the author discovered that the symptoms of the patients could be dramatically improved if the decoction of 9-12 grams of Radix Glycyrrhizae was combined with other medications. In *New Edition of Mei's Proved Recipes*, there was a prescription which can be used for the treatment of mastocarcinoma. The formula is:

Fructus Trichosanthis (peeled) 2
Radix Glycyrrhizae 15g
Radix Angelicae (parched with wine) 15g
Olibanum 4.5g
Myrrha 4.5g

All the herbs are pulverized and then decocted in 3000ml of wine in a casserole to 1000ml of decoction for oral administration three times a day, each time one third of the decoction.

CAULIS SACCHARI SINENSIS

It was reported in *Records of Famous Physicians* that: "The herb, sweet in taste, neutral in nature, and nonpoisonous, keeps *qi* flowing downward and harmonizes the functions of the stomach and the spleen."

Caulis Sacchari Sinensis is the dried stalk, skin, sprout and juice of *Saccharum sinensis Roxb.* of the family *Gramineae*, mainly containing elements such as calcium, sulfur, iron, aspartic acid, glutamic acid, serine, alanine, tyrosine, leucine, proline and lysine as well as many nutrients such as vitamins B and C.

ANTICANCER PHARMACOLOGICAL FUNCTIONS

The dregs of Caulis Sacchari Sinensis contains polysaccharides (mainly composed of pentose and hexose) that have inhibitive actions on Ehrlich's carcinoma and sarcoma-180 of mice. Every 2.6kg of the dregs produces 2.6 grams of such polysaccharides. The syrup extracted during the process of sugar production also consists of polysaccharides.

EXPERIMENTAL FORMULAS
For cardiac cancer:
The juice of Caulis Sacchari Sinensis (1000ml) and the juice of Rhizoma Zingiberis (120ml) are blended and divided into three portions for drinking. (*Mei's Collection of Proved Recipes*)
For esophageal cancer:

Caulis Sacchari Sinensis (juice) 1 cup
Nelumbinis Rhizomatis 1 cup
Succus Zingiberis 1 cup
Pear juice 1 cup
Pineapple juice 1 cup
Honey 1 cup
Semen Gingko 1 cup
Succus Bambosae 1 cup

The above ingredients are mixed, steamed warm and taken as a drink frequently. (*New Collection of Classic Prescriptions*)

HISTORICAL COMMENTS

It was reported in *Annotation on Shen Nong's Medicinal Herbs* that: "Caulis Sacchari Sinensis is a popular plant in the farm, the taste of which goes into the spleen so as to support the spleen-*qi*. Nowadays it is used to cure dysphagia, regurgitation, vomiting and constipation, with its actions to remove heat, produce body fluid and to moisten dryness."

In *Rest and Diet Recipes* it was described that: "The syrup extracted from Caulis Sacchari Sinensis is known as *Tiansheng Fumai Tang*, which functions to clear pharynx, strengthen muscles and bones, calm the endopathic wind to nourish the blood and invigorate the spleen-*yin*."

In *Selected Compilation of Materia Medica* it was commented that: "Long-term and over consuming of the plant will result in diseases characterized by phlegm, fullness, vomiting and coughing due to damp-fire."

RADIX KANSUI

Wu Yiluo of the Qing Dynasty put it: "The drug, bitter, cold and poisonous, goes directly to the locations of the retained body fluid and acts quickly to remove it."

Radix Kansui is the tuberous root of *Euphorbia kansui T.N. Lion ex T.P. Wang* of the family *Euphorbiaceae*, which is a perennial fleshy herb containing white juice in the whole plant and triterpenoids in the root, growing mainly in Shaanxi and Hubei Province.

ANTICANCER PHARMACOLOGICAL FUNCTIONS

The deproteinized water solution of Radix Kansui, when diluted with 5% glucose and injected intravenously, proved effective for squamous carcinoma, undifferentiated carcinoma and malignant melanotic carcinoma of the lung, and caused acute necrosis of cancer cells.

EXPERIMENTAL FORMULAS

For esophageal carcinoma:

Radix Kansui (15 grams, roasted with wheat flour before use) and Radix Aucklandiae (3 grams for patients with strong constitution and 1.5 grams for patients with weak constitution) are pulverized and mixed with wine for oral administration. (*Prescriptions for Strange Diseases*)

For ascites due to liver cancer:

1.5 gram of Radix Kansui and 0.5 gram of Moschus are ground into fine powder for external application on the navel once daily. (*Discourses on External Therapy*)

HISTORICAL COMMENTS

In *Synopsis of Prescriptions of the Golden Chamber* it was reported that: "The decoction of Rhizoma et Radix Rhei (60g), Radix Kansui (30g) and Colla Corii Asini (30g) cures female blood stasis with fullness in the lower abdomen and mild difficulty in urination due to the agglomeration of water and blood in the uterus."

In *Compendium of Medicinal Herbs* it was stated that: "The drug purges water and dampness retained in the Kidney Channel and its passages. It is also prescribed for dysphagia and obstruction caused by tumor mass."

In *Collection of Prescriptions for Life-saving*, Liu Hejian wrote: "For patients with edema who do not respond satisfactorily to other medications, powder of Radix Kansui is applied around the umbilicus, and decoction of Radix Glycyrrhizae is taken orally. This formula is very effective for relieving swelling."

In *New Materia Medica* it was commented that: "The drug cures fullness and mass in the abdomen, strangulated hernia, dyspepsia due to the heat of food retention, and epilepsy resulting from phlegm. Since the herb removes the retention of body fluid drastically and destroys the genuine *qi* very fast, it is prescribed as a temporary treatment for diseases of extreme excess and retention of fluid, and is not used in other conditions. Radix Polygolae and Radix Glycyrrhizae are not compatible with Radix Kansui. But Zhang Zhongjing, an ancient physician, administered Radix Kansui and Radix Glycyrrhizae together to treat chronic upper abdominal edema, taking the advantage of the opposing properties of the two herbs. When the powder of Radix Kansui is applied externally and the thick decoction of Radix Glycyrrhizae is taken orally, the combination is very effective for edema and pyrogenic infections. Though the two herbs counteract one another, the effect is mythical."

THE AUTHOR'S NOTE

Though a serious of animal experiments have been done in the recent years, the compatibility of Radix Kansui and Radix Glycyrrhizae still remains unknown:

1>. When Radix Kansui (2g/kg of body weight) and Radix Glycyrrhizae (6.5g/kg of body weight) were given together to guinea pigs through oral decoction, some of the guinea pigs showed severe toxic reaction and some even died. But no toxic reactions were seen in these animals when Radix Kansui was used alone.

2>. Rabbits did not show any abnormal responses no matter when Radix Glycyrrhizae (2.2g/kg of body weight) was administered alone in decoction or combined with Radix Glycyrrhizae (6.6g/kg of body weight).

3>. The half lethal dose experiment with mice revealed that when the two herbs were used together, the toxicity of Radix Kansui increased drastically, even when the ratio of Radix Glycyrrhizae to Radix Kansui was as low as 1:3.

4>. Experiments with rats indicated that no opposing effects would appear when the doses of the two herbs are the same or the dose of Radix Glycyrrhizae is less than that of Radix Kansui, but opposing effects would turn up when the dose of Radix Glycyrrhizae is larger than that of Radix Kansui.

There is a recipe in *Compendium of Medicinal Herbs* for the treatment of mass in the abdomen, which seams effective for tumors of the abdominal cavity. Crude Radix Kansui is wrapped in dough and boiled in water. Then remove the dough, parch it over small fire until it turns yellow and then grind it into powder for oral administration before bed-time with cold honey water. The dosage is 9 grams for adults and 3 grams for children. No fish, meat and anything greasy are eaten during the period of administration.

RADIX GENTIANAE

In *Origin of Medicine* it was reported that: "The drug, cold in nature and considerably bitter in taste, is indicative for lumps with intolerable pain."

Radix Gentianae is the dried root and rhizome of *Gentiana scabra Bge.*, or *Gentiana triflora Pall.* of the family *Gentianaceae*, containing such elements as gentianine. The plant grows all over China.

ANTICANCER PHARMACOLOGICAL FUNCTIONS

1. Total cellular volumetric method proved that the hot water extract of Radix Gentianae has an inhibitive rate of 52% on the growth of tumor cells, when injected intraperitoneally to male mice infected with ascitic sarcoma-180 for 5 days in succession with a dose of 100mg/kg of body weight daily.

2. Tests in vitro showed that the hot water extract of Radix Gentianae has an inhibitive rate of 70-90% on JTC-26.

3. *Huaai Dan* (Anticancer Pill), which consists of Radix Gentianae, was found having an antineoplastic effect after having been administered to mice with Ehrlich's ascites carcinoma.

EXPERIMENTAL FORMULAS

For nasopharyngeal carcinoma: Herbs of the following two formulas are decocted for oral administration:

1>. Radix Gentianae 15g
        Flos Chrysanthemi Indici 15g
        Fructus Xanthii 15g
        Radix Scrophulariae 15g
        Radix Pseudostellariae 15g
        Rhizoma Paridis 30g
        Radix Rubi Parvifolii 30g
        Radix Zanthoxyli 30g

(*New Traditional Chinese Medicine*, Vol. 11, 1977)

2>. Radix Gentianae 15g
        Ramulus Uncariae cum Uncis 15g
        Spica Prunellae 15g
        Radix Pseudostellariae Heterophyllae 15g
        Rhizoma Alismatis 50g
        Radix Rubi Parvifolii 100g
        Rhizoma Arisaematis 50-150g
        Rhizoma Paridis 50-100g

(*Practical Oncology*)

For pancreatic cancer:
        Radix Gentianae 15g
        Herba Artemisiae Capillaris 30g
        Rhizoma Coptidis 6g
        Spina Gleditsiae 2g

The herbs are decocted for oral medication daily. (*Data of New Medicine and Drugs*, Vol. 3, 1972)

For cancer of the gallbladder:
        Radix Gentianae 15g
        Spica Prunellae 15g
        Herba Solani Lyrati 30g
        Semen Euphorbiae Lathyridis 9g
        Squama Manitis 9g
        Corium Stomachichum Galli 9g
        Thallus Laminariae seu Eckloniae 9g
        Sargassum 9g
        Lapis Pumicis 9g
        Medulla Tetrapanacis 9g
        Resina Ferulae 1.5g
        Mylabris 1.5g

The herbs are taken daily in decoction. (*Treatment and Prevention of Tumors in Traditional Chinese Medicine*)

HISTORICAL COMMENTS

It was reported in *Records of Combined Traditional Chinese and Western Medicine* that: "The drug, bitter and slightly sour, is a sound drug for stomach diseases. Its bitterness keeps the stomach-*qi* descending and helps strengthen the build-up of the stomach, while the sourness supplements the gastric acid and aids digestion."

In *Materia Medica of Lu Chan Yan* it was pointed out that: "The drug cures hematochezia due to alcoholic poisoning."

In *Xue's Medical Records of Sixteen Types of Illnesses* it was commented that: "*Longdan Xiegan Tang*, a decoction of Gentiana for purging the liver-fire, is indicative for scrotal abscess, hematochezia, chancre, acute pyogenic infection of the perineum, abdominal pain and difficulty in micturition as well as woman's perineal itching, pain and man's infection of the penis with swelling or pus due to damp-heat of the Liver Channel."

THE AUTHOR'S NOTE

Longdan Xiegan Tang, a traditional prescription for fire syndrome of the excessive type and the damp-heat of the Liver Channel, has been used by some doctors in Japan in the recent years for benign and malignant tumors of the liver, the gallbladder and the productive system, with certain effect. The recipe being used in Japan is:

> Radix Angelicae Sinensis 5g
> Radix Rehmanniae 5g
> Caulis Aristolochiae Manshuriensis 5g
> Radix Scutellariae 3g
> Rhizoma Alismatis 3g
> Semen Plantaginis asiaticae 3g
> Radix Gentianae 1.5g
> Fructus Gardeniae 1.5g
> Radix Glycyrrhizae 1.5g

HERBA SOLANI NIGRI

Zhang Shanlei of the Republic of China described: "The herb is cold in nature with lubricating functions. It has soft and tender stalks and looks like a dragon."

Herba Solani Nigri is the dried plant of *Solanum nigrum L.* of the family *Solanaceae*, which is distributed all over China.

ANTICANCER PHARMACOLOGICAL FUNCTIONS

1. When administered to rats inoculated with cells of Ehrlich's ascites carcinoma, lymphatic leukemia-615, sarcoma-180 and sarcoma-37, the herb was found to have inhibitive effects on the strains.

2. Animal experiments in vivo with the herb revealed an inhibitive action on cancer cells of the stomach.

3. An inhibitive effect on cancer cells (leukemia) is proved with methylene-blue tube tests in vitro.

EXPERIMENTAL FORMULAS

For epithelial tumor of the urinary bladder:
> Herba Solani Nigri 30g
> Herba Solani Lyrati 30g

The herbs are decocted in water for oral administration daily. (*Diagnosis, Treatment and Prevention of Tumors*)

For postoperative chorioepithelioma:

        Herba Solani Nigri 45g

        Herba Scutellariae Barbatae 60g

        Radix Arnebiae 45g

The herbs are decocted in water for oral administration daily. (*Diagnosis, Treatment and Prevention of Tumors*)

For cancerous hydrothorax and ascites:

A dose of 500 grams of Herba Solani Nigri (fresh) is decocted in water for oral administration daily. (*Determination of Treatment Based on the Differentiation of Symptoms and Signs*)

For cancer of the liver:

        Herba Solani Nigri 60g

        Folium Ilecis 30g

The herbs are decocted in water for oral administration daily. (*Universal Prescriptions*)

For cervical cancer:

1>. Decoction: Herba Solani Nigri (30-60 grams when dry and 90-150 grams when fresh) is decocted twice on soft fire in 800ml of water. The two decoctions (approximately 300ml) are mixed for oral administration in three times. Fifteen days of administration make a therapeutic course.

2>. Injection: Herba Solani Nigri is decocted in water for two to three times and the decoction is condensed to 1:1 or 1:0.5. Then 1.5-fold alcohol is added and the sediment is filtered out repeatedly. After the alcohol is removed, certain amount of distilled water is added to the extract for filtering again. With some quantity of activated carbon, Tween-80 and benzyl alcohol added, the liquid is refined and then sealed by fusing for sterilizing at a temperature of 100°C for 30 minutes before use. (*Scientific Experiments*, Vol. 1, 1974)

For fibrosarcoma:

The decoction of Herba Solani Nigri (60-90g) is taken daily. (*Dictionary of Chinese Materia Medica*)

HISTORICAL COMMENTS

In *Compendium of Medicinal Herbs* it was described that the herb removes heat and blood stasis and cures erysipelas. Its seed is used to cure furuncle. Its root is used as a diuretic and its stalk, when pounded to pieces and mixed with soil, is indicative for furuncle and erysipelas through external application.

In *Illustrated Materia Medica*, Su Song pointed out: "The drug is effective for illnesses caused by wind. In addition, it nourishes the primordial *qi* of men and lochioschesis of women."

In *Comprehension of Materia Medica* it was reported that: "Herba Solani Nigri is administered either orally or externally as an antipyretic and diuretic, indicating for traumatic injury and blood stasis. It is also an effective drug particularly for relieving heat and resolving swelling."

THE AUTHOR'S NOTE

Herba Solani Nigri is one of the frequently used effective anticancer drugs. When combined with Herba Agrimoniae, Radix Sanguisorbae and other drugs, its antineoplastic actions can be multiplied and the astringing properties of Herba Agrimoniae and Radix Sanguisorbae are reduced with its lubricating attribute. When properly used, the effect is really satisfactory. Although being slightly poisonous, its toxicity can be reduced by decocting.

In *Anticancer Guidance*, Wang Youmin introduced a universal anticancer prescription of Quli Herbal Store in Shanghai, in which Herba Solani Nigri is used as the principal herb. The prescription includes the following herbs:

Herba Solani Nigri 45-60g
Herba Duchesneae 45-60g
Herba Solani Lyrati 45-60g

Based on the above recipe, a series of proved prescriptions against cancer have been introduced. They are:

For cancer of the throat:
Herba Clinopodii 20-30g
Rhizoma Fagopyri Cymosi 20-30g
Rhizoma Paridis 20-30g

For cancer of the plica vocalis:
Herba Salviae Sinensis 3g
Herba Ainsliaeae 3g
Radix Ophiopogonis 15g

For esophageal cancer:
Herba Salviae Chinensis 30g
Herba Scutellariae Barbatae 30g
Sargassum 30g
Folium Lycii 15g
Radix Clematidis 15g

For cancer of the stomach:
Herba Scutellariae 30g
Herba Salviae Chinensis 30g

For cancer of the breast:
Herba Taraxaci 30g
Fructus Fici Pumilae 30g
Rhizoma Paridis 30g

For lung cancer:
Radix Codonopsis Lanceolatae 15g
Radix Pecteilitis 15g
Herba Houttuyniae 30g

For cancer of the liver:
Herba Lobeliae Chinensis 15g
Herba Lysimachiae 45-60g

For ovary cancer:
Radix Coicis 30g
Herba Verbenae 30g
Herba Seneci 30g

For cancer of the urinary bladder:
Radix Coicis 30g
Herba Commelinae 30g
Radix Cayratiae 30g
Herba Lysimachiae 30g

For brain tumor:
Rhizoma Amorphophalli 30g
Rhizoma Paridis 30g
Rhizoma Dryopteris Crassirhizomae 30g
Herba Xanthii 45g

For tumor of the soft tissues:
Folium Ilecis 45-60g

Rhizoma Smilacis Glabrae 15g

Herba Galii Aprinis 15g

Herba Xanthii 45g

RHIZOMA PINELLIAE

Luo Guogang, a physician in the Qing Dynasty, pointed out: "The herb, acrid, warm and poisonous, acts on the Heart, Spleen and Stomach Channel, to eliminate dampness."

Rhizoma Pinelliae is the dried rhizome of *Pinellia ternate (Thunb.) Breit.* of the family *Araceae*, and those growing in Sichuan and Yunnan Province are the best. The crude herb has an exceedingly violent nature and is toxic, so it has to be processed with Rhizoma Zingiberis or Alumen before use.

ANTICANCER PHARMACOLOGICAL FUNCTIONS

1. Tests in vitro showed the herb has a slight inhibition on JTC-26 but does not cause any influence on the normal cells.

2. After intraperitoneal injection of the alcohol-precipitated hot water extract of Rhizoma Pinelliae to rats of ascitic sarcoma with a dose of 100ml/kg of body weight for 5 days in succession, the inhibitive rate on the growth of tumor cells was estimated to be 69% by total cellular volumetric method.

3. It has been proved that the herb has an inhibitive action on cervical cancer-14, sarcoma-180, solid liver cancer and Hela cells.

EXPERIMENTAL FORMULAS

For cancer of the stomach and the esophagus:

Rhizoma Pinelliae 8g

Fructus Gardeniae 3g

Radix Aconiti Lateralis Praeparata 0.5-1g

Poria 5g

Semen Armeniacae Amarum 4g

Radix Glycyrrhizae 2g

These herbs are decocted in water for oral administration daily. (*Explanation to Clinical Prescriptions of Traditional Chinese Medicine*)

For stomach cancer:

Rhizoma Pinelliae 5g

Radix Platycodi 3g

Radix Peucedani 3g

Carapax Trionycis 3g

Radix Ginseng 2g

Rhizoma Zingiberis 1g

Fructus Citri Aurantii 1g

Fructus Evodiae 0.5-1g

These herbs are decocted in water for oral administration daily. (*Explanation to Clinical Prescriptions of Traditional Chinese Medicine*)

For cervical cancer:

2 or 3 Rhizoma Pinelliae Pills (one pill contains 0.3 gram of the water soluble glue extracted with alcohol) are taken each time, three times daily. (*Bulletin of Medicinal Herbs*, Vol. 2, 1978)

For malignant lymphoma:

Rhizoma Pinelliae 120g

Bulbus Fritillariae Cirrhosae 180g

The above two herbs are pulverized, blended with Succus Zingiberis and made into boluses for oral administration, 3.6 grams each time, twice daily.

For cardiac cancer:

Equal portions of Rhizoma Pinelliae and Fructus Piperis are ground to powder, blended with Succus Zingiberis, and made into pills of the size of Fructus Firmianae. 30-50 pills are taken each time with ginger soup. (*Effective Prescriptions*)

For esophageal cancer (of *qi* deficiency type):

Rhizoma Pinelliae 10g
Radix Astragali 30g
Radix Codonopsis Pilosulae 20g
Radix Angelicae Sinensis 15g
Radix Paeoniae Alba 10g
Flos Inulae 10g
Haematitum 30g
Radix Clematidis 30g
Semen Impatientis 10g
Ramulus Cinnamomi 10g
Pericarpicum Citri Reticulatae 10g
Radix Rehmanniae 10g
Radix Rehmanniae Praeparata 10g

These herbs are decocted in water for oral administration daily. (*Oncology of Traditional Chinese Medicine*)

HISTORICAL COMMENTS

Zhang Shanlei commented: "With lots of foams, Rhizoma Pinelliae is quite smooth, very bitter in taste, stingy when licked with tongue and is thereupon used to disperse stagnation or accumulated pathogens."

In *Properties of Medicinal Herbs* it was reported that: "The crude herb is used to cure carbuncle and goiter."

Pearl Bag reported that the herb "resolves swelling and lumps".

In *Treatise on Properties of Drugs* it was expounded that: "The crude herb is applied externally to treat carbuncle as well as goiter."

In *Luo's Mirror of Medicine* it was stated that: "It cures sore and paralysis of the throat, regurgitation, vomiting, mass and goiter."

In *Synopsis of Prescriptions of Golden Chamber* it was recorded that: "*Da Banxia Tang* is effective for vomiting, regurgitation (The author's note: symptoms seen in cancer of the digestive system) and excessive fluid in the hypochondrium and epigastrium as well. The *Tang* is prepared with Rhizoma Pinelliae (45g), Ginseng (90g) and Mel (40ml), through decocting in 500ml of water to 150ml of broth for oral administration once daily, 40ml each time."

It was suggested in *Selection of Mysterious Prescriptions* that: "For the treatment of double tongue, swollen and rigid tongue (author's note: extremely like the signs of cancer of the tongue), Rhizoma Pinelliae is decocted in vinegar for gargling."

In *Handbook of Prescriptions for Emergencies* it was indicated that: "To cure carbuncle and cellulitis on the back and furuncle of the breast, powder of Rhizoma Pinelliae is mixed with egg white for application to the lesion."

Recorded in *Chinese Pharmacopeia* was the prescription of Zhang Zhongjing's Bitter Wine Decoction for the treatment of aphasia, aphonia due to pain of the *Shaoyin* Channel and sore throat. Seven pieces of Rhizoma Pinelliae are crushed and packed into an egg whose yolk has been taken out. Then fill the egg with some wine and place it in a cup for boiling over charcoal fire for a short time. The decoction is drunk slowly after its dregs have been removed. The prescription is very effective and should be repeated if the illness is not completely cured."

THE AUTHOR'S NOTE
To treat various types of obstinate vomiting, Zhang Xichun, an eminent doctor in Hebei Province, often makes preparations with Rhizoma Pinelliae himself and has achieved very good results. Perhaps, his preparations are also effective for cancer of the digestive system. The process of his preparations with Rhizoma Pinelliae is introduced in *Records of the Combination of Traditional Chinese and Western Medicine*. It says: "Several kilograms of Rhizoma Pinelliae, each piece being cleaved into two pieces, are put in a casserole with a lot of cool water for boiling, after having been soaked in hot water every day for a total of ten days. Then get the herb out and dry it under the sun before being stored for use. Each time, 30 grams of Rhizoma Pinelliae Praeparata is decocted in water to get two teapots of decoction for oral administering slowly after being mixed with 60 grams of Mel. The decoction is effective no matter how severe the vomiting is. If no Rhizoma Pinelliae Praeparata is available, Rhizoma Pinelliae (about 50g) obtained from herb stores is rinsed to get rid of the alum before being decocted."

Because Rhizoma Pinelliae is poisonous and a excessive dose may lead to death, care must be given to the processing procedures. Once poisoning occurs, the following approaches help to relieve the toxic reactions:

1>. Ask the patient to take some egg white, flour paste, fruit juice or diluted vinegar.

2>. Rhizoma Zingiberis (30g), Radix Ledebouriellae (60g) and Radix Glycyrrhizae (15g) are decocted in 4 bowls of water to 2 bowls of broth, half of which is for gargling and half for oral administration.

Rhizoma Zingiberis is really good for relieving poisoning of Rhizoma Pinelliae. According to a report in *Chinese Medicine* (Vol. 8, 1962), of the 4 persons who took Rhizoma Pinelliae by mistake and got poisoning, 3 were relieved by taking Rhizoma Zingiberis and 1 recovered spontaneously because he took a very small dose (0.1g).

HERBA LOBELIAE CHINENSIS

Li Shizhen of the Ming Dynasty remarked: "The herb is acrid, bitter and nonpoisonous. The plant blossoms in autumn with small reddish flowers looking like a half of lotus' flower."

Herba Lobeliae Chinensis is the dried whole plant of *Lobelia chinensis Lour.* of the family *Campanulaceae*, which is found growing in most places in China.

ANTICANCER PHARMACOLOGICAL FUNCTIONS
1. Screening tests in vitro with monolayer hela-cell culture proved that Herba Lobeliae Chinensis has an anticancer action.

2. Tests in vivo showed that the herb has an inhibitive action on sarcoma-37 of mice.

EXPERIMENTAL FORMULAS
For cancer of the kidney:

The decoction of Herba Lobeliae Chinensis (120g) is taken daily. (*Diagnosis, Treatment and Prevention of Tumors*)

For cancer of the nasal cavity:

The decoction of Herba Lobeliae Chinensis and Herba Geranii (60 grams each) is taken orally. (*Compilation of Herbal Exhibition in Wuhan*)

For liver cancer:

1>. Fresh Herba Lobeliae Chinensis is pounded to paste and made into poultice for application to the liver region.

2>. The decoction of the following herbs is taken daily:

      Herba Lobeliae Chinensis 30g

      Herba Scutellariae Barbatae 30g

      Herba Salviae Chinensis 30g

(*Anticancer Herbal Preparations*)

For cancerous ascites:

      Herba Lobeliae Chinensis 30g

      Herba Scutellariae Barbatae 30g

      Semen Coicis 30g

      Semen Plantaginis Asiaticae 12g

      Poria 12g

      Fructus Liquidambaris 12g

      Radix Salviae Miltiorrhizae 15g

      Herba Solani Nigri 15g

      Rhizoma Alismatis 9g

      Herba Eupatorii 9g

      Radix Glycyrrhizae 3g

The above herbs are decocted for oral administration daily. (*Essential Points of Oncology*)

HISTORICAL COMMENTS

In *Compendium of Medicinal Herbs* it was described that: "Juice of the herb cures snakebite."

In *Principal Toxic Plants in South China* it was amplified that: "An excessive dose of Herba Lobeliae Chinensis brings on salivation, nausea, headache, diarrhea, elevated blood pressure, initially slowed and then accelerated pulse, and even death due to paralysis of the respiratory center in severe cases. To relieve the conditions, emesis, gastrolavage, injection of glucose solution, and drinking thick tea are recommended. Folk doctors suggest to drink soybean milk, Radix Platycodi decoction, Radix Glycyrrhizae decoction, salty water or Succus Zingiberis."

THE AUTHOR'S NOTE

According to a report in *Journal of Combined Traditional Chinese and Western Medicine* (Vol. 4, 1984), Compound Antitumor Powder (Composed mainly of Herba Lobeliae Chinensis) was used for the treatment of 47 cases of cerebral glioma at early or intermittent stage, with complete recovery in 5 cases, remarkable effectiveness in 11, no changes or improvement in 16 and inefficacy in 15. The overall effective rate is calculated to be 68%. The symptoms and signs of the recovered cases disappeared completely and the tumor mass became veiled or calcified on CT scanning. Electronic microscopy in animal experiment revealed that the herb was capable of killing and inhibiting tumor cells, detoxifying poisonous effect, tonifying the brain and promoting the immunity of the body.

HERBA SCUTELLARIAE BARBATAE

It was reported in *National Collection of Medicinal Herbs* that: "The herb, slightly bitter and cool, is used as an antipyretic and detoxicant, as an agent to promote blood circulation to remove blood stasis, and as an antineoplastic."

Herba Scutellariae Barbatae is the dried whole plant of *Scutellaria barbata D. Don.* of the family *Labiatae*, which is mainly distributed over the areas south of the Yellow River and contains chemical elements such as alkaloids and flavones. Being a folk herb mainly used to treat cancer, it was not recorded in ancient literatures. Baicalein derived from Radix Scutellariae of the same family has been proved to be antineoplastically active.

ANTICANCER PHARMACOLOGICAL FUNCTIONS

1. Experiment in vitro has revealed that the hot water extract of Herba Scutellariae Barbatae has a very strong inhibitive action on JTC-26 (the rate is over 90%) but only a slight inhibition on normal cells.

2. This herb has been proved anticancer active in screening selection of anticancer herbs with bean sprout method.

3. An antiphagic action has been verified with bacteriophagic screening experiments in vitro.

4. Studies with the herb in vivo showed an inhibitive action on sarcoma-180, Ehrlich's ascites carcinoma and cerebroma-B_{22} in rats.

5. Methylene-blue tests revealed a mild inhibitive action on acute granular leukemia.

6. With cellular respirator method, the inhibition rate on blood cells of leukemia was calculated to be over 75%.

EXPERIMENTAL FORMULAS

For ovary cancer:

> Herba Scutellariae Barbatae 50g
> Herba Solani Nigri 50g
> Herba Solani Lyrati 30g
> Herba Oldenlandiae Diffusae 30g
> Carapax Trionycis 30g

These herbs are decocted in water for oral administration daily. If abdominal pain is present, the following herbs are added to the above formula:

> Radix Aucklandiae 6g
> Radix Polygoni Multiflori 9g
> Rhizoma Corydalis 9g

If abdominal distention is present, the following herbs are added:

> Pericarpium Arecae 9g
> Cortex Magnoliae 9g
> Fructus Citri Aurantii 9g

If ascites is present, the following are added:

> Semen Plantaginis Asiaticae 12g
> Rhizoma Alismatis 12g

(*Diagnosis, Treatment and Prevention of Tumors*)

For secondary pleural tumor:

> Herba Scutellariae Barbatae 120g
> Taraxaci 30g

The herbs are decocted in water and taken daily as tea. (*Diagnosis, Treatment and Prevention of Tumors*)

For nasopharyngeal carcinoma:

> Herba Scutellariae Barbatae 50g
> Rhizoma Typhonil 50g

The herbs are decocted in water and taken daily. (*New Compilation of Traditional Chinese Medicine*)

For malignant hydatidiform mole:

> Herba Scutellariae Barbatae 30g
> Herba Solani Nigri 30g

Radix Arnebiae 15g

The herbs are decocted in water and taken daily. (*National Collection of Medicinal Herbs*)

For cancer of stomach:

Herba Scutellariae Barbatae 30g

Rhizoma Imperatae 30g

The herbs are decocted in water and taken daily as tea. (*New Edition of Traditional Chinese Medicine*)

For cancers of the liver, the rectum and the lung:

Herba Scutellariae Barbatae 60g

Herba Oldenlandiae Diffusae 60g

The herbs are decocted in water and taken daily. (*Determination of Treatment Based on Differentiation of Symptoms and Signs*)

For fibroma of the breast or multiple neuroma:

Herba Scutellariae Barbatae 30g

Folium Laggerae Pterodontae 30g

Flos Chrysanthemi Indici 30g

Radix Angelicae Sinensis 12g

Corium Elephatis 9g

Squama Manitis 9g

Scorpio 6g

Scolopendra 2

The herbs are decocted for oral administration and 20-30 doses make a therapeutic course. (*New Collection of Materia Medica of Zhenan*)

For rectal cancer:

Herba Scutellariae Barbatae 30g

Herba Oldenlandiae Diffusae 30g

Caulis Sargentodoxae 15g

Herba Patriniae Scabiosaefoliae 12g

Semen Coicis 12g

Flos Lonicerae 12g

Radix Pulsatillae 12g

Corium Erinacei 9g

Radix Sophorae Flavescentis 9g

Squama Manitis 9g

The herbs are decocted in water to be taken orally every day. (*A Clinical Handbook for Doctors of Traditional Chinese*)

For esophageal cancer:

Herba Scutellariae Barbatae (30g) is decocted twice in water to be taken in the morning and in the afternoon or taken as a drink. (*Research of New Medicine and Drugs*, Vol. 2, 1971)

For lung cancer:

Herba Scutellariae Barbatae and Herba Solani Lyrati (30 grams each) are decocted in water and taken once daily. (*Research of New Medicine and Drugs*, Vol. 4 and 5, 1972)

For various cancers:

"Injection 442" is administered intramuscularly or locally with a dose of 2-4ml every day or every other day. To prepare Injection 442, equal portions of Herba Scutellariae Barbatae, Herba Solani Lyrati and Spica Prunellae are boiled in water three times, then the liquid is filtered and condensed. Two-fold 95% alcohol is added to the condensed liquid and is put aside for sedimentation. After alcohol is removed, pH of the fluid is adjusted to 5-7. Water for injection is used to dilute the liquid to make preparations that contains 10%, 20% and 100% of the crude herbs respectively. Finally 2% benzyl alcohol is added before sterilization. (*Diagnosis, Treatment and Prevention of Tumors*)

For various tumors:

1>.   Herba Scutellariae Barbatae 200g

Radix Sophorae Tonkinensis 100g

Nidus Vespae 100g

Cormus Iphigeniae 100g

The above herbs are ground to fine powder to make boluses of soybean-size. A dose of 15 boluses is taken each time after meal and 2-3 times a day. (*National Collection of Medicinal Herbs*)

2>. A dose of 10-20ml of "Herba Scutellariae Barbatae Syrup" is taken orally three times a day. The herb content in each 100ml of the syrup corresponds to the decoction of:

Herba Scutellariae Barbatae 5g

Cortex Phellodendri 5g

Fructus Meliae Toosendan 5g

Flos Lonicerae 5g

Carapax Trionycis 4g

Radix et Caulis Opuntiae 4g

Herba Orostachydis 20g

Flos Chrysanthemi Indici 20g

Fructus Crataegi 10g

Squama Manitis 2g

(*Anticancer Herbal Preparations*)

HISTORICAL COMMENTS

In *National Collection of Medicinal Herbs* it was reported that: "The herb is indicative for tumor, appendicitis, hepatitis, ascites due to cirrhosis and pulmonary abscess."

In *Handbook of Common Drugs* it was recorded that: "The herb cures cancer of the esophagus, the stomach and the uterus."

It was suggested in *Dictionary of Chinese Materia Medica* that: "The herb (15-30 grams when dried, or 30-60 grams when fresh) is taken in decoction. The juice squeezed out of the herb is used externally. The herb is contraindicative for patients with blood deficient syndrome and pregnant women."

It was pointed out in *Anticancer Consultant* that: "Herba Scutellariae Barbatae, used as an detoxicant, is effective for various types of tumors."

THE AUTHOR'S NOTE

The herb has a wide range of indications. According to a report by the Tumor Research Group of Jilin Second City Hospital in *Medicine and Drugs of Jilin*, (Vol. 2, 1973), among the 50 cases of primary cancer treated with the preparations of Herba Scutellariae Barbatae, 9 recovered shortly after the administration, 8 showed remarkable efficacy, 14 indicated efficacy, with an overall effective rate of 62%.

FOLIUM ARTEMISIAE ARGYI

It was stated in *Comprehension of Materia Medica* that: "The herb is acrid and warm, goes upwards and solidifies what it matches."

Folium Artemisiae Argyi is the dried leaf of *Artemisia argyi L. et V.* or *Artemisia vulgaris L.* of the family *Compositae*, both containing volatile oil and relatively abundant iodine, and being apt to absorb barium from the earth.

ANTICANCER PHARMACOLOGICAL FUNCTIONS

1. An anticancer activity of the herb has been proved with bean sprout screening method.

2. Bacteriophagic screening method for anticancer drugs confirmed that the herbs has an antiphagic action.

3. Artemisia vulgaris L. was found to have an inhibitive action on Hela-cells and on many types of transplanted tumors.

EXPERIMENTAL FORMULAS

For tumor of the thyroid:

1>. 3-6 Artemisia vulgaris L. Pills (each pill weighing 0.5 gram) are taken each time, three times a day.

2>. Folium Artemisiae Argyi is blended with wheat flour to make cakes for eating frequently. (*Anticancer Consultant*)

For bleeding due to cancer of the nasal cavity:

Ash of Folium Artemisiae Argyi is inhaled or the decoction of the drug is taken. (*Holy Prescriptions*)

HISTORICAL COMMENTS

In *Illustration of Materia Medica* it was reported that: "The herb, when pilled with steamed Fructus Chaenomelis or decocted in water, for oral administration on empty stomach, exceedingly nourishes patients of the deficiency type."

It was described in *Dictionary of Chinese Materia Medica* that: "To cure verruca vulgaris, fresh Folium Artemisiae Argyi is applied to the lesion several times daily until verruca vulgaris falls off spontaneously."

In *Records of Herbs in the Jin E Mountain* it was recorded that: "Folium Artemisiae Argyi is prescribed for goiter."

THE AUTHOR'S NOTE

Recently, the preparations of Artemisia vulgaris have been used in the management of cancers of the digestive system and the breast, with an overall effective rate of 58%. It is believed that the herb can relieve and improve the symptoms of the patients and prevent deterioration of their conditions.

HERBA SALVIAE CHINENSIS

In *Medicinal Herbs of Suzhou* it was reported that: "The herb, bitter and acrid in taste and neutral in nature, is used to cure dysphagia."

Herba Salviae Chinensis is the dried plant of Salvia chinensis Benth. of the family Labiatae, which is mainly distributed over areas south of the Yellow River.

ANTICANCER PHARMACOLOGICAL FUNCTIONS

1. An anticancer activity of Herba Salviae Chinensis has been observed with bean sprout method in vitro.

2. Studies in vivo showed an inhibitive action of the herb on sarcoma-180 in rats.

EXPERIMENTAL FORMULAS

For cancer of the nasal cavity:

The decoction of Herba Salviae Chinensis (30g) is taken three times a day. If the fresh plant is available, the juice of 60 grams is taken. (*Diagnosis, Treatment and Prevention of Tumors*)

For lung cancer:

        Herba Salviae Chinensis 60g

        Radix Arnebiae 30g

        Radix Adenophorae 12g

        Radix Ophiopogonis 12g

        Radix rehmanniae 12g

        Radix Stemonae 12g

        Radix Sanguisorbae 12g

        Fructus Schisandrae 6g

        Fructus Gardeniae 9g

        Semen Vaccariae 9g

        Herba Taraxaci 15g

These herbs are taken in decoction daily. (*Diagnosis, Treatment and Prevention of Tumors*)

For cervical cancer:

        Herba Salviae Chinensis 30g

        Herba Artemisiae Anomalae 30g

        Herba Patriniae Heterophyllae 30g

        Rhizoma Cyperi 15g

These herbs are taken in decoction, twice daily. (*National Collection of Medicinal Herbs*)

For various types of cancer:

1>. Herba Salviae Chinensis and Herba Scutellariae Barbatae (30 grams each) are decocted and taken frequently as a drink. (*Manual of Practical Anticancer Drugs*)

2>. An oral dose of 10ml of Herba Salviae Chinensis mixture (Each 100ml contains 200 grams of Herba Salviae Chinensis, 100 grams of Scutellariae Barbatae and certain amount of sucrose) is taken three times a day. (*Anticancer Herbal Preparations*)

For ulcerated cancer of the skin:

Certain amount of Herba Salviae Chinensis is ground to powder and mixed with lard for external application. (*Treatment and Prevention of Traditional Chinese Medicine*)

HISTORICAL COMMENTS

In *Compendium of Medicinal Herbs* it was recorded that: "The herb is used mainly to cure osteodynia, leprosy and carbuncle."

In *Records of Jiangsu Medicinal Plants* it was described that: "The herb cures scrofula."

It was commented in *New Collection of Materia Medica of Zhenan* that: "Being similar to Radix Salviae Mitiorrhizae in efficacy, Herba Salviae Chinensis is often used to treat chronic hepatitis and early cirrhosis, through promoting blood circulation and removing blood stasis. The dose for each administration is 9-15 grams and the herb is often used in compound recipes and taken in decoction."

RHIZOMA ACORI GRAMINEI

It was recorded in *Shen Nong's Medicinal Herbs* that: "The herb, acrid and warm, is used to supplement the five viscera and clear the nine orifices."

Rhizoma Acori Graminei is the dried rhizome of *Acorus gramineus Soland* of the family *Araceae*, which contains volatile oil, amino acids and organic acids in its rhizome and leaf."

ANTICANCER PHARMACOLOGICAL FUNCTIONS

1. The inhibitive rate of the herb has been found to be 92% on Aspergillus flavus, 97% on aspergillus, 100% on both aflatoxin B_1 and sporotrichosis.

2. Screening tests in vitro have preliminarily proved that the decoction of the herb kills cells of ascites carcinoma.

3. In addition, in vivo animal experiments verified that the herb has an active effect against cancer.

EXPERIMENTAL FORMULAS

For cervical cancer:

Equal portions of Rhizoma Acori Graminei and Fructus Psoraleae are parched into powder to be orally taken with a dose of 6 grams. At the same time, Rhizoma Acori Graminei is immersed in wine and taken daily. (*Effective Prescriptions for Women*)

For various types of cancer:

Rhizoma Acori Graminei (10g) is decocted in 200ml of water to be taken in three doses. (*Research Data of Medicinal Herbs*, Vol. 6, 1978)

HISTORICAL COMMENTS

It was described in *Compendium of Medicinal Herbs* that: "Rhizoma Acori Graminei is warm in nature and indicative for insufficiency of the heart-*qi*. It also supplements the liver for related disorders with its acrid taste."

In *Materia Medica of Southern Yunnan* reported that: "The herb cures nine kinds of the stomach diseases due to the disorder of its *qi* and relieves pain."

In *Essentials of Materia Medica* it was stated that: "The drug supplements the liver, nourishes the heart, promotes functional activity of the stomach and relieves epigastric distention."

THE AUTHOR'S NOTE

It has been confirmed in pharmacological experiments that volatile oil of the herb has a remarkable sedative effect, which indicates its proper application in treating cancer patients complicated with restlessness and unconsciousness. Besides, the volatile oil of the herb is actively antipyretic. To secure its curative efficacy, Rhizoma Acori Graminei is added later than other herbs for boiling and should not be decocted for a long time.

BULBUS LYCORIDIS RADIATAE

It was pointed out in *Illustration of Materia Medica* that: "The herb, acrid, warm and slightly poisonous, cures pyrogenic infections when applied on the affected lesion."

Bulbus Lycoridis Radiatae is the dried bulb of *Lycoris radiata (L Her.) Herb.* of the family *Amaryllidaceae*, which is mainly distributed in Hunan, Shaanxi, East China, South China and Southwest China, and contains a variety of alkaloids, chiefly, lycorine and lycoricidinol, both being antineoplastically active. The latter is also found inhibiting the growth of plants.

ANTICANCER PHARMACOLOGICAL FUNCTIONS

1. Tests both in vivo and in vitro showed that lycorine was capable of inhibiting aerobic and anaerobic glycolysis of cells of Ehrlich's ascites carcinoma in rats and inducing enlargement and dissolution of cancer cells.

2. Lycorine was also found to have inhibitive actions on ascitic hepatocarcinoma-AH130 and Yoshida's sarcoma, particularly on sarcoma-180 of mice.

3. Pseudolycorine, an acid alkaloid separated from Bulbus Lycoridis Radiatae, has a notable inhibitive effect on Walker's sarcoma-256 of rats.

4. As lycoramine carries positive charge, it can combine with the surface of tumor cells that carries obvious negative charge. The negatively charged hydroxybenzene ions can get into the inside of the positively charged tumor cells to produce antineoplastical effect.

EXPERIMENTAL FORMULAS

For cancerous hydrothorax and ascites:

Equal portions of Bulbus Lycoridis Radiatae and Semen Ricini are pounded into powder, mixed with water and spread on a piece of paper to be applied on the two soles before being covered with bandage. The process is repeated daily. Should phlycten occurs, the medication is withdrawn and honey is smeared on the feet. (*Prevention and Treatment of Tumors in Traditional Chinese Medicine*)

For cancer of the body surface:

Certain amount of Bulbus Lycoridis Radiatae is blended with Chinese onion, ginger and brown sugar and pounded into paste to be encased with a thin layer of cotton gauze and applied to the tumor lesion. (*Anticancer Herbal Preparations*)

For diverse sorts of tumors of the digestive system:

An intramuscular dribbling administration with a dose of 100-150mg of lycoramine injection is given after being diluted with 250-500ml of 1-5% glucose injection solution daily or every other day. A total dosage of 1500mg makes a therapeutic course and the therapy is continued after a week's interval. (*New Traditional Chinese Medicine*, Vol. 1, 1979)

HISTORICAL COMMENTS

In *Compendium of Medicinal Herbs* it was reported that: "For furuncle and malignant boils, the herb is administered either orally as decoction or externally as plaster."

It was recorded in *Supplement to Compendium of Medicinal Herbs* that: "To cure pulmonary abscess, the herb is decocted in wine for oral administration."

In *Dictionary of Chinese Materia Medica* it was indicated: "Persons who are weak and susceptible to nausea and vomiting and who have not be invaded by pathogenic factors of the excess type should not take the herb."

THE AUTHOR'S NOTE

Lycorine itself does not seem to have analgesic effects, but intensify analgesic actions of corydalis B and morphine, and hence is used to assist in relieving pains of cancer. (*Pharmaceutical Research*, Vol. 5, 1962). Mr. Ye Juquan has introduced in his *Practical and Effective Simple Recipes* the experience of applying Bulbus Lycoridis Radiatae and Semen Ricini on the soles for the treatment of ascites and edema induced by diverse causes, and commended that the effect is "incredibly effective".

SEMEN BENINCASAE

Yang Shitai of the Qing Dynasty pointed out: "The herb is sweet in taste and neutral in nature and used for eliminating heat accumulated in the Heart Channel."

Semen Benincasae is the dried seed of *Benincasa hispida (Thunb.) Cogn.* of the family *Cucurbitaceae*, which is cultivated in many places in China and is a dietetic medicinal herb.

ANTICANCER PHARMACOLOGICAL FUNCTIONS

1. The alcohol extract of Semen Benincasae was found having a weak anticancer effect on sarcoma-180 in rats with an inhibitive rate of 20.7%.

2. The hot water extract of the herb presented a stronger action against transplanted tumor in animals, with an inhibitive rate of 88.7% on sarcoma-180 without toxic reactions.

EXPERIMENTAL FORMULAS

For cancers of the rectum and the colon:

> Semen Benincasae 15g
> Radix et Rhizoma Rhei 12g
> Cortex Moutan 9g
> Semen Persicae 9g

The above herbs are decocted and then mixed with Natrii Sulfas (6g) for oral administration after the dregs have been removed. (*Synopsis of Prescriptions of Golden Chamber*)

HISTORICAL COMMENTS

It was recorded in *Ri Huan Zi Materia Medica* that: "Semen Benincasae nourishes the skin and removes its black color."

Compendium of Medicinal Herbs said that the herb "cures periappendicular abscess".

Illustrated Materia Medica regarded the herb as "a tonic to the liver."

In *Descriptions of Materia Medica* it was expounded that: "The herb is used for the treatment of heat accumulated in the Heart Channel, dribbling urination, rosacea, periappendicular abscess, abdominal stagnation and ulceration with pus and blood. It is the essential herb for removing stagnation of pathogenic factors in the abdomen."

It was pointed out in *Dietetic Materia Medica* that: "The meat of the plant has a better effect when taken hot. It reduces body weight when taken cold. Boiled meat of the plant strengthens the five viscera with its downward attribute. If you want to be slender, keep eating the plant and if you want to increase your body weight, never eat it."

THE AUTHOR'S NOTE

According to a report of an English journal, *Cancer Chemotherapy* (23, 1962), many plants of the family Cucurbitaceae contain cucurbitacin——a terpenes compound with strong anticancer activity.

CORDYCEPS

It was reported in *New Compilation of Materia Medica* that: "The drug, being sweet and neutral, is used to protect the lung and supplement the kidney."

Cordyceps is a complex of stroma of *Cordyceps sinensis (Burk.) Sacc.* of the family *Claricepitaceae* and corpse of larva of *Hepialus armori canus O.* of the family *Hepialidae*. In winter, the hyphae of *Cordyceps sinensis (Burk.) Sacc.* grows into the body of the larva of *Hepialus armori canus O.* in earth and as a result that the body of the larva is filled with hyphae and it dies finally. In summer, stroma grows out of earth and it is collected around the Autumnal Equinox when the amassed snow has not melted and the stroma are often above the snow. If collected too late, the stroma are difficult to be found, because of the overgrown weeds. Moreover, the larva corpse will wither and become improper for medicinal use. Cordyceps is mainly found growing in Sichuan, Qinghai and Guizhou and contains an effective anticancer component of 3-deoxyadenosine.

ANTICANCER PHARMACOLOGICAL FUNCTIONS

1. It has been proved that 3-deoxyadenosine has an inhibitive effect on cell division and cancer and is active in inhibiting the growth of cells of nasopharyngeal carcinoma (KB).

2. Both the complex and the hyphae of Cordyceps were found capable of elevating the phagocytic function of the macrophage in the abdominal cavity of mice and reducing rejection of T-lymphocytes.

3. The herb has a nonspecific immunofunction which can provoke and reinforce the anticancer power of the body, and prolongs the survival period of rats of Ehrlich's ascites carcinoma.

EXPERIMENTAL FORMULAS

For cancer patients who are weak or underwent radiotherapy and chemotherapy:

3 to 5 Cordyceps are filled into the cleaved head of an old male duck, the entrails of which have been removed, and the cleaved head is to be tied with a thread to prevent the leakage of the drug. Then the duck is steamed as usual with soy sauce, oil and wine, and the drug will defuse to the entire body of the duck. For weak patients after illness, one such duck is worthy of 30 grams of Ginseng. (*Supplement to the Compendium of Medicinal Herbs*)

THE AUTHOR'S NOTE

According to a report, Cordyceps Mixture was used for the treatment of 3 cancer cases (1 of the pubis, 1 of the lung and 1 of the prostate) for a course of 3 months and it was found very effective. (*Shanghai Journal of Medicinal Herbs*, Vol. 5, 1979)

HERBA AGRIMONIAE

It was stated in *Supplement to Compendium of Medicinal Herbs* that: "The herb is bitter in taste and neutral in nature, and enters the lung and the bowel and the stomach to resolve mass."

Herba Agrimoniae is the dried plant of *Agrimonia pilosa Ledeb.* of the family *Rosaceae*, which was first recorded in *Materia Medica for Saving the Starved* and then in *Supplement to Compendium of Medicinal Herbs* under the entry of Herba Salviae Chinensis. Nowadays, it is more often used as a hemostatic agent whereas in the old times it was considered to have diverse aspects of usage in addition to a tonic and a hemostatic.

ANTICANCER PHARMACOLOGICAL FUNCTIONS

1. The alcohol extract of the whole plant has an inhibition on sarcoma-180 of mice and subcutaneous liver cancer with a rate of over 50%.

2. An inhibition rate of 100% on JTC-26 was obtained through experiments in vitro. The methanol extract of the root exhibited a strong action against Hela-cells aggregation.

3. Under a content of $500\mu g/ml$, the herb did not cause damage to but, on the contrary, aid in the growth (100%) of normal cells, i.e, an action of reinforcing the body resistance.

4. The herb presented a notable analgesic effect under a dose of 100mg/kg of body weight when administered to domestic rabbits.

5. A daily oral administration of 1000mg/kg of body weight to guinea pig implanted with sarcoma-180 for successive 12 days, showed an inhibition rate of 37.24% on tumors.

6. With an intraperitoneal administration of 100mg/kg of body weight to mice implanted with sarcoma-180, the inhibition rate was calculated to be 18.5% for the hot water extract and 7.4% for the alcohol extract.

7. With Hela-cells aggregation method, a cytotoxic substance has been found in the root of Herba Agrimoniae, which is soluble in methanol and ether and is extremely active in the inhibition of Hela-cells aggregation.

8. When this cytotoxic substance was administered under a dose of $12.5\mu g/ml$ to mice implanted with Ehrlich's ascites carcinoma, the survival days were raised by 32% as compared with the control group. When the dose was elevated to $25\mu g/ml$, 4 mice among the 5 survived on average 60 days longer than those in the control group.

9. In addition, the above substance was found to have an action to facilitate agglutination of blood cells and its activity was greater than that of concanavalin A.

EXPERIMENTAL FORMULAS

For hematemesis caused by tumor of the digestive system:

The decoction of Herba Agrimoniae (30-60 grams) is taken twice daily. (*Diagnosis, Treatment and Prevention of Tumors*)

For lung cancer:

   Herba Agrimoniae 30g
   Herba Lysimachiae 30g
   Herba Euphorbiae Humifusae 30g
   Herba Oldenlandiae Diffusae 30g
   Cortex Mori 30g
   Herba Seu Radix Cirsii Faponici 15g
   Herba Cephalanoploris 15g
   Herba Gnaphalii Affinis 15g
   Semen Coicis 15g
   Radix Stemonae 6g
   Xihuang Xiaoxi Wan 6g

The above herbs are decocted and taken daily. (*Essential Points of Tumors*)

For esophageal cancer:

   Herba Agrimoniae 30g
   Radix Angelicae Sinensis 12g
   Xylotrupes 12g
   Herba Dendrobii 12g
   Radix Ophiopogonis 12g
   Radix Asparagi 12g
   Rhizoma Pinelliae 12g
   Caulis Bambusae in Taeniam 12g
   Flos Inulae 12g
   Haematitum 30g
   Radix Aucklandiae 9g
   Flos Caryophylli 9g
   Lignum Aquilariae Resinatum 9g
   Fructus Amomi Rotundus 9g
   Fructus Meliae Toosendan 9g
   Cortex Magnoliae 9g
   Radix Adenophorae 9g
   Radix Glehniae 9g
   Semen Impatientis 15g

The above herbs are decocted and the both is divided into two portions for oral administration in the morning and in the evening. (*Anticancer Herbal Preparations*)

For giant cell tumor of the bone:

4 to 8 pills of *Ping Xiao Dan* (0.5 gram each) are taken each time, three times daily. The recipe of *Ping Xiao Dan* consists of Herba Agrimoniae, Semen Strychni, Alumen, Radix Curcumae, Faeces Trogopterorl, Fructus Aurantii Immaturus and Lacca Sinica Exsiccata. (*Shaanxi Traditional Chinese Medicine*, Vol. 6, 1983)

HISTORICAL COMMENT:

It was described in *Mirro. of a Hundred Herbs* that: "The herb acts to keep the flow of *qi* downward, promote blood circulation, resolve abdominal mass with distention, and is used for the treatment of traumatic injury, hematemesis, severe diarrhea, and enterorrhagia. For acute mastitis, the early cases would be cured and the pyogenous cases would be relieved through ulceration with scarce blennorrhea. 30 grams of Herba Agrimoniae is decocted in half tea pot of white wine and the broth is taken after meal."

The herb was stated in *Treatise on Differentiation of False Drugs* "to cure scrofula".

In *New Collection of Materia Medica of Zhenan* it was said that: "The herb cures Meniere's syndrome, when 60 grams of it is decocted in water and taken daily."

In *Prescriptions of Ge's Ancestors* it was pointed out that: "The herb cures dyspepsia, abdominal distention, regurgitation, dysphagia, inflammation of the throat, pulmonary abscess, hemorrhoid and hematemesis with its downward attribute."

In *Supplement to Drug Mirror* Jiang Yi pointed out: "Herba Salviae Chinensis is effective for dysphagia and regurgitation which have been regarded as incurable illnesses. This herb, just like food for the starveling and clothes for the freezing, cures nine out of ten such patients."

In *Chinese Medical Dictionary* it was commented that: "The herb is the best drug for resolving and dissipating abdominal mass with distention and is well known for its wide indications."

THE AUTHOR'S NOTE

Herba Agrimoniae, in my opinion, is one of the herbs for the treatment of tumors. In recent years, the utilization of Herba Agrimoniae in simple or compound prescriptions for the treatment of all kinds of tumors except leukemia has virtually achieved certain effects. The basic recipes for cancer used clinically is as follows:

1 >. For pains due to various types of cancer: Herba Agrimoniae (120g) is decocted in water for 1.5 hours and the filtered liquid is steamed dry. The powder is taken with boiled water 6 times in 24 hours, and 45 days make a therapeutic course. This formula has been used by the author for many years and it takes effect 15 days after administration and is particularly effective for cancers of the bone, the liver and the pancreas with severe pain.

2 >. For various sorts of cancer (excluding leukemia):

Herba Agrimoniae 60g
Herba Solani Lyrati 25g
Semen Arecae 9g
Radix Glycyrrhizae 3g

The decoction is taken once daily.

A japanese scholar reported in *Journal of Pharmaceutics* (Vol. 2, 1980) that the herb contains anticancer substances. Most of the 11 kinds of substances separated from the root of Herba Agrimoniae were found to have antineoplastic effects. This has also been verified in studies in China.

RHIZOMA ATRACTYLODIS MACROCEPHALAE

In *Treatise on Properties of Drugs* it was recorded that: "The herb, being sweet and acrid, is used to remove edema caused by pathogenic wind and mass or swelling."

Rhizoma Atractylodis Macrocephalae is the dried rhizome of *Atractylodis macrocephala Koidz.* of the family *Compositae*, which is aromatic and somewhat mucous and is mainly produced in Xinchang District of Zhejiang Province. The ones grow in Yuqian District have the best quality, containing 1.4% of volatile oil and vitamin A.

ANTICANCER PHARMACOLOGICAL FUNCTIONS

1. The inhibition rate on sarcoma-180 of mouse was calculated to be 22.8% for the alcohol extract and 32.1% for the water extract.

2. Screening tests in vivo showed an active anticancer effect of the volatile oil.

EXPERIMENTAL FORMULAS

For tumor of thymus gland:

Rhizoma Atractylodis Macrocephalae 25g

Radix Salviae Miltiorrhizae 25g

Flos Carthami 25g

Radix Astragali 25g

Radix Codonopsis Pilosulae 25g

Rhizoma Dioscoreae 25g

Rhizoma Pinelliae 15g

Radix Po 15g

Rhizoma Scirpi 15g

Rhizoma Zedoariae 15g

Radix Bupleuri 15g

The above herbs can be reduced and increased according to the symptoms and are taken in decoction daily. (*New Traditional Chinese Medicine*, Vol. 11, 1983)

For lung cancer:

Rhizoma Atractylodis Macrocephalae 10g

Poria 10g

Rhizoma Arisaematis 10g

Radix Ginseng 10g

Rhizoma Curculiginis 10g

Fructus Psoraleae 10g

Nidus Vespae 10g

Bombyx Batryticatus 10g

Radix Astragali 30g

Radix Pseudostellariae Heterophyllae 30g

Radix Codonopsis Lanceolatae 30g

Fructus Schisandrae 9g

Rhizoma Zingiberis 6g

Cordyceps 3g

The above herbs can be increased and decreased in amount according to the symptoms and are taken in decoction daily. (*Oncology of Traditional Chinese Medicine*)

HISTORICAL COMMENTS

It was stated in *Annotation on Shen Nong's Herbs* that: "The herb is extremely aromatic in smell, truly sweet in taste and completely positive in nature and is the supreme drug for curing wind arthralgia and tranquilizing the stomach and the spleen."

In *Ri Huan Zi Materia Medica* it was described that: "The herb is capable of curing all kinds of illnesses caused by pathogenic wind, such as regurgitation, hiccup, fragile bone and muscle, mass beside umbilicus, and cold abdominal mass in women."

THE AUTHOR'S NOTE

According to *Explanation to Clinical Prescriptions of Traditional Chinese Medicine* written by a Japanese scholar: "If fire-assuaging drugs are not effective for tumors of ears, *Huoxiang Zhengqi San* may be tried." The recipe is as follows:

Rhizoma Atractylodis macrocephalae 3g

Rhizoma Pinelliae 3g

Poria 3g

Cortex Magnoliae 2g

Pericarpium Citri Reticulatae 2g
Radix Platycodi 1.5g
Radix Angelicae Dahuricae 1.5g
Folium Perillae 1g
Pericarpium Arecae 1g
Fructus Ziziphi Inermis 1g
Rhizoma Zingiberis 1g
Radix Glycyrrhizae 1g

AGKISTRODON ACUTUS

Miao Xiyong of the Ming Dynasty reported: "The drug is sweet and salty in taste and extremely poisonous in nature."

Agkistrodon acutus is the dried or fresh slough or the flesh of Crotalidae, *Agkistrodon acutus (Guenther)* of the family *Reptilia*, which contains components such as protein, fat and saponin. Agkistrodon acutus lives on the leaves and flowers of *Photinin Serrulata Lindl*. The poisonous gland in the head can secrete hemorrhagic hemotoxin.

ANTICANCER PHARMACOLOGICAL FUNCTIONS
Assessed by fluorescent microscopy in vitro, the drug was found to have an antagonistic action on cells of leukemia.

EXPERIMENTAL FORMULAS
For lymphosarcoma and lymphadenoma:
60 grams of the flesh of Agkistrodon acutus (parched before being immersed in wine), 45 grams of Cornu Rhinoceri (pounded into powder), 15 grams of Semen Pharbitidis (half parched and half not), and 15 grams of Pericarpium Citri Reticulatae Viride are ground to powder for oral administration 6 grams, once daily with glutinous rice soup. (*Prescriptions Based on Three Categories of Pathogenic Factors*)

For cancer of the middle ear:
Agkistrodon acutus (9g) and Aranea (3g) are parched, powdered, mixed with Borneol (0.3g) and powdered again. The powder is administered through puffing into the ear. (*Treatment and Prevention of Tumors*)

For metastasis of chorioepithelioma:
Agkistrodon acutus 2
Scolopendra 2
Nidus Vespae 6g

The drugs are pulverized and taken once daily with a dose of 6 grams. (*Diagnosis, Treatment and Prevention of Tumors*)

For cancers of the liver, the lung, the breast and the digestive tract and for leukemia:
Agkistrodon acutus 75g
Bufo 5g
Carapax Trionycis 150g
Rhizoma Polygonati 60g
Radix Salviae Miltiorrhizae 60g
Rhizoma Scirpi 60g
Rhizoma Zedoariae 60g
Bombyx Batryticatus 60g

Indigo Naturalis 60g

All the above herbs are ground into fine powder to be mixed with water before being made into pills and coated with Haematitum. The pill is called *Yan Zhong Wan* and 6 grams is taken each time, three times a day. (*Diagnosis, Treatment and Prevention of Tumors*)

HISTORICAL COMMENTS

It was expounded in *Compendium of Materia Medica* that: "Agkistrodon acutus penetrates the bone to expel the pathogenic wind and alleviate convulsion and is the essential drug for wind arthralgia, convulsion, scabies and malignant scabies because it travels everywhere, outward to the skin and inward to the viscera. Persons who drink snake wine should protect themselves from being exposed to wind."

In *Amplified Materia Medica* it was described that: "The nose of most snakes grow downwards, but that of Agkistrodon acutus grows upwards."

It was described in *Prescriptions of Materia Medica* that: "Patients with wind-stroke syndrome of the deficiency type are alerted not to take Agkistrodon acutus."

It was pointed out in *Practical Materia Medica* that: "Agkistrodon acutus is incompatible with iron."

In *Illustrated Materia Medica* it was recorded that: "Agkistrodon acutus has a quicker effect in treating wind syndrome than that of other snakes. For scabies that does not respond to any drugs, people living in the jungle use Agkistrodon acutus. They catch such a snake, cut it into equal pieces to be placed on a brick which had been burnt red and poured with vinegar to cause evaporation. Finally the pieces of the snake are covered with a basin. After three repetitions of the process, the flesh and the bone of the snake are removed and five flavors are added to the slough for boiling. After taking the slough, the patient is asked to sleep for a day and a night and the scabies will disappear on the waking of the patient."

THE AUTHOR'S NOTE

Agkistrodon acutus, as an anticancer drug, is very popular among the folks. In 1983, I collected a proved recipe for the treatment of esophageal cancer in Jichun, Hubei Province: A chicken is fed with the flesh of Agkistrodon acutus and the chicken's feces is then collected, parched dry and ground into powder for oral administration with hot water 2-3 times daily, 3-6 grams each time. In the Second Affiliated Hospital of Hubei Medical College, *Longshe Xiaoliu Wan* was used to treat 8 cases of stomach cancer, among whom 3 was found effective and 2 very effective. The recipe of *Longshe Xialiu Wan* is as follows:

Syngnathus 1
Agkistrodon acutus 2
Rhizoma Polygonati 6g
Nidus Vespae 6g
Hirudo 6g
Tabanus 6g
Scorpis 9g
Unguis Hominis 6g
Olibanum 6g
Myrrha 6g
Fructus Meliae Toosendan 6g
Radix Gentianae 15g

These drugs are powdered and mixed with a decoction of Flos Lonicerae to make boluses to be coated with 30 grams of Realgar.

HERBA OLDENLANDIAE DIFFUSAE

It was quoted in *Folk Medicinal Herbs of Southern Fujian* that: "The herb is bitter in taste, neutral in nature, poisonous and used as an antipyretic, detoxicant and analgesic."

Herba Oldenlandiae Diffusae is the dried whole plant of *Oldenlandia diffusa (Wild.) Roxb.* of the family *Rubiaceae*, which is distributed over areas south of the Yangtze River. The herb was not recorded in ancient literatures and first appeared in *Herbal Records of Guangxi* published after 1949. The book says: "The herb is used to cure child malnutrition, snakebite and tumor, and when used externally it is effective for vesicles and ichthyosis." The herb is low in toxicity, with a half lethal dose of 104 grams of the crude drug per kilograms of the body weight when injected intraperitoneally to rats. At Changning Central Hospital in Shanghai, 36 patients with liver and stomach cancer were treated with the herb and the result was remarkably effective in 4 cases and effective in 10 cases. In Guangxi and Fujian, *Oldenlandiae corymbosa L.*, *Oldenlandiae tenelliflora (Bl.) Oldenlandiae Kize* and *Oldenlandiae pinifolia (Wall.) K. Schum.* of the same family are used as the substitutes of the herb which contains ursolic acid, oleanolic acid, ß-coumaric acid, stigmasterol, ß-sitosterol and glucoside etc..

ANTICANCER PHARMACOLOGICAL FUNCTIONS

1. Methylene-blue tube method in vitro (corresponding to 6g/ml of crude drug) proved that the drug has strong inhibition on acute lymphatic, granulocytic, monocytic and chronic granulocytic leukemia.

2. Determined by War's respirator, the herb was active in inhibiting acute lymphatic and granulocytic leukemia.

3. Methylene-blue tube method (0.5-5g/ml of the crude herb) showed an inhibitive action on Yoshida's sarcoma and Ehrlich's ascites sarcoma.

4. A decoction of the herb has been proved to have inhibitive effects on uterine cancer-14, sarcoma-180 and ascitic lymphosarcoma-1 of mice to varying degrees.

5. The herb functions to promote the proliferation of the reticuloepithelial system, the formation of antibodies and the phagocytic power of leukocytes.

EXPERIMENTAL FORMULAS

For cancer of the stomach:

A decoction of Herba Oldenlandiae Diffusae (90 grams), Rhizoma Imperatae (60 grams) and certain amount of white sugar is taken daily. (*New Edition of Traditional Chinese Medicine*)

For cancers of the esophagus, the rectum and the stomach:

> Herba Oldenlandiae Diffusae 70g
> Semen Coicis 30g
> Rhizoma Dioscoreae Bulbiferae 9g
> Radix Linderae 3g
> Herba Solani Nigri 3g
> Fructus Mume 6g
> Radix Notoginseng 1.5g

The decoction of the above herbs is taken daily. (*National Collection of Medicinal Herbs*)

For lymphosarcoma:

A decoction of equal shares of Herba Oldenlandiae Diffusae and Herba Scutellariae Barbatae is taken. (*Medicine and Drugs of Fujian*, Vol. 2, 1976)

For esophageal cancer:

> Herba Oldenlandiae Diffusae 60g
> Herba Scutellariae Barbatae 60g
> Folium Cycis Revolutae 60g
> Rhizoma Imperatae 60g

Radix Gossypii Hirsuti 60g

The decoction of the above herbs is taken daily. (*New Collection of Materia Medica of Zhenan*)

For rectal cancer:

Herba Oldenlandiae Diffusae 60g

Herba Solani Nigri 60g

Caulis Lonicerae 60g

Herba Scutellariae Barbatae 15g

Herba Violae 15g

The decoction of the above herbs is taken daily. (*New Collection of Materia Medica of Zhenan*)

For cervical cancer:

Herba Oldenlandiae Diffusae 60g

Radix Sophorae Subprostratae 30g

Umbilicus 30g

Rhizoma Dryopteris Crassirhizomae 30g

Cortex Phellodendri 30g

The decoction of the above herbs is taken three times daily. (*Selection of the Simple and Proved Recipes of Medicinal Herbs in Zhejiang Province*)

For various types of cancer:

1>. Herba Oldenlandiae Diffusae 250g

Lumbricus 30g

Scolopendra 30g

Nidus Vespae 30g

Herba Taraxaci 30g

Radix Isatidis 30g

Scorpio 30g

Periostracum Serpentis 30g

These herbs are pounded into fine powder, blended with honey and made into pills (each weighing 6g) for oral administration in the morning and in the evening. (*Herbal Handbook*)

2>. A dose of 20-30ml of Herba Oldenlandiae Diffusae Syrup is taken after meal three time a day and each 100ml of syrup contains 70g of the crude drug. The syrup contains:

Herba Oldenlandiae Diffusae 70g

Herba Scutellariae Barbatae 35g

Sargassum 85g

Thallus Laminariae Seu Eckloniae 85g

Semen Alpiniae Katsumadai 5g

Salmiacum 0.17g

Fructus Mume 85g

(*Anticancer Herbal Preparations*)

For cancers of rectum and breast:

A decoction of Herba Oldenlandiae Diffusae and Rhizoma Curculiginis (120 grams each) is taken daily. (*Data of New Medicine and Drugs*, Vol. 2, 1972)

HISTORICAL COMMENTS

It is described in *Chaozhou Annals* that: "The juice squeezed from the stem and the leaf of the plant is taken for the treatment of cecitis and all kinds of intestinal disorders."

It was recorded in *Materia Medica of Quanzhou* that: "As an antipyretic, detoxicant, antipyogenic and an agent to alleviate blood stasis, the herb is used in the treatment of carbuncle, cellulitis, scrofula and other external diseases as well as pneumonia and pulmonary infections."

THE AUTHOR'S NOTE

An intramuscular administration of Herba Oldenlandiae Diffusae injection (100%) was given to one case of cervical cancer, one of stomach cancer and one of liver cancer and the condition of these patients became improved. In Jiangsu, an overall effective rate of 82.6% was reported in the treatment of 23 cases of lymphosarcoma with a Herba Oldenlandiae Diffusae preparation. In Nanchang, a compound recipe of Herba Oldenlandiae Diffusae was used to treat 81 cases of stomach cancer, with complete recovery in 15 cases and an overall effective rate of 75.3%. The drug was also administered in 3 cases of rectal cancer and it was found all effective.

RHIZOMA IMPERATAE

It was reported in *Comprehension of Materia Medica* that: "The herb, cold and very sweet, is used to eliminate pathogenic heat of the blood without causing dryness."

Rhizoma Imperatae is the dried rhizome of *Imperata cylindrica Beauv. var. major (Nees) C.E. Hubb.* of the family *Gramineae*, which is found growing in a majority of places in China and contains large amount of sucrose, glucose, fructose, xylose, malic acid and citric acid. It was also reported to contains anemonin.

ANTICANCER PHARMACOLOGICAL FUNCTIONS

Bacteriophagic method has proved an antiphagic effect of the herb, and this suggests that the herb is active in inhibiting tumor cells.

EXPERIMENTAL FORMULAS

For esophageal cancer:

        Rhizoma Imperatae 60g
        Herba Oldenlandiae Diffusae 60g
        Radix Adenophorae 15g
        Rhizoma Polygonati Odorati 15g
        Radix Ophiopogonis 9g
        Flos Inulae 9g
        Rhizoma Dioscoreae 24g

These herbs are decocted in 2000ml of water to a volume of 600-800ml of broth to be mixed with 120 grams of honey after the dregs being removed for further decoction. The broth is divided into four equal portions for oral administration four times a day, each time one portion. (*New Traditional Chinese Medicine*, Vol. 4, 1972)

For tumor of the sellae:

        Rhizoma Imperatae 15g
        Herba Solani Lyrati 15g
        Semen Strychni 1.5g
        Flos Albiziae 4.5g
        Radix et Rhizoma Cynanchi 9g
        Sargassum 9g
        Bombyx Batryticatus 9g
        Semen Astragali Complanati 9g
        Rhizoma Ligustici 9g

The above herbs are decocted for oral administration daily. (*Journal of Zhejiang Traditional Chinese Medical College*, Vol. 2, 1980)

For nasopharyngeal carcinoma:

Rhizoma Imperatae 12g
Radix Codonopsis Pilosulae 12g
Radix Asparagi 12g
Radix Ophiopogonis 12g
Radix Adenophorae 10g
Radix Rehmanniae 10g
Rhizoma Atradylodis Macrocephalae 10g
Poria 10g
Radix Scrophulariae 9g
Flos Lonicerae 9g
Rhizoma Polygonati Odorati 9g
Herba Oldenlandiae Diffusae 30g
Herba Solani Lyrati 20-30g
Radix Salviae Miltiorrhizae 12-15g
Radix Glycyrrhizae 3g

The herbs are decocted and taken as a drink three times a day. (*Journal of Combined Traditional Chinese and Western Medicine*, Vol. 2, 1985)

HISTORICAL COMMENTS

It was described in *Prescriptions Worth a Thousand Gold* that: "For regurgitation and vomiting food, Rhizoma Phragmitis and Rhizoma Imperatae (60 grams each) are cut to slices and decocted in 160ml of water to 80ml of broth for oral administration at a draught."

In *Understanding of Canon of Materia Medica* it was expounded that: "The herb cures, without side effect, toothache, gingival swelling, ulcerative gingivitis, sores of the mouth and the tongue, asphyxia due to stagnated lung-heat, sore and pus of the throat."

ALUMEN

In *Essentials of Materia Medica* it was stated that: "The drug is sour and salty in taste and cold and astringent in nature."

Alumen is the large or fragmented colorless transparent octahedral crystals coated with white powder and soluble in water, and is chiefly produced in Hubei, Anhui, Zhejiang and Fujian, containing a chemical element called aluminum potassium sulfate. The water solution of Alumen can make protein and colloid coagulate. Melted by heat, Alumen expands due to the loss of moisture stored in the crystals, becomes light and soft like a sponge and is referred to as alumen exsiccatum.

ANTICANCER PHARMACOLOGICAL FUNCTIONS

Studies in vitro at Osaka Research Institute of Traditional Chinese Medicine in Japan showed:

1. Under a dose of 500µg/ml, the hot water extract of Alumen has an inhibitive action on JTC-26 with a rate as high as over 90%.

2. Alumen Exsiccatum has an inhibition rate of 70-90% on JTC-26.

EXPERIMENTAL FORMULAS

For stomach cancer:

Pulverized Alumen Exsiccatum (9g) is stewed together with white vinegar (180g) for 5 minutes and the broth is taken at a draught. This prescription is very effective clinically. (*Guangdong Traditional Chinese Medicine*, Vol. 3, 1960)

For nasopharyngeal sarcoma:

Alumen is burnt, pounded into powder and blended with lard to make a paste for filling the nostrils with cotton balls. (*Essential Prescriptions Worth a Thousand Gold*)

For cancer of the tongue:

Alumen and Malachitum (3 grams each) are grounded to powder for external application, and at the same time, warm vinegar is given as a gargle. (*Shen's Works on Longevity*)

For tumors of the abdominal cavity:

Alumen and Realgar (60 grams each) are pulverized and mixed up with flour paste to make plaster for external application. (*New Collection of Classic Prescriptions*)

For nasopharyngeal carcinoma:

Calcined Alumen (6g) and Salmiacum (1.5g) are crushed into fine powder to be inhaled in small amount. (*Comprehended Medicine*)

For ulcerative cancer of the stomach:

  Alumen 210g
  Os Sepiae 210g
  Rhizoma Bletillae 180g
  Semen Pharbitidis 240g
  Sodium Bicarbonate 240g
  Gecko 90g
  Concha Arcae 90g
  Pericarpium Citri Reticulatae 60g
  Rhizoma cyperi 60g

The above herbs are ground into fine powder and taken before meal with a dose of 12-18 grams. (*Talks on Drugs and Prescriptions*)

HISTORICAL COMMENTS

It was reported in *Amplified Materia Medica* that: "It is used as a hemostatic and analgesic for healing wound and promoting granulation."

It was recorded in *Compendium of Medicinal Herbs* that: "It cures carbuncle, cellulitis, furuncle and malignant boils."

In *Treatise on Origin of Materia Medica* it was said that: "Alumen is used as a purgative to clean the stomach and the bowels."

Prescriptions of Chen's Teachers stated that: "Alumen is mixed with wax to make boluses for the effective treatment of pyrogenic infections."

It was announced in *Holy Prescriptions* that: "Equal shares of powdered Alumen and Semen Longan are placed under the tongue to relieve swollen and rigid tongue."

It was described in *One-From-A-Hundred Prescriptions* that: "Three portions of Alumen plus one and half portions of Radix Glycyrrhizae powder are parched and wrapped in a piece of cloth for application to the vulva to relieve pains."

Medical Secrets from an Official indicated that: "The drug cures nebula, when crushed into pieces of the size of broomcorn millet and placed in the eyes to cause tears dropping day after day. Once the filthy tears are all driven out, the condition is cured."

THE AUTHOR'S NOTE

In *New Edition of Mei's Proved Recipes*, there was a simple recipe for the treatment of regurgitation and vomiting which may be tried on patients with cancer of the stomach. Half unprocessed and half processed Alumen are mixed with cold water for oral administration. Doctors of traditional Chinese medicine often use Alumen in the treatment of internal and external diseases and diseases of women and children. When curing tumors of the digestive system, the author often adds Alumen (20g) and yeast (20 pills) to other herbs to make a decoction, which seems to have certain effect.

HERBA SOLANI LYRATI

Zhang Shouyi of the Republic of China pointed out: "The herb has a light smell and is cool in nature, and is used to remove heat and dampness to clear the water channels and ease joint movement. In addition, it is able to clear away phlegm and blood stasis with its action to regulate the circulation of *qi* and remove stagnation caused by pathogenic factors."

Herba Solani Lyrati is the dried whole plant and root of *Solanum lyratum Thunb.* of the family *Solanaceae*, which is mainly found growing in areas south of the Yellow River. It should be distinguished from *Aristolochia mollissima Hance.* of the family *Aristolochiaceae*.

ANTICANCER PHARMACOLOGICAL FUNCTIONS

1. Experiments in vitro showed the hot water extract of the herb has a very strong inhibitive action (100%) on cells of JTC-26 but does not affect the normal cells.

2. Experiments in vivo showed the herb has an inhibition rate of 14.57% on sarcoma-180 in rats.

3. The decoction of equal portions of Herba Solani Lyrati and Fructus Ziziphi Inermis has been verified to be active in inhibiting solid and ascitic types of Ehrlich's ascites carcinoma of mouse and of fusocellular sarcoma. Clinically, it was found also effective for cervical cancer.

4. The alcohol extract of the drug with ß-soladulcamaridine as an effective anticarcinogen has been found to have inhibitive actions on sarcoma-180 in rats in addition to its remarkable effect on Walker's cancer-256.

EXPERIMENTAL FORMULAS

For lung cancer:

The decoction of Herba Solani Lyrati and Herba Sedi Sarmentosi (30 grams each) is taken daily. (*National Collection of Medicinal Herbs*)

For esophageal cancer:

Herba Solani Lyrati 30g

Herba Solani Nigri 30g

Herba Oldenlandiae Diffusae 15g

Herba Scutellariae Barbatae 15g

The herbs are decocted in water and taken daily. (*Information of Science and Technology*, Vol. 5, 1976)

For cancer of the plica vocalis:

Herba Solani Lyrati 30g

Herba Solani Nigri 30g

Herba Duchesneae 15g

Herba Solviae Chinensis 15g

Rhizoma Fagopyri Cymosi 15g

The herbs are decocted in water and taken daily. (*National Collection of Medicinal Herbs*)

For cavernous hemangioma:

Herba Solani Lyrati 30g

Radix Astragali 30g

Fructus Fici Pumilae 30g

Rhizoma Smilacis Glabrae 30g

Radix Codonopsis Pilosulae 12g

Radix Paeoniae Alba 12g

Radix Arnebiae 9g

Cortex Moutan 9g

The herbs are decocted in water and taken daily. (*Shanghai Journal of Traditional Chinese Medicine*, Vol. 6, 1979)

HISTORICAL COMMENTS

In *Supplement to Compendium of Medicinal Herbs* it was told that: "A decoction of the herb is taken for the treatment of dysphoria with smothery sensation, rubella, erysipelas, cold and fever caused by malignant malaria and fever in children."

It was stated in *Supplement to Compendium of Medicinal Herbs* that: "To cure tinea versicolor, the herb is boiled together with beef before administration."

In *Chinese Medical Dictionary* it was recorded that: "The herb is indicative for edema, migratory arthralgia, stranguria complicated with hematuria, lower abdominal pain related to *qi*, rheumatic arthralgia, abdominal pain due to ascariasis in children, pain due to pus and blood in the ear."

THE AUTHOR'S NOTE

The drug has a good analgesic effect on cancer. The Anticancer Single Blade Sword created by the author with Herba Solani Lyrati is capable of reducing and relieving pains of cancer.

According to an article reported in *Medicine and Drugs of Beijing* (Vol. 2, 1980), pharmacological experiments on Ehrlich's ascites carcinoma in rats with *Fufang Baishe Jiu*, a comprehensive prescription of wine, showed that the wine has an inhibitive rate of 66.2% on the growth of cancer cells. The formula is:

Herba Solani Lyrati 30g
Herba Solani Nigri 30g
Herba Duchesneae 30g
Radix Salviae Miltiorrhizae 30g
Radix Angelicae Sinensis 15g
Radix Curcumae 9g
Toads 10
Millet wine 1.5kg

Once the cancer cells become depressed, the contents of 3', 5'-cAMP in the cancer cells begin to increase obviously. Further experiments proved that the herbal component of *Fufang Baishe Jiu* has an inhibitive rate of 36.7%, while the toad wine has a rate of 26.2%, with no remarkable difference in concentration and activity of cAMP in the cancer cells of both groups.

HERBA CHELIDONII

It was recorded in *Common Medicinal Herbs in Beijing* that: "The herb, being bitter in taste, cold in nature and poisonous, is used as an anodyne, antitussive, antiseptic and diuretic."

Herba Chelidonii is the dried whole plant of *Chelidonium majus L.* of the family *Papaveraceae*, which mainly contains alkaloids and flavonoids. The fresh plant owns thick yellowish juice which also contains alkaloids.

ANTICANCER PHARMACOLOGICAL FUNCTIONS

1. Chelidonine contained in Herba Chelidonii is a mitotic toxin, which inhibits mitosis of fibroblast in experiments in vitro.

2. Chelidonine prevents the growth of malignant tumor and has inhibitive actions on sarcoma-180 and Ehrlich's ascites carcinoma of mice. But the side and toxic reactions of chelidonine are also great.

3. 40% Methanol extract of Herba Chelidonii has an anticancer effect with relatively low toxic and side reactions.

4. Herba Chelidonii contains chelerythrine, a cytotoxic substance, which acts to remove verrucous vegetation of skin, and coptisine.

EXPERIMENTAL FORMULAS
For stomach cancer:
Herba Chelidonii (stalk and leaf, 2.5g) is decocted in 300ml of water for oral administration three times a day. (*Research Data of Medicinal Herbs*, Vol. 6, 1978)
For esophageal cancer:
10ml of the syrup prepared with the following herbs are taken twice daily: Herba Chelidonii (10g), Herba Scutellariae Barbatae (10g) and Radix Actinidiae Chinensis (30g) are decocted in water to make syrup after the dregs have been removed. (*Clinical Essentials of Tumors*)

HISTORICAL COMMENTS
It was reported in *Chinese Medicinal Flora* that: "The herb cures pains and ulcer of the stomach and the intestine; and it is used to treat tinea and scabies, remove swelling when the juice extracted from the plant is externally applied."
It was described in *Dictionary of Chinese Materia Medica* that: "The juice squeezed from the fresh plant was applied to flat wart three times daily, each time 5 to 15 minutes. Among the 18 cases treated, 4 cases were fully recovered, 3 remarkably improved, 4 improved and half of the cases had irritation symptoms such as pain and itching after administration of the drug."

CORTEX DICTAMNI

Huang Gongxiu of the Qing Dynasty pointed out: "The herb is bitter and salty in taste, cold and nonpoisonous in nature and is used to open the senses and remove heat by promoting the flow of the fluid."
Cortex Dictamni is the root-bark of *Dictamnus dasycarpus Turcz.* or *Dictamnus angustifolius G. Don* of the family *Rutaceae*, which is yellowish white with solid kernel. With sebaceous glands, the plant smells exceptionally aromatic.

ANTICANCER PHARMACOLOGICAL FUNCTIONS
1. Experiments in vitro with bean sprout method showed a cytotoxicity of Cortex Dictamni.
2. Experiments in vivo proved certain inhibitive actions on sarcoma-180 of mice.

EXPERIMENTAL FORMULAS
For drastic itching due to malignant lymphoma:
    Cortex Dictamni 30g
    Fructus Kohiae 30g
    Herba Artemisiae Capillaris 30g
    Radix Salviae Miltiorrhizae 30g
    Radix Sophorae Flavescentis 15g
    Radix Stemonae 10
The decoction of the herbs is taken daily. (*Clinical Essentials of Tumors*)
For cancer of vulva:
    Cortex Dictamni 15g
    Semen Coicis 15
    Caulis Aristolochiae Manshuriensis 9g
    Semen Sojae Germinatum 9g

Radix Gentianae 9g
Rhizoma Dioscoreae 9g
Cortex Moutan 6g

The decoction of the herbs is taken daily. (*Concise Dermatology in Traditional Chinese Medicine*)

HISTORICAL COMMENTS

It was noted in *Compendium of Medicinal Herbs* that: "It is an essential drug for jaundice of diverse causes and wind arthralgia. Some doctors have a superficial understanding of the herb and only use it for the skin and the external diseases."

Zhang Shanlei pointed out: "Men of these days are using the herb solely for diseases of the skin and the hair and have forgot many of its actions such as to remove stagnation syndrome and free the channels."

It was reported in *Handbook of Prescriptions for Emergencies* that: "To treat ulcerated scrofula complicated with pus and blood, 40ml of the decoction of Cortex Dictamni is taken."

In *Supplement to Handbook of Prescriptions for Emergencies* it was also reported that: "40ml of the water decoction of Cortex Dictamni is administered for the treatment of ulcerated scrofula that has festered with bleeding."

It was alerted in *Annotation on Shen Nong's Herbs* that: "Those who have cold of deficiency type in the lower part of the body must not take this herb, even though they have dampness syndrome."

THE AUTHOR'S NOTE

In Tieling People's Hospital of Liaoning Province, an injection was prepared from Cortex Dictamni for intramuscular administration with a dose of 2-4ml each time, twice daily. When used for the treatment of 7 cases of malignant tumorous pleuritis through thoracic medication, hydrothorax almost disappeared in 4 cases and remarkably reduced in 3 cases.

In curing lung cancer and osteocarcinoma, the author often prescribes the following recipe:

Cortex Dictamni (added later) 50g
Herba Oldenlandiae Diffusae 100g
Herba Aristolochiae Mollissimae 25g
Fructus Ziziphi Inermis 30 pieces

The decoction of the herbs is taken once dose daily at 4 or 5 o'clock in the morning.

BOMBYX BATRYTICATUS

It was reported in *On Properties of Drugs* that: "The drug is slightly warm and somewhat poisonous, and is used for curing unceasing metrorrhagia of women."

Bombyx Batryticatus is the dried corpse of larva of *Bombyx mori L.* of the family *Bombycidae*, which died after having been infected with *Beauveria bassiana (Bals.) Vaillant*. The white powder of the body contains ammonium oxalate. The alcohol and the water extract of Bombyx Batryticatus has hypnotic actions on mise and rabbits.

ANTICANCER PHARMACOLOGICAL FUNCTIONS

1. The alcohol extract of Bombyx Batryticatus was found having inhibitive actions on sarcoma-180 of mouse through experiments in vivo.

2. Experiments in vitro proved that the herb has an inhibitive action on cells of human liver cancer.

EXPERIMENTAL FORMULAS

For malignant lymphoma:

The decoction of the powdered Bombyx Batryticatus is taken with hot water twice daily with a dose of 1.5 grams each time. (*Essential Prescriptions Worth a Thousand Gold*)

For tumor in the saddle:

> Bombyx Batryticatus 9g
> Folium Ilecis 9g
> Fructus Ligustri Lucidi 9g
> Spica Prunellae 9g
> Radix Dipsaci 9g
> Rhizoma Ligustici 15g
> Folium Mori 6g
> Rhizoma Pinelliae 6g
> Flos Chrysanthemi Indici 6g
> Scolopendra 1
> Scorpio 4

The decoction of the above drugs is taken daily. (*Journal of Zhejiang Traditional Chinese Medical College*, Vol. 2, 1980)

For tumor of the brain:

> Bombyx Batryticatus 15g
> Otolithum Sciaenae 15g
> Semen Livistonae 30g

The drugs are pounded into powder and 6 grams is taken each time, twice daily. (*Handbook of Practical Anticancer Drugs*)

For stomach cancer:

> Bombyx Batryticatus 60g
> Scolopendra 24g
> Squama Manitis 24g
> Semen Strychni (sliced after being soaked & peeled) 12g
> Sulfur 4.5g

The herbs are grounded into fine powder to be mixed with honey to make bolus of the size of Arillus Longan. A bolus is taken daily until the symptoms complete vanish. (*Journal of Traditional Chinese Medicine*, Vol.7, 1963)

For hematemesis caused by intestinal cancer:

Bombyx Batryticatus (30 grams, parched with its mouth & feet taken away) and Fructus Mume (30g, Baked) are ground into powder, blended with rice to make boluses of the size of Semen Firmianae. A dose of 100 boluses is taken three times daily with water before meal. (*Health Problems*)

HISTORICAL COMMENTS

In *Compendium of Medicinal Herbs* it was indicated that: "The herb is used to treat subcutaneous nodes caused by wind-phlegm, scrofula, and intermittent fever due to phlegm and mass in the abdomen."

It was described in *New Collection of Classic Prescriptions* that: "For aching, hard, movable or unmovable cancer in the abdomen, Bombyx Batryticatus (30g) is powdered and mixed with one bowl of horse urine for oral administration and application to the painful regions. The effect is fantastic."

It was noted in *Classic Prescriptions of Jide Tang* that: "To cure double tongue or swollen and rigid tongue (author's note: cancer of tongue), Bombyx Batryticatus (3g) and honey-parched Rhizoma Coptidis (6g) are pounded into powder and applied on the tongue."

THE AUTHOR'S NOTE

It was reported that Bombyx Batryticatus and Semen Strychni were powdered and taken orally for the treatment of esophageal cancer, and that a case of liver cancer was healed by taking boluses made from Bombyx Batryticatus and horse urine in combination with *Xiaoyao San*. A Military Hospital in Beijing claimed that the decoction of Calyx Kaki, Bombyx Batryticatus and Caulis Bambusae in Taeniam was used in the treatment of tumor patients. Most of patients were relieved and the tumor mass in some patients became reduced in size and it was found effective for cancers of the lung, the stomach and the esophagus.

Chrysalis Batryticatus derives from the dried chrysalis that dies due to the infection of Beauveria bassiana (Bals.) Vaillant. Since pharmacological experiments have proved that it surpasses Bombyx Batryticatus in hypnotic and anticonvulsive actions, it has been used to replace Bombyx Batryticatus. In addition, Chrysalis Batryticatus has an inhibitive action on sarcoma-180 of mise. With a daily dose of 0.2ml of 50% decoction of Chrysalis Batryticatus perfused into the stomach of mice, the effect is remarkable with an inhibitive rate of 71.4% (P < 0.05). (*Bulletin of Medicinal Herbs*, 1972)

BORNEOLUM

In was recorded in *Materia Medica of the Tang Dynasty* that: "The drug, bitter, acrid and slightly cold, is used to dispel pathogenic factors in the chest and the abdomen."

Borneolum is a crystalline substance obtained from *Dryobalanops aromatica Gaertner* of the family *Dipterocarpaceae*, or synthesized with Camphor and Oleum Terebinthinae. Its principal component is d-Borneol.

ANTICANCER PHARMACOLOGICAL FUNCTIONS

1. The low-temperature-dried substance of Borneolum dissolved in hot water was found to have an inhibition rate of 50-70% on JTC-26 in experiments in vitro.

2. *Fufang Yingguang Ji* (composed of Borneolum, Flos Carthami, etc.) was found active in suppressing cancer in experiments in vitro.

EXPERIMENTAL FORMULAS
For cancer of throat:
      Realgar 1g
      Alumen 150g
      Natrii Sulfas 45g
      Borax 45g
      Calculus Bovis 1g
      Radix Angelicae Duhuricae 0.1g
      Borax 3g
      Herba Menthae 0.2g
      Cortex Phellodendri 0.1g
      Pollen Typhae 0.1g
      Radix Glycyrrhizae 0.5g
      Borneol 1g

The above herbs are ground into fine powder for insufflation into the throat. (*Clinical Essentials of Tumors*)

For cancer of breast:

1>. Crucian carp, after the entrails being removed, is fried, pulverized and mixed with some Borneolum for application to the lesion. (*Journal of Jiangsu Traditional Chinese Medicine*, Vol. 7, 1960)

2>. Equal shares of live crucian carp and peeled Rhizoma Dioscoreae are ground into paste to be mixed with little amount of Moschus and Borneolum for application to the lesion. Should itching arise, do not scratch but tenderly stroke it. The paste is changed weekly. (*Journal of Jiangsu Traditional Chinese Medicine*, Vol. 1, 1958)

HISTORICAL COMMENTS

It was reported in *Amplified Materia Medica* that: "Borneolum can drastically relieve epigastric obstruction due to pathogenic heat. Its aromatic flavor is preeminent among all the herbs. If a bit of it is added to tea, the taste of the tea will become better. But too much will spoil the taste."

It was described in *Descriptions of Materia Medica* that: "It is a bitter-tasted drug used for dispersing. Any kind of excess syndrome of stroke, constipation, dysuria and stagnation of *qi* can be cured."

BULBUS LILII

Huang Gongxiu of the Qing Dynasty reported: "The herb, sweet and flat in taste and slightly cold, functions to benefit the lung and the heart and to astringe *qi*."

Bulbus Lilii is the dried bulb of *Lilium brownii F.E. Brown var. colchesteri Wils.*, *Lilium tenuifolium Fisch.*, *Lilium longiflorum Thunb.*, *Lilium concolor Salisb.* or *Lilium lancifolium Thunb.* of the family *Liliaceae*. Its different species are found growing all over China.

ANTICANCER PHARMACOLOGICAL FUNCTIONS
The herb is found to inhibit sarcoma-180 of mice and cervical cancer-14.

EXPERIMENTAL FORMULAS
For cancers of the lung and the breast:
A poultice is prepared by pulverizing Bulbus Lilii with olivary oil or an adhesive plaster is made with Bulbus Lilii, resin and dear fat for external application. (*Bulletin of Medicinal Herbs*, Vol. 6, 1974)
For rectal cancer with continuous bleeding:
Bulbus Lilii is parched slightly with wine and ground into powder for oral administration with water. (*Compendium of Medicinal herbs*)
For lung cancer:

> Bulbus Lilii 15g
> Radix Rehmanniae 15g
> Flos Lonicerae 15g
> Radix Adenophorae 12g
> Radix Glehniae 12g
> Radix Asparagi 9g
> Radix Ophiopogonis 9g
> Rhizoma Imperatae 30g
> Radix Scutellariae 9g
> Herba Oldenlandiae Diffusae 30g
> Herba Houttuyniae 30g
> Folium Cycis Revolutae 30g
> Semen Coicis 15g
> Pericarpium Citri Reticulatae 9g

The decoction of the herbs is taken daily. (*Journal of Shanghai Medicinal Herbs*, Vol. 3, 1979)

HISTORICAL COMMENTS

It was described in *Origin of Herbs* that: "Bulbus Lilii can supplement the spleen to keep the lung pure, arrest cough and promote diuresis. Zhang Zhongjing combined Bulbus Lilii and Radix Rehmannae to remove blood stasis."

In *Mirror of a Hundred Herbs* it was expounded that: "Lilium with white flower is of medicinal properties; Lilium with red flower or with yellow flower is solely an ornamental plant. Lilium can be sweet or bitter. The sweet one, with its root and base removed, is the best drug for inducing diuresis and curing constipation. Patients with collapse due to *qi* deficiency should not take it."

THE AUTHOR'S NOTE

The bulb of Bulbus Lilii contains a variety of alkaloids, such as colchicine, which has been verified to have an inhibitive action on mitosis of cells at the metaphase. Tissue culture in vitro proved the herb has an anticancer function even with a concentration of $0.1\mu g/ml$. (*Studies on Effective Components of Medicinal Herbs*)

HERBA GERANII ET ERODII

It was pointed out in *Materia Medica of Southern Yunnan* that: "The herb, slightly warm in nature and acrid, and bitter in taste, acts to expel pathogenic wind, promote blood circulation and eliminate toxic materials."

Herba Geranii et Erodii is the dried herb of *Erodium stephanianum Willd.* or *Geranium nepalense Sweet* or many other plants of the family *Geraniaceae*, containing tannic substances, gallic acid, succinic acid, quercetin, calcium salt, betaine, purine and arginine.

ANTICANCER PHARMACOLOGICAL FUNCTIONS

1. Bacteriophagic tests in vitro showed an active biological effect of the herb against tumor.

2. The inhibition rate of the hot water extract of Erodium of the family *Geraniaceae* on sarcoma-180 is 45%.

3. Geraniol contained in Erodium has a very strong inhibition on carcinogenic fungus--Aspergillus flavus.

EXPERIMENTAL FORMULAS

For cervical cancer:

1>.　　Herba Geranii et Erodii 12g
　　　　Semen Cassiae Torae 15g

The two herbs are decocted for oral administration daily. (*Collection of Herbal Prescriptions of Gynecology*)

2>.　　Herba Erodii 15g
　　　　Semen Plantaginis Asiaticae 9g
　　　　Herba Houttuyniae 9g
　　　　Semen Cassiae 15g
　　　　Fructus Catalpae 15g

The above herbs are decocted into a bowl of broth to be divided into three portions for oral administration with a portion daily. (*Collection of Herbal Prescriptions of Gynecology*)

For cancers of the lung, the rectum, the throat, the prostate and the breast and leukemia:

The liquid extract of Herba Geranii is taken orally with an arbitrary dose. (*Bulletin of Medicinal Herbs*, Vol. 6, 1974)

For various types of cancer:

Herba Geranii et Erodii (10g) is decocted in 200ml of water for oral administration three times a day. (*Research Data of Medicinal Herbs*, Vol. 6, 1978)

HISTORICAL COMMENTS

It was expounded in *Supplement to Compendium of Medicinal Herbs* that: "The herb functions to expel the wind, dredge the channel to promote blood circulation and free the collaterals. For treatment of injuries, arthralgia syndrome, numbness and skin paralysis, it is immersed in wine and taken frequently."

In *Herbology* it was recorded that: "Because the herb is an antipyretic and detoxicant, it is indicative for carbuncle, cellulitis, sores and swelling."

THE AUTHOR'S NOTE

Mr. Ye Juquan strongly advocated the use of Erodium in the treatment of uterine tumor and other difficult and complicated cases of woman's diseases, because "Erodium seems to contain a kind of substance like vitamin E". Mr. Ye used a recipe consisting of Semen Cassiae, Herba Erodii and Herba Houttuyniae which were decocted and taken as a drink for the treatment of uterine and vaginal illnesses, and achieved effective results. The three herbs have been verified in recent years to have anticancer activities to various degrees.

HERBA ELEPHANTOPI

It was reported in *New Collection of Materia Medica of Zhenan* that: "The herb, bitter in taste and slightly cold in nature, is used as an antipyretic and diuretic, and as a drug to calm the liver and keep the lung pure."

Herba Elephantopi is the dried plant of *Elephantopus scaher L.* or *Elephantopus tomentosa L.* of the family *Compositae*, which is largely distributed over Guangdong, Guangxi, Fujian, Yunnan and Guizhou and contains sesquiterpenes——elephantopin and elephantin. Additionally, *Elephantopus scaher L.* shows reactions of alkaloids, flavones, phenols and amino acids.

ANTICANCER PHARMACOLOGICAL FUNCTIONS

1. Elephantopin is found having inhibitive actions on Walker's carcinosarcoma, lymphatic leukemia-120 and lymphocyte-388.

2. Elephantin is effective for WM. In abroad, it also has been confirmed that the drug has an anticancer effect.

3. Bacteriophagic methods proved that Elephantopus scaher L. has antiphagic effects and this suggests an anticancer activity.

EXPERIMENTAL FORMULAS

For lymphogenous metastasis of cancer:

Herba Elephantopi is mixed with salt and vinegar, pulverized and applied on the affected lesion. (*Collection of Medical Records*)

For various types of tumors:

Herba Elephantopi (6 to 9 grams) is soaked in water and taken three times daily. (*Diagnosis, Treatment and Prevention of Tumors*)

HISTORICAL COMMENTS

It was described in *Collection of Experience Gained in Prevention and Treatment of Diseases* that: "30 grams of Herba Elephantopi was decocted and taken orally for 3 days on average for the treatment of stomatitis and pharyngolaryngitis in 22 cases. 18 cases recovered and no recurrence was observed during the follow-up for three months."

It was expounded in *New Edition of Materia Medica* that: "To cure ascites caused by cirrhosis, fresh Herba Elephantopi (60g) is simmered with lean pork or a cuttlefish and taken orally, or Herba Elephantopi (30g) is pulverized, mixed up with an egg, fried done and divided into two portions for oral administration each a portion with a decoction of Radix Codonopsis Pilosulae (15g), Poria (15g) and Radix Angelicae Sinensis (9g)."

THE AUTHOR'S NOTE

The whole plant of Herba Elephantopi has inhibitive actions on a variety of bacteria, for example, Staphylococcus aureus, Bacillus subtilis and Bacillus typhosus. Its decoction has certain effects on experimental arthritis of guinea pigs. The herb may cause enterogastric malaise and should be combined with drugs for tonifying the spleen.

HERBA ARISTOLOCHIAE MOLLISSIMAE

In *Yin Pian Xin Can* it was stated that: "The herb, bitter and neutral, is used to dissipate migratory arthralgia and clears the channels."

Herba Aristolochiae Mollissimae is the dried rhizome or the whole plant of *Aristolochia mollissima Hance* of the family *Aristolochiaceae*, which is found mainly growing in areas south of the Yellow River and should be discriminated from *Solanum lyratum Thunb*. of the family *Solanaceae*.

ANTICANCER PHARMACOLOGICAL FUNCTIONS

1. In Experiments with mice that were fed with forage adulterated with the powder of Herba Aristolochiae Mollissimae, observed was an obvious inhibitive action on Ehrlich's ascites carcinoma in mice, and the cells of ascites and the subcutaneous Ehrlich's cancer. Oral administration of the decoction of the plant was also effective.

2. The effective anticancer component is soluble in water and alcohol, but not in trichloromethane and cannot be destroyed by heat.

.3. Animal experiments showed inhibitive actions of Herba Aristolochiae Mollissimae on sarcoma-37 in mice and the alkaloid it contains has a notable anodyne effect.

EXPERIMENTAL FORMULAS
For osteosarcoma:

> Herba Aristolochiae Mollissimae 30g
> Herba Solani Lyrati 30g
> Radix Rumei Crispi 30g
> Fructus Psoraleae 15g

The decoction of the herbs is taken daily. (*Manual of Practical Anticancer Drugs*)

For pains caused by stomach cancer:

1 >. A dose of 9 grams of Rhizoma Aristolochiae Mollissimae is taken daily after being decocted or chewed.

2>. Rhizoma Aristolochiae Mollissimae (6g), Radix Schisandra Sphenantherae (15g) and Os Sepiae (15g) are dried in the sun and ground into powder. A dose of 6 grams is taken three times daily. (*Collection of Medicinal Herbs*)

For cancers of the lung and the uterus and tumor of the bone:

An intramuscular medication of Herba Aristolochiae Mollissimae Injection with a dose of 2-4ml is given twice daily.

For postoperative local recurrence of breast cancer:

Herba Aristolochiae Mollissimae 24g
Radix Astragali 24g
Radix Asparagi 15g
Radix Ophiopogonis 15g
Radix Paeoniae Rubra 12g
Radix Paeoniae Alba 12g
Flos Lonicerae 12g
Radix Rehmanniae 12g
Herba Artemisiae Annuae 12g
Cortex 9g
Fructus Forsythiae 9g
Radix Glycyrrhizae 3g
Pollen 24g
Semen Coicis 24g
Semen Coicis 24g
Spina Gleditsiae 12g

The above herbs are immersed in water for an hour and then decocted on slow fire, for oral administration. At the same time, powder of Bulbus Fritillariae Cirrhosae is taken three times daily, each time 2 grams; and 4 grams of the powder of Cormus Iphigeniae is divided into three portions and taken separately. (*Journal of Traditional Chinese Medicine*, Vol. 1, 1985)

HISTORICAL COMMENTS

It was reported in *Folk Medicinal Herbs of Nanjing* that: "The whole plant is soaked in water and taken for the treatment of pains of the muscles and the bones and the stomach."

In *Supplement to Compendium of Medicinal Herbs* it was indicated that: "It is used to promote blood circulation, drive the pathogenic wind and eliminate damp-heat."

It was described in *Dictionary of Chinese Materia Medica* that: "To cure gastralgia, the decoction of 9 grams of Herba Aristolochiae Mollissimae is taken. The therapy is continued daily till the patient is fully recovered. The therapy was prescribed for over 400 cases of stomach cancer and achieved certain effect. A case of duodenal ulcer had his pain relieved after taking 6 doses of the drug and no relapse occurred in the following several months."

THE AUTHOR'S NOTE

Herba Aristolochiae Mollissimae is mainly indicative for osteocarcinoma and lung cancer. Aristolochic acid isolated from plants of the same species was found capable of inhibiting the growth of the experimental tumor cells, but it is unknown whether Herba Aristolochiae Mollissimae has this chemical component. Poisoning tests showed that the drug has extremely low toxicity and no side effects. No abnormalities such as proteinuria and change of the number of leukocytes and erythrocytes as compared with the control group, were observed in domestic rabbits who received perfusion of the decoction of the herb with a dose of 5g/kg of body weight (corresponding to 250 grams of an adult dose) for 24 days. (*Collection of Papers of Academic Conference of Shanghai First Medical College in 1959*)

SCORPIO

It was recorded in *Kai Bao Materia Medica* that: "Being sweet, acrid and poisonous, scorpio is indicative for treating wind syndrome and rash."

Scorpio is the dried body of *Buthus martensii karsoh* of the family *Buthidae*, which contains buthotoxin, a sulfurous toxic protein like neurotoxin of snakes, in addition to lecithin, trimethylamine and taurine. Li Shizhen described the shape of Scorpio vividly: "Scorpio is an arthropod animal with eight feet and a long tail, green in color, looking like a water turtle."

ANTICANCER PHARMACOLOGICAL FUNCTIONS

1. Experiments in vitro showed that the alcohol preparations of Scorpio was capable of inhibiting cellular respiration of human liver cancer.

2. With methylene-blue method, the water extract and the alcohol extract of Scorpio were found to inhibit cells of colon cancer and liver cancer.

EXPERIMENTAL FORMULAS

For lung cancer:

      Scorpio 10

      Scolopendra 4

      Squama Manitis 9g

      Cinnabaris 1.5g

      Olibanum 6g

      Myrrha 6g

      Dinodon (calcined) 1

The above drugs are pulverized and capsulized. One capsule each time, three times a day. For more severe cases, 5-6 Mylabris with its head and feet removed are added to the above formula. (*Shanghai Journal of Medicinal Herbs*, Vol. 10, 1984)

For fibroadenoma of breast:

Scorpio (160g) is incased in 25 Fructus Trichosathi for parching without changing the nature and crushing into powder. 3 grams of the powder is taken three times daily for 1 month in succession. (*Effective Prescriptions for Women*, Vol. 5, 1982)

For hematemesis due to intestinal caner:

A dose of 1.5 grams of powdered Scorpio (60g, slightly parched) and Alumen (90g) is taken with warm rice soup before meal. (*Holy Prescriptions*)

HISTORICAL COMMENTS

It was reported in *Yujiu's Annotation on Medicinal Herbs* that: "Scorpio is able to get into the muscles and the bones to expel pathogenic factors, remove dampness and eliminate pathogenic wind."

Zhang Shouyi wrote: "The tail of scorpio was often used in ancient prescriptions, probably because its medical properties mainly exist there."

THE AUTHOR'S NOTE

Some people use the venom squeezed from the stinger of Scorpio to cure cancer, and others use a bolus prepared with scorpio venom, Periostracum Serpentis, Nidus Vespae with Mel for treating malignant tumors. It was reported that a patient with cancer of the ascending colon took Scorpio, Scolopendra and Mylabris and the tumor mass disappeared finally.

RADIX ARISTOLOCHIAE CINNABARIAE

In was pointed out in *Records of Herbs in Guangxi* that: "The herb, being bitter and acrid in taste and cold in nature, removes blood stasis to kill pain."

Radix Aristolochiae Cinnabariae is the dried tuberous root of *Aristolochia cinnabaria C.Y. Cheng Mss.* or *Aristolochia tuberosac F. Liang et S.M. Huang* of the *Aristolochiaceae* family, which is an analgesic drug usually used by folks of Sichuan, Guangxi, Yunnan and other places. Radix Aristolochiae Cinnabariae was mistakenly categorized into the family *Lobiatae* in *Records of Herbs in Sichuan* and was corrected later with the name of *Aristolochia cinnabarina C.Y. Cheng Mss.*. Radix Aristolochiae Cinnabariae produced in Guangxi was once erroneously regarded as *Aristolochia kaempferi Wild* which was verified to be a new breed named *Aristolochia tuberosac F. Liang et S.M. Huang*. The morphological and histological characteristics of *Aristolochia cinnabarina C.Y. Cheng Mss.* and *Aristolochia tuberosac F. Liang et S.M. Huang* are not remarkably different. (*Pharmaceutic Journal*, Vol. 7, 1982)

ANTICANCER PHARMACOLOGICAL FUNCTIONS

1. Aristolochic acid C contained in Radix Aristolochiae Cinnabariae has actions against cancer and increases phagocytic functions.

2. The anodyne effect of the extract of Radix Aristolochiae Cinnabariae is greater than that of morphine, and it is inferred that it might be the magnoflorine that works.

EXPERIMENTAL FORMULAS

For pains caused by various cancer:

Radix Aristolochiae Cinnabariae powdered by scraping is taken with boiled water or wine with a daily dose of 1-2 grams, Or chewed together with 3-5 fresh leaves. The dose can be increased. (*Sichuan Traditional Chinese Medicine*, Vol. 1, 1985)

HISTORICAL COMMENTS

It was reported in *Dictionary of Chinese Materia Medica* that: "The herb, as an antipyretic, anodyne and an agent to resolve swelling, eliminates blood stasis. Weak people should not take it."

THE AUTHOR'S NOTE

It was reported that Radix Aristolochiae Cinnabariae, powdered and made into pills of 0.25 gram, is taken orally three times a day, each time 0.5 gram, for pains caused by cancers of the biliary tract and the gastrointestinal canal. 23 cases took the pill and 21 showed improvement. In Guangxi Province, a preparation made of the total aristolochic acids of the herb, named *She Bai Ling*, was administered to 254 cases of leukemia and was found having an effective rate of 89.3%, which is better than currently available leukogenic drugs.

CAULIS HELIANTHI ANNUI

It was recorded in *Folk Medicinal Herbs of Fujian* that: "The flower disc is sweet, warm, nonpoisonous and is used to induce diuresis, remove damp-heat, clear the orifices and expel the wind."

Caulis Helianthi Annui is the dried seed, tuberous root, floral disc, pericarp, flower and leaf of *Helianthus annuus L.* of the family *Compositae*, growing all over China and contains an anticancer component of polyose——hemicellulose.

ANTICANCER PHARMACOLOGICAL FUNCTIONS

1. The hemicellulose extracted from the floral disc was found to have inhibitive actions on sarcoma-180 and Ehrlich's ascites carcinoma of mouse.

2. The hemicellulose extracted from the stem pulp has a weaker inhibition on cells of the above two strains than the extract from the floral disc.

EXPERIMENTAL FORMULAS

For stomach cancer:

The decoction of the stem pulp of Caulis Helianthi Annui is taken as a drink with a daily dose of 4.5-6 grams and one year is a therapeutic course. (*Collection of Data on Treatment of Tumor with Herbs in Anhui*, Vol. 65, 1971)

For trophocytic tumor:

The floral disc of Caulis Helianthi Annui (90g), Herba Pteridis Multifidae (60g) and Radix Adinae (60g) are decocted in water for 1 to 2 hours into semi-colloid broth for oral administration daily. 30-60 doses make a course. (*Zhejiang Bulletin of Tumors*, Vol. 3, 1972)

HISTORICAL COMMENTS

In *Collection of Herbs*, Wang Lianren said: "The seed is used to promote flow of *qi* and boost pyogenesis."

It was reported in *Illustration of Chinese Medicinal Plants* that: "The bitter leaf and flower is used to reinforce the function of the stomach."

It was noted in *Collection of Common Folk Medicinal Herbs* that: "The decoction of the pericarp is used to cure tinnitus."

It was recorded in *Herbal Records of Sichuan* that: "The root is used as a remedy for pains in the stomach, intestine, chest and hypochondrium and as a purgative and laxative."

It was indicated in *Materia Medica of Quanzhou* that: "To restore constipation and bradyuria, the juice squeezed from the fresh seeds of Caulis Helianthi Annui is mixed with honey for oral administration with a dose of 15-30 grams."

THE AUTHOR'S NOTE

It has been pinpointed out in a report that the seed of the herb contains a carcinogen called 3.4-benzopyrene, and that its oil, fed to mice after being heated at a temperature of 110-300°C, was able to increase the carcinogenicity of some carcinogens in guinea pigs. This report is only for reference.

According to a report in *Botanical Chemistry* (Vol. 8, 983), a yellowish oleaginous substance with the molecular formula of $C_{20}H_{26}O_7$ has been obtained from the tender leaves and the upper stem of Caulis Helianthi Annui, which inhibits the growth of plant. Experiments in vivo on the synthesis of DNA and RNA in the cells of Ehrlich's ascites carcinoma, with a dose of 20ug/ml, revealed that the above substance has an inhibition on DNA synthesis with a rate of 5% and on RNA synthesis with a rate of 75%.

In one of the recent studies in Japan, it has been analyzed and further proved that the pollen of Caulis Helianthi Annui contains coumarinic acid, ferulic acid, caffeic acid, glyceryl palmitate and quercitrin, some of which are found having certain activities against cancer.

TESTA ORYZAE

It was reported in *Chinese Pharmacopeia* that: "The herb is acrid, sweet and hot, and is used to cure dysphagia."

Testa Oryzae is the dried seed crust of *Oryza Sativa L.* of the family *Gramineae*, which is mainly produced in the Southern provinces of China and contains sitosterol glyceride, squalene, polysaccharide and glucoside.

ANTICANCER PHARMACOLOGICAL FUNCTIONS

1. A substance extracted from the stem, husk or chaff of *Oryza Sativa L.* is found active in inhibiting Ehrlich's sarcoma-180 and sarcoma-180 of mouse.

2. In foreign countries, an anticancer substance (23.6μg/kg) has been extracted from *Oryza Sativa L.* and it is probably a kind of polyoses (primarily, pentose and hexose) which is soluble in water but not in general organic solvents.

EXPERIMENTAL FORMULAS

For esophageal cancer:

1>. The decoction of Testa Oryzae, Radix Ginseng and Fructus Nelumbinis (3 grams each) is taken three times daily. (*Records of Holy Relief*)

2>. A marble-sized bolus made by blending finely-powdered Testa Oryzae with honey is sucked, not swallowed. (*Holy Prescriptions*)

3>. The following herbs are taken in decoction. (*Comprehension of Medicine*):

> Radix Adenophorae 9g
> Radix Salviae Miltiorrhizae 9g
> Poria 3g
> Bulbus Fritillariae Cirrhosae 4.5g
> Fructus Amomi 1.2g
> Folium Nelumbinis 2
> Radix, Curcumae 1.5g
> Testa Oryzae 1.5g

For cancer of the large intestine: A dose of 3 to 16 grams of Testa Oryzae is taken daily. The herb also prevents cancer of the large intestine through increasing the bowel movement. (*On Cancer Prevention and Treatment*)

HISTORICAL COMMENTS

It was pointed out in *Chinese Pharmacopeia* that: "Sucking Testa Oryzae perlingually or taking Testa Oryzae in decoction cures dysphagia."

In *Compendium of Medicinal Herbs* it was reported that: "Testa Oryzae is burned, pulverized and taken with water to help delivery."

It was expounded in *Origin of Herbal Canon* that: "Crushed Testa Oryzae heals the dysphagic because it is capable of removing the stagnancy of undigested food, and is particularly effective for extremely severe cases."

THE AUTHOR'S NOTE

A recipe called *Jiao Long Zheng* in *New Collection of Classic Prescriptions* written by Bao Xiang Ao of the Qing Dynasty, can be used to treat tumors of the abdominal cavity. The formula suggests the administration of large dose of Testa Oryzae. Recorded in *New Edition of Mei's Proved Recipes* was Testa Oryzae Bolus, which is prepared with the fine powder of Testa Oryzae after being mixed with honey and made into pills of the size of a marble, and is taken through sucking frequently. The bolus may have certain effect on esophageal cancer.

FLOS CARTHAMI

It was reported in *Essentials of Materia Medica* that: "The herb, acrid, bitter or sweet in taste and warm in nature, enters the Lung Channel to remove blood stasis."

Flos Carthami is the dried tubular flower of *Carthamus tinctorius L.* of the family *Compositae*, with an orange color and a special flavor. It contains carthamin and mainly grows in Henan, Zhejiang and Sichuan provinces.

ANTICANCER PHARMACOLOGICAL FUNCTIONS

1. The decoction of the plant was found having an inhibition on JTC-26 with a rate of 90%.
2. An inhibitive activity was revealed on sarcoma-180 of mouse.
3. Experiments in vitro showed an inhibitive effect on cells of leukemia.

EXPERIMENTAL FORMULAS

For cervical cancer:

Flos Carthami (6g), Alumen (6g) and Herba Orostachydis (30g) are decocted for washing the vulva once or twice daily, each time 30 to 60 minutes.

For esophageal cancer:

1>.   Flos Carthami 9g
       Radix Savlviae Miltiorrhizae 9g
       Radix Paconiae Rubra 9g
       Radix Rehmanniae 9g
       Radix Angelicae Sinensis 9g
       Caulis Spatholobi 30g
       Rhizoma Chuanxiong 3g

The herbs are decocted and taken daily. (*Collection of Data on Tumor*, Vol. 2, 1978)

2>.   Flos Carthami 6g
       Rhizoma Acori Graminei 6g
       Caulis Spatholobi 6g
       Catechu 4.5g
       Cormus Iphigeniae 18g

The herbs are taken daily in decoction. (*Prevention and Treatment of Tumors in Traditional Chinese Medicine*)

For skin abscess caused by acute granular leukemia:

       Flos Carthami 30g
       Olibanum 30g
       Myrrha 30g
       Radix Ardisiae 15g
       Fructus Gardeniae 60g
       Herba Phyllanthi Vrinariae 150g

The herbs are powdered, mixed with egg white or boiled water and applied on the lesion. (*New Traditional Chinese Medicine*, Vol. 4, 1977)

For pancreatic cancer:

       Flos Carthami 10g
       Semen Persicae 10g
       Rhizoma Scirpi 10g
       Faeces Trogopterori 10g
       Pollen Typhae 10g
       Rhizoma Picrorhizae 10g
       Cortex Phellodendri 10g
       Radix Linderae 10g
       Rhizoma Corydalis 10g
       Endothelium Corneum Gigeriae Galli 10g
       Radix Angelicae Sinensis 10g
       Squama Manitis 10g
       Radix Salviae Miltiorrhizae 30g
       Cortex Moutan 30g

Herba Chelidonii 30g

Rhizoma Zedoariae 15g

Herba Oldenlandiae Diffusae 20g

The herbs are taken in decoction. (*Clinical Essentials of Tumors*)

For various types of cancer:

Flos Carthami (5g) is decocted three times in 200ml of water and the broth is divided into three portions for oral administration in the morning, at noon and in the evening. This is a folk prescription in Japan. (*Research Data of Medicinal Herbs*, Vol.6, 1978)

HISTORICAL COMMENTS

It was explained in *Supplement to the Amplified Materia Medica* that: "The herb, in large dose, removes blood stasis and in small dose nourishes blood."

It was also stated in *Descriptions of Materia Medica* that: "The herb, decocted in water, nourishes blood and decocted in wine removes blood stasis."

It was described in *Medical Secrets of an Official* that: "To cure chronic ceruminosis with unceasing fetid pus, a small amount of pulverized Flos Carthami (0.3g) and Alumen (30g) is filled into the ear."

THE AUTHOR'S NOTE

The decoction of Flos Carthami is similar to that of Stigma Croci in actions on the circulatory system, but the toxicity of the former is far less than that of the latter. No side and toxic reactions appeared in mice fed with forage containing 6% of Flos Carthami, but reactions did appear in mice fed with only 2% of Stigma Croci.

FLOS TRIFOLII

In *National Collection of Medicinal Herbs* it was reported that: "The herb, bitter and cold, is used as an antiinflammatory agent, diuretic, antipyretic and as an agent to improve the acuity of vision."

Flos Trifolii is the dried inflorescence and flowering shoot of *Trifolium pratense L*. of the family *Leguminosae*, which is widely distributed over Northeast China and contains isoflavones, which possesses estrogen-like actions and the activity of 100 grams of the dried plant corresponds to 0.55-$0.565\mu g$ of estradiol, in addition to its anticancer active carotene (richest in florescence) and vitamin E.

ANTICANCER PHARMACOLOGICAL FUNCTIONS

The water extract of Flos Trifolii was found having anticancer actions. The oral or intraperitoneal administration to rats inhibits the growth of sarcoma-45, but not Ehrlich's ascites carcinoma. The extract takes effect only after being sterilized and stored under 4°C for at least 100 days, hence the anticancer constituent in it was presumed to be some kind of denatured protein and not alkaloids.

EXPERIMENTAL FORMULAS

For breast cancer:

Some amount of Flos Trifolii is taken as a drink with boiled water daily. (*Bulletin of Medicinal Herbs*, Vol. 6, 1974)

For diverse cancers:

A decoction of equal portions of Flos Trifolii, Folium Violae Verecundae and Radix Rumei Crispi is taken daily. (*Bulletin of Medicinal Herbs*, Vol. 6, 1974)

HISTORICAL COMMENTS

It was recorded in *Economic Flora of the Northeast* that: "The flower, stem, seed and root all can be used to prepare ointment, plaster, paste, decoction or tea against tumor, hard mass and cancer, with indications for cancerous ulcer, stomach cancer, breast cancer, intestinal cancer and so on." Also recorded was that: "The flower and the seed of *Trifolium repens L.* of the same species can also be used as anticancer and antitumor drugs."

LIGNUM AQUILARIAE RESINATUM

In *Origin of Herbal Canon* it was reported that: "The herb is warm but not dry, flowing but not astringing. It is used to tonify the spleen, act on the kidney, and send back the pathogenic heat to its origin."

Lignum Aquilariae Resinatum is the resinous wood of *Aquilaria agallocha Roxb.* or *Aquilaria sinensis (lour.) Gilg* of the family *Thymelaeaceae*, the former being the primal plant of imported Lignum Aquilariae Resinatum and the latter, the inland Lignum Aquilariae Resinatum.

ANTICANCER PHARMACOLOGICAL FUNCTIONS

1. The hot water extract of Lignum Aquilariae Resinatum was found in experiments in vitro to have an inhibition rate of 70-90% on JTC-26.

2. Studies in vitro on the cells of lymphocytic leukemia-388 showed that the two cytotoxic components separated from the wood exocarp became activated only at the contents of $0.8\mu g/ml$ and $0.0022\mu g/ml$ respectively, which exceeded the criterion of $ED_{50} < 4\mu g/ml$ laid down in the previous experiments of this system.

EXPERIMENTAL FORMULAS

For constipation due to cancer:

> Radix Angelicae Sinensis 9g
> Fructus Aurantii 9g
> Semen Armeniacae Amarum 9g
> Herba Cistanches 9g
> Radix Asteris 30g

The above herbs are decocted and the broth is mixed with the juice of Lignum Aquilariae Resinatum (2.4g) for oral administration. (*Orthodox Recipes*)

For unceasing hiccup caused by stomach cancer:

> Lignum Aquilariae Resinatum 3g
> Folium Perillae 3g
> Fructus Amomi 3g

1.5-2.1 grams of the powder of the above herbs is taken with *Shidi Tang* (Calyx Kaki Decoction). (*Huo Ren Xin Tong*)

HISTORICAL COMMENTS

In *Ri Huan Zi Materia Medica* it was reported that: "The herb functions to regulate the middle-*jiao*, invigorate the five viscera, replenish the vital essence, reinforce *yang*, remove pathogenic wind and resolve abdominal mass."

It was described in *Interpretation of Drugs* that: "The herb has very powerful functions, ascending with its positiveness, descending with its heaviness, dispersing with its bitterness and pushing with its forcefulness. It is used to clear the channels and collaterals, promote blood circulation and eliminate phlegm by moving *qi*, cure all cases of itching."

It was stated in *New Compilation of Materia Medica* that: "It is contraindicative for those with extreme heat due to deficiency of *yin*."

FRUCTUS CHEBULAE

In *Ocean Materia Medica* it was reported that: "The herb, being sour, astringent and warm, functions to dissipate stagnation of *qi* in the diaphragm and chest, and abdominal pain of insufficiency type."

Fructus Chebulae is the dried ripe fruit, green fruit, leaf or kernel of *Terminalia chebula Retz.* of the family *Combretaceae*, containing large quantities of tannic substances (approximately 23.6-37.36%) in addition to shikimic acid, quinic acid, fructose, amino acids and sennoside A in the fruit.

ANTICANCER PHARMACOLOGICAL FUNCTIONS

1. Experiments in vitro showed that the hot water extract works on JTC-26 with an inhibiting rate of 100% under a content of 500μg/ml, while the inhibiting rate of the alcohol extract is also 100%.

2. Studies in vivo showed that the hot water extract inhibits sarcoma-180 of mouse with a rate of 29.9%, and the alcohol extract with 7.6%.

3. In addition, the herb was also found inhibiting Ehrlich's ascites carcinoma of mouse and fusocellular sarcoma.

EXPERIMENTAL FORMULAS

For cancer of the esophagus and the stomach:

> Fructus Chebulae 9g
> Fructus Trapae Bispinosae 9g
> Caulis Wisteriae 9g
> Semen Coicis 9g

The decoction of the herbs is taken three times daily. (*Medicinal Food and simple Recipes*)

For aphasia due to cancer of the throat:

> Fructus Chebulae 4
> Radix Platycodi 30g
> Radix Glycyrrhicae 60g

The above herbs are ground into powder and a dose of 6 grams is taken with water. (*Xuanming's Treatise on Prescriptions*)

For hematemesis caused by intestinal cancer:

Fructus Chebulae (5kg) is soaked in wine, wrapped in a piece of cloth, then simmered and crushed before being mixed with the following herbs:

> Radix Angelicae Dahuricae 30g
> Radix Ledebouriellae 30g
> Radix Gentianae Macrophyllae 30g

All the herbs are parched, pulverized and blended with rice to make pills of the size of Semen Firmianae. A dose of 9 grams is taken in the morning and in the evening. (*Compilation of Materia Medica*)

HISTORICAL COMMENTS

It was reported in *Amplified Materia Medica* that: "For persons who are insufficient of *qi*, it is also applicable but the dose should be small and the herb should be simmered under a soft fire slowly until it is done."

In *Compendium of Medicinal Herbs* it was reported that: "Combined with Fructus Mume and Galla Chinensis, it astringes; with Pericarpium Citri Reticulatae and Cortex Magnoliae, it flows *qi* downward; and with Radix Ginseng, it acts to supplement the lung and relieve cough."

It was expounded in *Properties of Materia Medica* that: "The ripe plant is capable of clearing the lung and promoting the circulation of *qi*, while the simmered ones act to warm the stomach and consolidate the bowel."

THE AUTHOR'S NOTE

In 1959, a Japanese scholar began to conduct anticancer researches with a recipe (named WTTC) consisting of the following Chinese herbs:

Fructus Chebulae 10g
Caulis Wisteriae 10g
Fructus Trapae Bispinosae 10g
Semen Coicis 10g

All the above herbs are decocted for oral administration three times a day. Comparison was made with a control group that received X-ray and radium. The result was satisfactory in regard to degeneration of cancer cells and the intracellular substances, repression of the division of cancer cell and hyperblastosis. Animal experiments indicated that the herb was active in inhibiting the growth of tumors.

GANODERMA

In was reported in *Classic Herbs* that: "The herb is sweet and warm, and acts as a sedative and a drug to replenish vital essence and energy."

Ganoderma is the dried fructification of the fungi *Ganoderma japonica (Fr.) Llogd* or *Ganoderma lucidum (leyss. ex Fr.) Karst.* of the family *Polyporaceae*, the former containing ergosterol, fumaric acid, aminoglucose and mannitol, and the latter, coumarins, alkaloids, lactone and diverse enzymes.

ANTICANCER PHARMACOLOGICAL FUNCTIONS

1. The hot water extract of *Ganoderma lucidum (leyss. ex Fr.) Karst.*, administered subcutaneously for successive 10 days to the right inguen of female mice that had been vaccinated with sarcoma-180 for 7 days, showed an inhibiting rate as high as 95.6-98.5%.

2. The herb is found to have an action to promote the immunological function and to raise the quantity of leukocytes.

EXPERIMENTAL FORMULAS

For various types of cancer:

Ganoderma (15-20g) is decocted in 250ml of water and taken three times daily. (*Research Data of Medicinal Herbs*, Vol.6, 1978)

For esophageal cancer:

Ganoderma 10g
Herba Elsholtiziae Blandae 40g
Lasiosphaera seu Calvatia 7g
Calculus Bovis 4.5g
Moschus 2.5g

The above herbs are ground into fine powder and taken with warm water three times daily with a dose of 1.2-1.8 grams each time. (*Selection of Data on National Exhibition of New Medicinal Herbs*)

For arrest of the bone marrow following chemotherapy:

Ganoderma 9g
Radix Codonopsis Pilosulae 9g
Radix Astragali 9g
Radix Angelicae Sinensis 9g
Radix Paeoniae Alba 9g
Radix Aucklandiae 9g
Caulis Spatholobi 12g
Herba Bidens Triparititae 15g

The above herbs are made into powders and taken daily in two separate doses. (*Shanghai Journal of Medicinal Herbs*, Vol. 1, 1980)

HISTORICAL COMMENTS

In *Medicinal Flora of Hangzhou* it was told that: "For chronic stomach diseases with a history of many years, Ganoderma (1.5g) is cut to pieces and soaked in wine for oral administration daily."

In *Variorum of Classic Herbs*, it was expounded that: "Rhizoma Dioscoreae is a conductant drug for Ganoderma which should not be combined together with Radix Dichroae, Azurite and Herba Artemisiae Scopariae."

It was described in *Dictionary of Chinese Materia Medica* that: "The herb was administered to 52 cases of leukopenia caused by chemical and physical factors, drugs or chronic diseases, and showed remarkable efficacy in 11 cases, improvement in 12 and betterment in 21, with a contemporary effect of 84.6%."

THE AUTHOR'S NOTE

The anticancer effect of Ganoderma has been verified through animal experiments of mouse. In a Japanese hospital, repeated experiments with the extract of Ganoderma decoction indicated that administered alone, the herb seems to have little anticancer effect, but when combined with cryosurgery and adjusted in duration of medication, it inhibits proliferation of cancer cells and promotes the immunity.

The experiment was conducted through implanting cancer cells on the back of mice and then administering orally and intraperitoneally the extract of Ganoderma decoction to the mice. The result of the intraperitoneal administration was that under a dose of 100mg/kg of body weight, the herb arrested proliferation of cancer cells with a rate of 96.5%, and under a dose of 500mg/kg of body weight, with a rate of 98.6%. Oral administration showed a different result. Under a dose of 500ml/kg of body weight, the effective rate was only 24.5% and under a dose of 2.5kg/kg of body weight, the effective rate was 23.5%. But when combined with cryosurgery, oral administration of the herb can obtain the same result as that of intraperitoneal administration. The extract of Ganoderma could markedly increase immunological functions. (*News of Japanese Agriculture*, Dec. 26, 1984)

SEMEN ARMENIACAE AMARUM

In *Selected Materia Medica* it was reported that: "The drug, sweet or bitter in taste and warm in nature, functions to clear the lung."

Semen Armeniacae Amarum is the dried seed of *Prunus armeniaca L., Prunus armeniaca L. var. ansu Maxim., Prunus Mandshurica (Maxim.) Koehne* or *Prunus sibirica L.* of the family *Rosaceae*, the first two of which are more often used medically. The seed can be sweet or bitter, the bitter ones being preferred for medicinal purpose. The seeds of *Prunus sibirica L., Prunus Mandshurica (Maxim.) Koehne or wild Prunus armeniaca L. var. ansu Maxim.* are bitter while those of *Prunus armeniaca L., Prunus armeniaca L. var. ansu Maxim.* and those cultivated in orchard may be bitter or sweet. The major component of the seed is amygdalin, which can be hydrolysed by emulsin to form a toxic substance called hydrocyanic acid.

ANTICANCER PHARMACOLOGICAL FUNCTIONS

1. Experiments in vivo showed that the hot water extract of Semen Armeniacae Amarum has an inhibiting rate of 50-70% on JTC-26.

2. Experiments in vitro proved that the dried powder of Semen Armeniacae Amarum can completely inhibit the growth of strong carcinogenic fungi, i.e., aspergillus flavus and aspergillus. The effective element of the powder was found to be benzaldehyde.

EXPERIMENTAL FORMULAS

For intolerable itching caused by cervical cancer:

Peeled Semen Armeniacae Amarum is moderately burnt without changing its nature, cloaked with cotton and applied to cervix. (*Meng Shen, Chong Ju Fang*)

For warty tumor:

Peeled Semen Armeniacae Amarum is ground into powder, mixed with egg white, applied on the affected lesion at night and washed away in the morning with warm wine. (*Meng Shen, Sheng Mian You Mu Fang*)

For lung cancer:

Semen Armeniacae Amarum 9g
Nodus Nelumbinis Rhizomatis 9g
Folium Eriobotryae 9g
Radix Astragali 9g
Pollen Trogopterorl 9g
Radix Rhapontici Uniflori 15g
Radix Adenophorae 12g
Mel 12g
Fossilia Spiriferis 20g
Herba Scutellariae Harbatae 60g

The decoction of these herbs is taken twice daily. (*Selected Clinical Recipes of Medicinal Herbs*)

For esophageal cancer:

Semen Armeniacae Amarum 4g
Poria 5g
Rhizoma Zingiberis 2g
Radix Glycyrrhizae 2g

The decoction of these herbs is taken daily. (*Explanation to the Clinical Prescriptions of Traditional Chinese Medicine*)

For esophageal and cardiac cancer:

Equal portions of Semen Armeniacae Amarum, Semen Sojae Praeparatum, Massa Medicata Fermentata, Rhizoma Zingiberis, Fructus Corni, Pericarpium Zanthoxyli Bungeani are crushed to powder, mixed with honey for rubbing on the chest several times a day. (*External Therapy*)

For tumor of uterus and its appendages:

Semen Armeniacae Amarum 15g
Semen Persicae 60g
Radix et Rhizoma Rhei 9g
Hirudo 30
Tabanus 30

The herbs are decocted in two bowels of water to the content of one bowel and divided into three portions for oral administration daily three times, each time one portion. (*Collection of Herbal Prescriptions of Modern Gynecology*)

HISTORICAL COMMENTS

It was reported in *Compendium of Medicinal Herbs* that: "Because of its dispersing and descending attributes, Semen Armeniacae Amarum is used to expel pathogenic factors from the muscles and the skin, drive out pathogenic wind, keep *qi* flowing downward, eliminate dryness, relieve stagnation of *qi* and used with other drugs for traumatic injuries; And because of its toxicity, it is used as an agent for treating sores and as an anthelmintic."

Li Gao said: "Semen Armeniacae Amarum cures asthma because it adjusts the travelling of *qi*, and Semen Persicae cures mania because it regulates blood circulation. Both Semen Armeniacae Amarum and Semen Persicae are effective for constipation caused by either *qi* or blood. Constipation during daytime is caused by *yang qi* and constipation at night is caused by *ying* blood. Hence, Semen Armeniacae Amarum and Pericarpium Citri Reticulatae are administered to patients of the insufficient type with pulse floating on *qi*, who can not tolerate strong purgation. Semen Persicae and Pericarpium Citri Reticulatae are prescribed for those with pulse sinking to the blood. Pericarpium Citri Reticulatae is used in both cases because constipation is both an external disease of the Large Intestine Channel of Hang-*Yangming* and an interior disease of the Lung Channel of Hand-*Taiyin*."

It was recorded in *Health Preservation* that: "To relieve diarrhea and exceeding bitterness of the mouth caused by poisoning of Semen Armeniacae Amarum, juice of Fructus Mume is given."

It was cautioned in *Annotation on Classical Herbs* that: "For cough due to insufficiency of *yin*, heat of the deficiency type and heat-phlegm, Semen Armeniacae Amarum is prohibited."

HERBA AINSLIAEAE

It was reported in *National Collection of Medicinal Herbs* that: "The herb is acid, bitter, and cold. It is used to remove heat, resolve mass, cool blood and remove toxic materials."

Herba Ainsliaeae is the dried plant of *Ainsliaea fragrans Champ.* of the family *Compositae*, which is mainly grown in East China, Southern Central China and the Southwest. Its capitulum is streaked and its flower is white and tubular with a flavor similar to apricot kernel.

ANTICANCER PHARMACOLOGICAL FUNCTIONS

Screened with fluorescent microscope method, the herb exhibited an antagonistic effect on the growth of cells of leukemia.

EXPERIMENTAL FORMULAS

For early cases of lung cancer:

1 >. Herba Ainsliaeae (60 grams) and Folium Photiniae (30 grams) are decocted and taken with millet wine. Two doses of the formula is taken daily and ten days makes a therapeutic course. (*Dictionary of Chinese Materia Medica*)

2 >. The decoction of Herba Ainsliaeae (90g) is taken frequently as a drink. (*Determination of Treatment Based on Differentiation of Symptoms and Signs*)

HISTORICAL COMMENTS

It was stated in *Supplement to Compendium of Materia Medica* that: "The herb, bitter, cold and nonpoisonous, is most effective in cooling blood and promoting blood circulation, clearing lung-heat, curing hematemesis and consumptive diseases."

It was suggested in *Wu Puren's Prescriptions* that: "To cure hectic fever caused by consumptive diseases, a chicken steamed with Herba Ainsliaeae is taken."

RADIX PAEONIAE RUBRA

It was reported in *Classic Herbs* that: "The herb, being bitter in taste and neutral in nature, is used to resolve solid mass and periumbilical colic and mass due to invasion of the cold and the heat."

Radix Paeoniae Rubra is the dried root of *Paeonia lactiflora Pall.*, *Paeonia obovata Maxim.* or *Paeonia veitchii lynch* of the family *Ranunculaceae*, which contains paeoniflorin.

ANTICANCER PHARMACOLOGICAL FUNCTIONS

1. 70% alcohol extract of the herb has an apparent inhibition on solid sarcoma-180 of mice.

2. After the administration of the herb, the phagocytic index was found elevated through assessing the function of the reticuloepithelial system. This is very useful for anticancer research.

3. It is known that the cAMP level is generally low in cancer cells. But after using the extract of Radix Paeoniae Rubra, cAMP in cells of ascitic sarcoma-180 had been elevated by 60%.

EXPERIMENTAL FORMULAS

For squamous carcinoma of the sole:

> Radix Paeoniae Rubra 9g
> Radix Salviae Miltiorrhizae 9g
> Radix Achyranthis Bidentatae 9g
> Bombyx Batryticatus 9g
> Flos Lonicerae 9g
> Radix Rehmanniae 12g
> Radix Angelicae Sinensis 12g
> Semen Phaseoli 60g
> Herba Taraxaci 30g
> Herba Oldenlandiae Diffusae 30g
> Radix Stephaniae 30g
> Poria 30g
> Bufo 6g
> Olibanum 4.5g
> Myrrha 4.5g
> Radix Glycyrrhizae 4.5g

The herbs are taken in decoction. (*Journal of Shanghai Medicinal Herbs*, Vol. 1, 1984)

For tumor of the thyroid:

> Radix Paeoniae Rubra 15g
> Radix Bupleuri 9g
> Rhizoma Zedoariae 9g
> Rhizoma Scirpi 9g
> Radix Aucklandiae 9g
> Semen Persicae 9g
> Flos Carthami 9g
> Cortex Moutan 9g
> Fructus Gardeniae 12g
> Radix Curcumae 12g
> Spica Prunellae 30g

Carpapax Trinycis 30g

Corcha Ostreae 30g

The decoction of herbs is taken daily or every other day. (*Journal of Traditional Chinese Medicine*, Vol. 7, 1979)

HISTORICAL COMMENTS

In *Treatise on Properties of Drugs* it was stated: "The herb cures pathogenic wind in the lung, severe abdominal pain, and stagnation of blood and *qi*."

It was reported in *Materia Medica of Southern Yunnan* that: "It is used to promote blood circulation, eliminate blood stasis, dissipate blood clot, and relieve abdominal pain."

It was indicated in *Extensive Notes of Medical Practice* that: "To cure incessant epistaxis, a dose of 4.5 grams of the powder of Radix Paeoniae Rubra is taken with water."

FRUCTUS XANTHII

In *Dictionary of Chinese Materia Medica* it was recorded: "The herb, bitter, acrid, cold and poisonous, is used as an antipyretic, detoxicant, anthelmintic and as a drug to eliminate the pathogenic wind."

Fructus Xanthii is the dried stalk, leaf, fruit or root of *Xanthium sibiricum Patr*. of the family *Compositae*. The whole plant contains xanthostrumarin, and derivatives of chalcone and organic acids, while the root contains a glucoside which is an active anticarcinogen with a melting point of 242 °C. Fructus Xanthii is poisonous and the toxin is a water soluble substance.

ANTICANCER PHARMACOLOGICAL FUNCTIONS

1. The water or the methanol extract of Radix Xanthii (glucoside) was found capable of prolonging the survival period of mice vaccinated with Ehrlich's ascites carcinoma.

2. A remarkable inhibitive effect of the hot water extract of Fructus Xanthii on ascitic sarcoma-180 has been prove to be 50.2%.

3. When frozen and dried, the hot water extract of Fructus Xanthii exhibited an inhibitive rate of 50-70% in studies in vitro.

EXPERIMENTAL FORMULAS

For diverse types of cancer:

Fructus Xanthii (or the leaf, or the stalk, 9 grams) is decocted three times in water and taken in three times. (*Research Data of Medicinal Herbs*, Vol. 6, 1978)

For nasopharyngeal cancer:

Flos Magnoliae 15g

Fructus Xanthii 7.5g

Radix Angelicae Dahuricae 30g

Folium Menthae 1.5g

The herbs are ground into powder and taken with tea after vegetarian meals with a dose of 6 grams. (*Complete Works of Zhang Jingyue*)

For tumor of the brain:

Folium Xanthii 30g

Rhizoma Dryopteris Crassirhizomae 30g

Rhizoma Amorphophalli 30g

Radix Typhae 15g

Rhizoma Paridis 15g

The decoction of the herbs is taken daily. (*Manual of Practical Anticancer Drugs*)

HISTORICAL COMMENTS

In *Tian Bao Materia Medica*, Fructus Xanthii was described "to eliminate pathogenic wind and remove toxic materials".

In *Essential Drugs in Prescriptions* Fructus Xanthii was stated to be used "for the treatment of nasal polyp".

It was reported in *Dietetic Materia Medica* that: "For nail-shaped boil, sleepiness and heaviness, Radix Xanthii is crushed in the urine of a child and the liquid is taken in cold three times a day."

ALOË

In *Annotation on Classic Herbs* it was pointed out that: "Aloë, with its cold nature to remove heat and its bitter taste to eliminate dampness, is used as an anthelmintic."

Aloë is the dried solid residue obtained through evaporating the juice from the leaves of *Aloe vera L.*, *Aloe ferox Mill* or *Aloe vera L. var. chinensis (Haw.) Berger* of the *family Liliaceae*. All plants of the family Liaceae contain derivatives of anthraquinone, especially aloin, and among all the purgative herbs that contains chrysophanein, Aloë is the most powerful.

ANTICANCER PHARMACOLOGICAL FUNCTIONS

1. Experiments in vivo proved that the alcohol extract of Aloë (1:500) was capable of inhibiting the growth of sarcoma-180 of mice and Ehrlich's ascites carcinoma.

2. One of the substances separated from the above extract was found to have an even stronger anticancer effect, the median lethal dose of mice being 5g/kg of body weight.

EXPERIMENTAL FORMULAS

For constipation caused by intestinal cancer:

Finely crushed Aloë (21g) and Cinnabaris (15g) are blended with rice and wine to make boluses. A dose of 9 grams is taken with wine. (*Annotation on Classic Herbs*)

For cancers of the rectum and the anus:

Aloë is ground into powder in white wine and mixed with a small amount of Borneol for external application. (*Essential Points of Materia Medica*)

For chronic granular leukemia:

Danggui Luhui Wan (consisting of Radix Angelicae Sinensis, Aloë and Indigo Naturalis) is taken twice a day with a dose of 6 grams. The dose can be increased to 30 grams. Side effects are abdominal pain and diarrhea. (*Oncology of Traditional Chinese Medicine*)

HISTORICAL COMMENTS

It was reported in *Compilation of Materia Medica* that: "It is certainly the drug for febrile diseases of the liver."

In *Origin of Herbal Canon* it was recorded that: "Abdominal mass can not be resolved unless this herb is administered."

THE AUTHOR'S NOTE

In *Anticancer Herbal Preparations* it was introduced that in the Hematology Institute of Chinese Academy of Medical Sciences, *Danggui Luhui Wan* was administered to 28 cases of chronic granular leukemia, 16 of which were relieved and 6 improved, with a total effective rate of 78.6%. It was also found that illnesses of short duration have the best effect.

FLOS GENKWA

It was stated in *Records of Famous Physicians* that: "The herb, being bitter, slightly warm and somewhat poisonous, is used to eliminate phlegm and fluid retention in the chest."

Flos Genkwa is the dried bud, leaf or root of *Daphne genkwa Sieb. et Zucc.* or *Wikstroemia chamaedaphne Meisn.* of the family *Thymelaeaceae*, which contains flavonoid glycosides, apigenin, sitosterol, benzoic acid and pungent oleaginous substance in its flower, ß-sitosterol, yuankanin and yellow crystal substance in its root and skin. Genkwanin is the substance that has anticancer activities.

ANTICANCER PHARMACOLOGICAL FUNCTIONS

1. Injection of the water solution of the volatile oil of Flos Genkwa to the base of rectal cancer causes rapid necrosis of the tumor.

2. The methanol extract of Flos Genkwa was found to have a notable inhibitive action on lymphatic leukemia-388.

EXPERIMENTAL FORMULAS

For cervical cancer:

      Flos Genkwa 30g

      Radix Angelicae Sinensis 30g

      Semen Longan 30g

The herbs are pounded into fine powder, blended with cooked rice to make pills of the size of Semen Firmianae. A dose of 10 pills is taken with warm wine before meal. (*Holy Prescriptions*)

For malignant hydatidiform mole:

Radix Genkwa (90g) is parched yellow and then ground into powder. A dose of 3 grams is taken with the decoction of Semen Persicae. (*Holy Prescriptions*)

For tumor of the skin:

1>. Decocted paste of Radix Glycyrrhizae is applied around the pen-shaped tumor; Then the powder of equal shares of Flos Genkwa, Radix Euphorbiae Pekinensis and Radix Kansui (blended with vinegar) is applied on the top of the tumor. The mass will contract and become crisp spontaneously after several times of medication. (*Inherited Formulas*)

2>.   Flos Genkwa 60g

      Rhizoma et Radix Rhei 60g

      Sargassum 60g

      Thallus Laminariae seu Eckloniae 60g

      Rhizoma Pinelliae 30g

      Galla Chinensis 30g

      Rhizoma Alismatis 30g

      Calcaria 60g

The first four of the above herbs are decocted in charcoal water mixed with vinegar and the rest of the herbs are added in for further decoction. The extract of the decoction is applied topically on the affected lesion. (*External Therapy*)

For lymphosarcoma and lymphadenoma:

The decoction of Radix Genkwa is taken. (*Collection of Simplified Recipes of Binhu*)

HISTORICAL COMMENTS

It was described in *Original of Materia Medica* that: "A thread soaked in the decoction of Flos Genkwa is tied around the hemorrhoid to make it fall off. The same therapy can be given to tumors."

It was stated in *Records of Famous Physicians* that: "The drug is indicative for lumbago caused by cold in the lower part of the body, malignant boils, tinea and scabies."

In *Zhi Zhi Fang* it was expounded that: "To cure hypochondrial lumps, Flos Genkwa is needed and it can also nourish the stomach when fluid retention has been relieved."

It was told in *New Compilation of Materia Medica* that: "Flos Genkwa is bitter and warm and used for the treatment of accumulated phlegm and fluid retention in hypochondrium, edema of the five viscera and distention of the skin. It is very poisonous with rapid action. Patients with symptoms of dampness may die after taking the drug."

In *Proved Recipes of Zhong Fu Tang* it was written that: "Fresh Radix Genkwa is washed and pounded into juice in a wood or stone utensil (without exposure to iron). Then a thread, after being immersed in the juice for half a day or a night, is tied around the tumor for a day and the tumor will drop off itself. If the tumor does not fall off, the therapy is repeated. After that, the powder of Fissilia Ossis Mastodi and Fructus Chebulae is applied on the wound."

It was noted in *Variorum of Classic Herbs* that: "Semen Cassiae is a conductant drug for Flos Genkwa which cannot be used together with Radix Glycyrrhizae."

BITTERN

Canon of Materia Medica reported that: "The drug, bitter in taste and cold in nature, is effective for treating sweltering fever, easing thirst and mania, and eliminating pathogenic factors."

It is the crystal bittern mainly composed of magnesium and some trace elements such as chloride, silicon dioxide, germanium and fluorine. In *Canon of Materia Medica* it is called salty bittern.

ANTICANCER PHARMACOLOGICAL FUNCTIONS
The substance rich in magnesium seems to improve the immunity of rats against carcinoplasia, while on the other hand, deficiency of magnesium reduces the vitality of lymphocytes and makes rats susceptible to malignant tumor.

EXPERIMENTAL FORMULAS
For osteoblastosarcoma:

  Refined bittern powder 100g
  Starch 10g
  Distilled water 100ml
  Magnesium stearate 1ml

The four ingredients are put together and made into tablets each 0.5 gram. A therapeutic course lasts 15 days and the drug is taken twice a day, each time two tablets. From the second course, the dosage is doubled. Usually the formula is continued for 5 courses. (*Journal of Integrated Traditional Chinese and Western Medicine*)

For pulmonary cancer:

Journal of Diagnosis, Prevention and Treatment of Tumor reported oral administration of 2 grams of bittern powder three times daily.

For carcinodermatoulcer:

It is reported in *Journal of Diagnosis, Prevention and Treatment of Tumor* that 30 grams of bittern powder, is blended with paraffin liquid and mixed with 100 grams of vaseline to make a paste for application to the ulcer after disinfection.

HISTORICAL COMMENTS
In *Records of Renowned Doctors*, it is said that: "Bittern is effective in clearing up accumulated heat in the five viscera, the intestines and the stomach, dispersing stagnation of vital energy, easing hiccup, vomiting and rapid respiration, improving vision and curing ophthalmalgia."

Journal of Jilin Chinese Medicinal Herbs reports that: "The drug functions to cordialize, tranquilize, promote digestion, resist convulsion, relieve inflammation and cure tumors."

In *Dictionary of Chinese Medicinal Herbs*, it is reported that: "The drug, according to the literatures from various regions of the country, is used clinically to treat pulmonary cancer and cervical cancer, as a preliminary approach."

CONCHA OSTREAE

Wang Ang of the Qing Dynasty commended that: "The drug is salty for softening hard lumps, astringent for curing dysentery and lightly cold for clearing up heat and replenishing water."

Concha Ostreae is an animal of *Ostrea gigas Thunbery* genus of the *Ostreidae* family. Its shell and body are for medical use. The shell, composed of an outer and an inner layer, has an oblate and irregular leaf-like shape, looking like the scale of flakes. The inner shell is somewhat caved inwardly, while the outer one, 6 to 10 centimeters long, is as oblately flat as a cover. The surface, due to the reflection of light, appears to be grayish brown or greenish blue, while the inside layer being opalescent and lustrous. The meat is dietetic and tasty. Concha Ostreae is produced and cultivated in all the provinces along the coast of China Sea. The shell contains 80-95% of calcium carbonate, calcium phosphate, calcium sulfate, magnesium, plumbum, silicon and magnesium oxide. Its flesh is rich in protein, fat and vitamins.

ANTICANCER PHARMACOLOGICAL FUNCTIONS

1. The crude extract of the animal, gained from grinding, extraction with disinfected water, separation and centrifugalization, is capable of inhibiting sarcoma-180 and Kreb's tumor-2 in a similar way as the snail and the cuttlefish.

2. Pharmacological sensitivity test shows that Concha Ostreae can inhibit the growth of cancer cells.

3. The liquid substance extracted from its meat, when injected into tumor body, is found effective against tumors of rats induced by viruses A-12 and SV-40.

4. Its meat contains an element called paolin, which is effective in inhibiting the growth of some oncocytic strains through neutralizing cytovirus. The molecular weight of paolin is between 8000 to 15000 and it may lose its effect after being heated.

5. The anticancer mechanism of paolin lies in its cellular toxic effect or a certain kind of enzyme which destroys the metabolic substance that is essential to oncocyte.

EXPERIMENTAL FORMULAS

For Mesothelioma of the abdominal cavity:

        Concha Ostreae 60g
        Roast Carapax Trionycis 60g
        Sargassum 60g
        Squama Manitis 30g
        Radix Salviae Miltiorrhizae 20g
        Scorpio 30g
        Nidus Vespae 30g
        Flos Carthami 15g
        Radix Aucklandiae 15g

The formula is taken one dosage daily in decoction. (*Exchange of Medical Information*, Vol. 9, 1974)

For massive metastatic mucinous adenocarcinoma of the abdominal wall:

Concha Ostreae 30g
Radix Codonopsis Pilosulae 9g
Rhizoma Atractylodis Macrocephalae 9g
Poria 9g
Radix Glycyrrhizae
Pericarpium Citri Reticulatae 9g
Rhizoma Pinelliae 9g
Carapax Trionycis 15g
Spica Prunellae 15g
Rhizoma Alismatis 12g
Lumbricus 9g
Radix Sophorae Tonkinensis 15g
Herba Scutellariae Barbatae 30g
Fructus Ligustri Lucidi 15g
Fructus aurantii immaturus 12g

The formula is taken one dosage daily in decoction. (*Exchange of Medical Information*, Vol. 9, 1974)

For pulmonary cancer:
Concha Ostreae 30g
Herba Oldenlandiae Diffusae 15g
Rhizoma Imperatae 15g
Semen Coicis 15g
Spica Prunellae 15g
Semen Citri Reticlatae 9g
Exocarpium Citri Rubrum 9g
Sargassum 18g
Thallus Laminariae seu Eckloniae 18g
Radix Stemonae 18g
Flos Hibisci Mutabilis 18g
Rhizoma Paridis 18g
Radix Rehmanniae 12g
Radix Scrophulariae 12g

The formula is taken one dosage daily in decoction.

For osteocytoma:
Concha Ostreae 90g
Spica Prunellae 30g
Herba Dendrobii 30g
Radix polygoni Multiflori 30g
Fructus Logustri Lucidi 30g
Cortex Eucommiae 30g
Radix Angelicae Sinensis 30g
Rhizoma Atractylodis Macrocephale 30g
Radix Astragali 30g
Fossilia Ossis Mastadi 30g
Rhizoma Drynariae 30g
Rhizoma Scirpi 15g
Olibanum 15g
Myrrha 15g
Radix Rehmanniae 15g

Mel 500g

The herbs are simmered into a paste to be taken orally 3-5 times daily with 2-3 spoonful each time.

For Malignant lymphoma and thyroedoma:
Concha Ostreae
Radix Scrophulariae
Bulbus Fritillariae Cirrhosae

Equal amount of the three ingredients is ground into powder and made into honey-coated pills for oral administration twice daily with warm water, 9g each time.

For gastrocancer:
Concha Ostreae 15g
Concha Haliotidis 15g
Sargassum 15g
Thallus Laminariae seu Eckloniae 15g
Gecko 15g
Thallus Porphyrae 15g

The formula is taken one dosage in decoction. (*Chinese Marine Biology*)

For neurofibroma:
Concha Ostreae 50g
Radix Bupleuri 15g
Radix Paeoniae Alba 15g
Radix Paeoniae Rubra 15g
Poria 15g
Thallus Laminariae seu Eckloniae 15g
Spica Purnellae 15g
Herba Oldenlandiae Diffusae 25g
Sargassum 25g
Rumulus Vncariae Cum Vncis 25g

The formula is taken one dosage daily in decoction or made into honey-coated pills with 15g for each, two pills each time and three times a day.

For pancreatic cystadenoma:
Concha Ostreae 35g
Spica Prunellae 20g
Thallus Laminariae seu Eckloniae 15g
Sargassum 15g
Rhizoma Cyperi 15g
Fructus Aurantii 15g
Semen Persicae 15g
Radix Scutellariae 15g
Radix Bupleuri 15g
Rhizoma Pinelliae 15g
Flos Carthami 10g
Radix Platycodi 10g

The formula is taken in decoction. (*New Traditional Chinese Medicine*, Vol. 12, 1982)

For mammocancer:
Concha Ostreae 4g
Radix Angelicae Sinensis 5g
Radix Paeoniae 3g
Radix Glycyrrhizae 3g

Radix Syringae Vulgaridis 3g
Rhizoma et Radix Rhei 1.5g
Flos Lonicerae 1.5g
Rhizoma Cimicifugae Foetidae 2g
Radix Glycyrrhizae 0.1g

Modification of the dosage of Rhizoma et Radix Rhei is decided with respect to whether the patient's defecation is normal or not. For those detesting the bitter taste of Rhizoma Cimicifugae Foetidae, the dosage may be reduced to 0.5-1g.

For Esophagocancer:
Concha Ostreae 60g
Radix Scrophulariae 15g
Radix Rehmanniae 15g
Radix Ophiopogonis 15g
Radix Paeoniae Alba 15g
Semen Trichosanthis 15g
Radix Trichosanthis 15g
Semen Arecae 18g
Herba Dendrobii 18g
Lapis Pumicis 30g
Radix Glycyrrhizae 6g
Fructus Forsythiae 9g

(Note: *Yangjiecao* refers to a certain kind of grass eaten by sheep but remains undigested in the stomach and combines with forge, saliva and gastric juice to form a hard mass, blackish brown in color, warm and non-toxic in nature, foul in smell, effective in clearing up heat and toxic materials, eliminating phlegm and stasis, promoting digestion and relieving dyspepsia. It is frequently used in treating maldigestion, gastralgia, dysphagia, eructation and infantile malnutrition due to improper feeding.) (*New Traditional Chinese Medicine*, Vol. 1, 1978)

HISTORICAL COMMENTS

In *Decoction of Materia Medica*, it is commented that: "The drug is effective in eliminating the feeling of fullness and rigidity of the hypochondrium, scrofula and all kinds of furuncles."

In *Compendium of Materia Medica*, it is recorded that: "The drug eliminates phlegm, softens hard lumps, relieves cardiosplenalgia, due to stagnation of vital energy and leucorrhea with reddish discharge, and cures stasis, goiter and tuberculosis."

In *Golden Prescriptions*, it is recommended: "In treating ulcerous paronychia, phalangeal polyp with pyorrhage, the thick part of the head of Concha Ostreae is ground into powder and taken 6 grams each time with alcohol decoction of Flos Carthami. The decoction is taken three times a day and applied to the lesion at the same time."

In *Proved Recipe of Yiao Zhenghe*, it is said that: "The drug can be used to draw pus out of painful swelling without festering, when the powder is blended in water and applied to the affected part frequently."

In *Prescriptions Worth a Thousand Gold* it is suggested that: "Carbuncle can be cured by sprinkling the powder of Concha oxtreae on the affected part and applying egg white around it. Frequent application will ensure high efficacy."

In *Chinese Pharm...copedia*, it is mentioned that: "The cooked meat of Concha Ostreae has the function of curing consumptive disease, inflammatory disease and menoxenia, and regulate the middle-*jiao*. When taken rawly with ginger and vinegar, it can cure inflammatory disease and relieve thirst and irritation caused by drinking."

In *Comparison of Traditional Chinese Medicine with Western Medicine*, it is reported that: "Concha Ostrae is effective in softening hard lumps, dispelling phlegm, eliminating scrofula, relieving hiccup, restoring sperm, and curing metrorrhagia and leukorrhagia."

THE AUTHOR'S NOTE

At the 33rd East Asian Medical Symposium held in Japan, Muratakofu reported that, by testing the substance extracted from the shells and the soft body of ten varieties of shellfish, it is found that only Concha Ostreae shell can obviously increase the number of antibody in the spleen, and this indicates that it can reinforce the immune effect. In *Chinese Prescriptions* compiled by Otsukakersuke from Japan, it was reported that a 28 year old employee had the recurrence of wart in the back of the thigh three years after the first operation to remove a growth diagnosed as wart. He took a second operation and not long after that, a large tumor appeared on the very region. The patient was again hospitalized in a state-run hospital for operation and six tumors of ball size were removed. Pathological examination proved that it was "black sarcoma", and the patient was regarded as an incurable case. Radix Syringae Vulgaridis and Concha Ostreae Decoction was prescribed. (Concha Ostreae 4g, Radix Angelicae; Sinensis 5g, Radix Paeomiae 3g, Rhizoma Chuanxiong 3g, Radix Syringae Vulgaridis 3g, Flos Lunicerae 1.5g, Rhizoma Cimicifugae Foetidae 2g, Radix Astraali 2g, Radix Astragali 2g and Radix Glycyrrhizae 1g). After two months of treatment, the local tumor disappeared and no oncocytes were found in further examination. The doctors in the hospital became surprised and found it hard to understand. Radix Syringae Vulgaridis, therefore, seems to have extraordinary curative effect.

HERBA SEDI

Su Song of the Song Dynasty defined: "Being sweet in taste, cold and slightly toxic in nature, the plant crawls on stones of the southern side of a mountain and it is tender and lustrous like Herba Portulacae."

It is the whole herb of *Sedum lineare Thunb.* of *Crassulaceae* family, and grows in the south provinces of China. In Zhejiang Province alone, there exists nine kinds of the plant. All have the function of clearing up pathogenic heat and toxic materials, but the one with four leaves is used for the treatment of internal lesion due to trauma with its acrid taste and warm nature.

ANTICANCER PHARMACOLOGICAL FUNCTION

It is proved through internal screening tests in animal that Herba Sedi possesses the function of inhibiting tumor.

EXPERIMENTAL FORMULA:

For Stomatocancer, cheilocancer and linguocancer:

      Herba Sedi (fresh) 12g

      Flos Rosae 30g

      Myrrha 6g

      Borneol 15g

The ingredients are ground into powder and sprinkled on cotton gauze for application to the lesion and the therapy is repeated frequently. The formula is especially effective for cancerous ulcer.

For cancer of the mouth cavity, the lips and the tongue:

      Herba Sedi 30-60g

      Thallus Laminariae seu Eckloniae 15g

      Sargassum 15g

      Radix Scutellariae 9g

Fructus Gardeniae 9g
Flos Lonicerae 12g
Gypsum Ribrosum 30g
Cortex Mori 15g
Spica Prunellae 15g
The formula is taken one dosage a day.
For esophageal and cardiac cancer:
Herba Sedi (fresh) 6-12g
Herba Capsellae 9-18g
Take one dosage a day in decoction. (*Determination of Treatment Based on Differentiation of Symptoms and Signs*)

HISTORICAL COMMENTS

It is reported in *He Han Textual Research* that: "The juice extracted from the fresh leaves can cure lesions caused by poisonous insect sting or by scald."

It is recorded in *Supplement to Compendium of Materia Medica* that: "Herba Sedi cures furuncles, abnormal defecation, jaundice and membranous pharyngitis."

It is said in *New Compilation of Materia Medica* that: "Herba Sedi can be used for emergency management of various restless conditions due to various pyogenic diseases, septicemia and hematotoxicosis, when a lot of its fresh juice is taken orally."

It is suggested in *Dutch Medical Reflection* that: "The leaves of Herba Sedi are salty in taste, astringent in nature and as cool as Natrii Sulfas. It is effective in removing filthy and malignant toxic materials. Its raw juice alone, or with sugar and syrup can relieve asthenic and sweltering fever, ease restless thirst, subside pharyngitis, laryngitis, stomatic and lingual inflammation, and cure diarrhea or diarrhea with blood stool. If patients have developed thick callus, callosity and corn, apply fresh Herba Sedi leaves to the lesion after the herb being rinsed in vagina, and the polyp will gradually become soft and disappear eventually."

It is mentioned in *Survival from Bitter Sufferings* that: "Blended with old Chinese ink to make a juice for gargling 4-5 times daily, Herba Sedi can cure membranous pharyngitis."

It is recommended in *Collection of Medical Information* that: "When pounded with a little salt, and applied around the lesion, Herba Sedi can cure unbearable headache."

It is reported in *Chinese Medical Dictionary* that: "Herba Sedi is effective in curing laryngitis, pharyngitis, carbuncles, inflammation, furuncle, inflammatory diseases, scald, snake bite, jaundice and dysentery."

SPINA GLEDITSIAE

It is recorded in *Compendium of Materia Medica* that: "Spina Gleditsiae is acrid in taste and warm in nature, effective in treating carbuncle, inflammation and galactostasis."

This medicinal herb is the spine of *Gleditsia sinensis Lam.* of *Leguminosae* family, the main components of which are flavonoid glycosides and amino acid.

ANTICANCER PHARMACOLOGICAL FUNCTIONS

1. In vitro experiment shows that the inhibiting rate of the hot water extract of the herb on JTC-26 is 50-70%.

2. Experiments in vivo prove that the herb can actively inhibit sarcoma in rats.

EXPERIMENTAL FORMULAS:

For mammocancer:

Spina Gleditsiae 15g
Squama Manitis 15g
Rhizoma Bletillae 15g
Rhizoma Pinelliae 15g
Bulbus Fritillariae 15g
Pollen 20g
Rhizoma Anemarrhenae 20g
Olibanum 10g
Flos Lonicerae 25g

The formula is taken in decoction. (*Orthodox Surgery*)

For nasopharyngeal carcinoma:

360 grams of Spina Gleditsiae and Ramulus Gleditsiae is decocted to a broth similar to yellow rice wine in color, for oral administration for two days, three times a day. (*Collection of Chinese Herbal Therapy*)

For obstinate abdominal pain after enterocancer operation:

30 grams of Radix Astragali and 30 grams of Spina Gleditsiae are decocted into a broth, filtered before being blended with rice porridge for further decoction, and taken daily. (*Anticancer Consultation*)

HISTORICAL COMMENTS

In *Zhi Zhi Prescriptions* it is said that: "For curing female mammary abscess, 30 grams of Spina Gleditsiae (slightly burned) and 3 grams of Anodonta Pulveratum are ground to powder for oral administration with warm wine, 3 grams each time."

In *Origin of Materia Medica*, it is reported that: "For treating serious disease caused by severe pathogenic wind, falling of eyebrow and collapse of nose, 1500 grams of Spina Gleditsiae is burnt into ashes both for application to the lesion and for oral administration of 3 grams each time with Rhizoma et Radix Rhei Decoction after meal."

CORIUM STOMACHICHUM GALLI

It is defined in *Ri Hua Zhi Materia Medica* that: "The drug is mild and nontoxic, effective in curing emission and blood urine."

This drug is the dried inner membrane of chicken crop of *Phasianidae* family, containing vitamin B_1, B_2, C and a kind of globin.

ANTICANCER PHARMACOLOGICAL FUNCTIONS

Experiments in vitro showed that Corium Stomachichum Galli is effective in inhibiting oncocytes.

EXPERIMENTAL FORMULAS

For Esophagocancer:

1>. Corium Stomachichum Galli 10g
Radix Adenophorae 10g
Flos Inulae 10g
Rhizoma Pinelliae 10g
Spica Prunelae 30g
Radix Arneliae 30g
Herba Scutellariae Barbatae 60g
Fructus Ziziphi Inermis 15g

The above ingredients are decocted, filtered, and mixed with 120 grams of honey to make a paste for oral administration three times a day. (*Clinical Approaches to Tumor*)

2>. Realgar 30g

Scolopendra 15g

Scorpio 15g

Radix Salviae Miltiorrhizae 15g

Semen Strychii 15g

Corium Stomachichum Galli 15g

The above ingredients are ground into powder, made into honey-coated pills of Semen Firmianae Size and taken three times a day with warm boiled water, 5-10 grams each time. (*Chinese Anticancer Herbal Preparations*)

For stomach cancer:

Corium Stomachichum Galli 10g

Rhizoma Dioscoreae 30g

Radix Rehmanniae 15g

Radix Scrophulariae 15g

Radix Paeoniae Alba 15g

Fructus Lyxii 15g

Fossilia ossis Mastodi 15g

Concha Ostreae 15g

Rhizoma Anemarrhenae 12g

Radix Salviae Miltiorrhizae 12g

Haematitum 6g

Rhizoma Zedoariae 6g

Rhizoma Atractylodis 6g

The formula is taken in decoction. (*Hubei Journal of Traditional Chinese Medicine*, Vol. 4, 1980)

For Cardiac cancer:

1>. Corium Stomachichum Galli is burnt and taken with wine, 3 grams each time. (*Prescriptions Worth a Thousand Gold*)

2>. 10 to 20 grams of dried Corium Stomachichum Galli is decocted in 200ml of water and the broth is divided into three portions for oral administration. (*Research Data of Traditional Chinese Medicine*)

HISTORICAL COMMENTS

Records of Combined Traditional Chinese and Western Medicine says: "The drug is effective to remove any kind of stagnation in the internal organs. Long administration will cure mass in the hypochondrium in males and abdominal mass in females."

Zhengnan Materia Medica records: "The drug functions to benefit the spleen and the middle-*jiao*, in addition to the promotion of digestion, appetite, the muscles and the bones."

In *Herbs Growing in the Mountains* it is reported: "The drug helps to promote the growth of the muscles and the growth of new tissues, hence, it is effective for ulcers."

CAULIS MILLETTIAE

It is reported in *Revised Reference of Processed Medicinal Herbs* that: "The drug, being bitter, astringent, fragrant and slightly sweet, is effective for the removal of blood stasis and the manufacture of the blood."

The herb is the dried stem of *Spatholobus suberectus Dunn.* and *Millettia dielsiana Harms ex Diels* of family *Leguminosae*, which contains friedelin, taraxerone, camphesterol, stigmasterol and sitosterol. A 100% decoction of the herb is specially effective for experimental anemia.

ANTICANCER PHARMACOLOGICAL FUNCTIONS
1. Tests in vitro with a dose of 500μg/ml of its water extract showed an inhibitory rate of 94.4% on JTC-26.
2. Screening tests with bacteriophages for anticancer drugs proved the herb has an antiphagic function.

EXPERIMENTAL FORMULAS
For giant dermatokeras before canceration:
Liaoning Journal of Traditional Chinese Medicine (March, 1979) reported bath with the decoction of the following herbs once daily and 20 minutes each time:

>   Caulis Millettiae 25g
>   Spica Prunellae 30g
>   Rhizoma Scirpi 15g
>   Rhizoma Zedoariae 15g
>   Cortex Lycii Radicis 50g
>   Cortex Dictamni 50g
>   Cortex Pseudolaricis 50g

For radiation leukemia:
Dictionary of Traditional Chinese Medicine recommends oral administration of the decoction of 30 grams of Caulis Millettiae daily on a long term basis.

HISTORICAL COMMENTS
Supplement to Compendium of Materia Medica says: "The herb activates blood, warms the lumbus and the knee and cures paralysis caused by wind pathogen."
Shunning Fu Annals recorded: "When combined with Flos Carthami, Radix Angelica Sinensis and Fructus Oryzae germinatus, and cooked into paste, the herb is a sacred drug for blood diseases."
Chinese Medicinal Herbs reports: 2kg of Caulis Millettiae is decocted into a broth of 500ml to be mixed with 800 grams of sugar, filtered, added with 100ml of water for oral administration three times daily, each time 10 to 20ml. The preparation is effective for malnutrition and loss of blood and anemia."

HERBA LYCOPI

It is reported in *Essentials of Materia Medica* that: "The bitter taste of the herb helps to expel pathogenic heat, the sweet flavour to tonify the blood, the sour flavor to benefit the liver and the warm nature of the drug to promote the circulation of the blood."

This is the dried stem or leaf of *Lycopus lucidus Turcz.* of the family *Labiatae*, or of *L. lucidus Turcz. var. taiwanensis Hayata, L. lucidus Turcz. var. hirtus Reg.* and *Eupatorium formosanum* and *E. japonicum. T* of the family *Compositae*.

ANTICANCER PHARMACOLOGICAL FUNCTIONS
1. The herb inhibits cells of human nasopharyngeal carcinoma and Walker's carcinoma-256 in rats.
2. Eupatorin extracted from Eupatorium has a cytotoxic effect on human nasopharyngeal and epithelial carcinoma.

3. Eupatorin, which belongs to sesquiterpenes, inhibits Henle's cells.

EXPERIMENTAL FORMULAS
For pelvic malignant tumors complicated with ascites:

Prevention and Treatment of Tumors recommend the oral administration of the decoction of the following herbs once daily:

        Herba Lycopi 9g
        Herba Euphorbiae Lunulatae 9g
        Herba Solani Nigri 30g
        Herba Scutellariae Barbatae 30g
        Herba Lobeliae Chinese 30g
        Semen Coicis 30g
        Radix Salviae Miltiorrhizae 15g
        Rhizoma Smilacis Glabrae 15g
        Semen Plantaginis 12g
        Caulis Aristolochiae Manshuriensis 3g

For Liver cancer:

Essential Points of Oncology records the administration of the following herbs in decoction once daily:

        Herba Lycopi 9g
        Rhizoma Scirpi 9g
        Rhizoma Zedoariae 9g
        Radix Angelicae Sinensis 9g
        Herba Ardisiae Japonicae 15g
        Radix Salviae Miltiorrhizae 15g
        Radix Actinidiae Valvatae 30g
        Herba Scutellariae Barbatae 30g
        Radix Diospyros Rhombifoliae 60g

HISTORICAL COMMENTS
Practical Materia Medica says: "The drug disintegrates masses in the abdomen and edema. When administered together with other tonics, it can carry out disintegration and tonification at the same time without causing damage to the vitality. Hence, it is a wonderful drug."

Compendium of Materia Medica says: "The herb is particularly effective for diseases of the blood system."

Prescription of Materia Medica comments: "The drug is contraindicative for deficiency of the blood."

HERBA EUPHORBIAE LUNULATAE

Dictionary of Chinese Medicinal Herbs says: "The drug, acrid and bitter in flavor and cold in nature, promotes the circulation of body fluid, clears away phlegm, kills parasitic worms and removes toxin."

It is the herb of *Euphorbia* genus of the family *Euphorbiaceae*, which mainly contains hemolytic phasin, flavones and euphorbin. The juice of the herb contains rubber hydrocarbon and resin.

ANTICANCER PHARMACOLOGICAL FUNCTIONS

Experiments on animals showed that the drug has an inhibitory effect on sarcoma-180, sarcoma-37 and leukemia-L16.

EXPERIMENTAL FORMULAS

For lymphosarcoma:

Anticancer Herbal Preparations reports the administration of the following herbs in decoction once daily:

> Herba Euphorbiae Lunulatae 15g
> Rhizoma Arisaematis 30g
> Rhizoma Smilacis Glabrae 30g
> Squama Manitis 9g

For cervical cancer:

Shaanxi Journal of Medicinal Herbs reported the administration of the following therapy once daily. Boil three eggs together with 100 grams of Herba Euphorbiae Lunulatae and then eat the eggs and drink the soup.

For cancer of the esophagus:

Data of New Medicine (Vol. 2, 1972) reported the intramuscular injection of 2ml of 20% steroidal saponins extracted from the herb daily. A course included 15 days and the effect would appear after 3 to 5 days of the injection.

For cancer of the stomach:

Supplement to the Handbook of Prescriptions recommends the following prescription:

> Herba Euphorbiae Lunulatae 120g
> Semen Lepidii 60g
> Radix et Rhizoma Rhei 60g

All the following herbs are put together, ground into fine powders and then made into pills of the size of Semen Firmianae and taken three times a day, each time two pills.

HISTORICAL COMMENTS

Collected Comments on Materia Medica Says: "The drug has the same functions as Radix Euphorbiae Pekinensis, but somewhat milder. It seldom damages the vitality, but may cause purgation, so being contraindicative for patients with deficiency of the stomach."

Explanations to the Herbs in Chang Sha says: "The bitter taste of the herb is good for removing water retention, so it is indicative for cough caused by retention of phlegm."

HERBA SELAGINELLAE

Canon of Materia Medica reports that: "The drug, acrid in flavor and mild in nature, is effective for diseases of the five solid organs, such as masses, hematoma and so on."

This is the herb of *Selaginella tamariscina (Beauk) Spring* of the family *Selaginellaceae*, which contains trehalose, biflavone, amentoflavone, hinokiflavone, isocryptomerin and sotetsuflavone.

ANTICANCER PHARMACOLOGICAL FUNCTIONS

1. Measured with dissolving and depositing method of the total cells, the hot water extract of the herb is found to have an inhibitory rate of 61.2% on sarcoma-180 in rats, while the ether extract has an inhibitory rate of 18.6%.

2. Clinical observations have detected that the herb has a better effect on tumors of small size.

3. Experiments in vitro proved that its homogeneous plant, *S. doederleinii Hieron*, has a better anticancer action.

4. Experiments in vivo showed that the herb has certain inhibitory action on Ehrlich's ascites carcinoma and prolongs the survival period of animals who have received tumor transplantation.

EXPERIMENTAL FORMULAS
For nasopharyngeal carcinoma:

Bulletin of Chinese Medicinal Herbs (Vol. 6 and 7, 1970) reported the following therapy for the tumor: 30 to 60 grams of Herba Selaginellae (90 t0 120 grams, if fresh) and 50 to 100 grams of lean pork are boiled in six to eight bowls of water to a broth of one or one and a half bowl. The soup is taken in one or two times. The therapy is repeated daily and a course includes 15 to 20 days.

For liver cancer:

Exchange of Medical Information (Vol. 9, 1974) reported the administration of the decoction of the following herbs:

> Herba Selaginellae 30g
> Radix Rhodomyrtis Tomentosae 30g
> Squama Menitis 9g
> Poria 9g
> Herba Oldenlandiae Diffusae 9g
> Radix Salviae Chinensis 30g
> Hippocampus 3g

For malignant reticulosis:

Progress in Management of Malignant Reticulosis reported the administration of the following herbs:

> Herba Selaginellae 20g
> Herba Verbenae Officinalae 15g
> Radix Isatidis 15g
> Rhizoma Pinelliae Cordatae 15g
> Herba Crotalariae 3g
> Radix Rumicis 10g
> Radix Cynanchi Paniculati 10g
> Radix Berberidis Virgetora 10g
> Radix Aucklandiae 5g
> Rhizoma Paridis 30g

For cancer of the lungs:

Determination of Treatment Based on Differentiation of Symptoms and Signs recommended the administration of the following herbs in decoction once daily:

> Herba Selaginellae 60g
> Herba Oldenlandiae Diffusae 30g

HISTORICAL COMMENTS

Canon of Materia Medica says: "The drug is indicative for the diseases of the five solid organs, dysmenorrhea, female abdominal mass and abdominal pain due to cold and heat."

Ri Hua Zi Materia Medica commented that: "The herb removes blood stasis when administered fresh and stops bleeding when used as moxa."

Practical Materia Medica recorded that: "The fresh herb, being cold in nature, can remove blood stasis, activate the channels and collaterals and cure masses in the abdomen."

Ren's Preserved Prescriptions says: "For hemorrhage of the large intestine, equal portions of Herba Selaginellae, Folium et Ramulus Biotae and Fructus Trachycarpi are burnt and ground for oral administration with wine, 9 grams each time."

Carefully Selected Prescriptions says: "To treat chronic hemorrhage, equal portions of Herba Selaginellae and Radix Sanquisorbae are baked and 30 grams of the baked herbs is decocted in a cup of water for a short period of time for oral administration."

THE AUTHOR'S NOTE
The drug, one of the effective anticancer agents that have been discovered in the recent years, is effective for all tumors that respond to anticancer chemical agents and radiation therapy and has a better effect if the size of the tumor is small. When used together with chemotherapy and radiotherapy, it can reduce the course of the treatment and increase the speed of shrinkage and disappearance of the tumor mass. Clinically it is used to treat chronic epithelioma, nasopharyngeal carcinoma, lung cancer and liver cancer. The anti-laryngocarcinoma tablets available in the market is extracted from Herba Selaginellae and it is fond inhibiting cancer cells in animal tests.

RADIX SOPHORAE FLAVESCENTIS

Canon of Materia Medica recorded that: "The herb, bitter in flavor and cold in nature, is mainly indicative for knotted syndromes and mass in the chest and abdomen."

The drug is the dried root of the *Sophora flavescens* of the family *Leguminosae*, which contains various alkaloid such as matrine, oxymatrine, sophocarpine and flavones.

ANTICANCER PHARMACOLOGICAL FUNCTIONS
1. Matrine, oxymatrine and dehydromatrine have an inhibitory rate of 35% on sarcoma-180 in rats on average.

2. The anti-abdominal mass alkaloid, composed of different alkaloids extracted from the herb at different ratio, has an inhibitory rate of 61.38% on sarcoma-180 in rats when given with a dosage of 113mg per kilo of body weight. The effective rate is higher than that of mitomycin and 323.5% higher than that of the total matrine.

3. The anti-abdominal mass alkaloid has an inhibitory rate of 40% on sarcoma-37 and cervical cancer-14 on average.

4. *Xianseng Puohe Yu*, prepared with Radix Sophorae Flavescentis and leaves of Pelargonium Grareolens L'hent, can directly inhibit transplanted tumors in animals and the cells of stomach cancer in human.

EXPERIMENTAL FORMULAS
For cervical cancer:
Prevention and Treatment of Tumors reported the administration of the following herb:

        Radix Sophorae Flavescentis 60g
        Fructus Cnidii 30g
        Flos Chrysanthemi Indici 30g
        Flos Lonicerae 30g
        Cortex Phellodendri 15g
        Radix Angelicae Dahuricae 15g
        Fructus Kochiae 15g
        Rhizoma Acori Graminei 15g

The decoction of the herbs is applied to the tumor mass with a piece of gauze.
For cancer of the urinary bladder:
Essential Points of Oncology reported the administration of the following herbs in decoction once daily:

Radix Sophorae Flavescentis 15g

Radix Rehmanniae 15g

Flos Lonicerae 12g

Herba Seu Radix Cirsii Japonici 12g

Herba Cephalanoploris 12g

Rhizoma Alismatis 9g

Rhizoma Dioscoreae Steptemlobae 9g

Cortex Phellodendri 6g

Succinum 1.5g (Taken separately)

For cancer of the large intestine:

Handbook of Common Anticancer Drugs offers the decoction of the following herbs, one dose daily:

Radix Sophorae Plavescentis 15g

Caulis Sargentodoxae 30g

Fructus Ziziphi Inermis 10g

For malignant lymphoma:

Prescriptions for Emergent Cases recommends the administration of the pills processed in the following way, three times a day after meals, each time 10 pills: 120 grams of Radix Sphorae Flavescentis are smashed into fine powder and then pilled with Radix Achyranthis Bidentatae into the size of Semen Firmianae.

HISTORICAL COMMENTS

On Properties of Drugs says: "The drug is indicative for mass in the chest and abdomen."

Ri Hua Zi Materia Medica commented: "The drug is effective for enterorrhagia."

Canon of Materia Medica says: "The drug is contraindicative for deficiency of the kidney without fever."

THE AUTHOR'S NOTE

Chinese Forum of Medical Science reported in January 25, 1985 that Shanxi Medical Research Institute tested the clinical effect of anti-abdominal mass alkaloid through administering it to 94 cases with cancer of the digestive system (84.2% of which were in the advanced stage). Respondence turned up in 41 cases and the effective rate was 43.16%. The subjective symptoms of the patients were generally relieved and the appetite was improved. The tumor lesion was progressing slowly and the white blood cell count was not reduced, but instead it became increased by 5.79%. The blood cell count in the control group which took chemotherapy, however, was reduced by 36.3%.

HERBA ET SEMEN SOPHORAE ALOPECUROIDITIS

Dictionary of Chinese Medicinal Herbs recorded that: "The herb is bitter in taste and cold and poisonous in nature. It clears away pathogenic heat, eliminates pathogenic dampness, relieves pain and kills parasites."

The drug is the dried herb, root or seed of *Sophora alopecuroides* of the family *Leguminosae*, which grows mainly in the Inner Mongolia, Xinjiang and Tibet. The portion of the herb above earth contains 6.11-9.03% of alkaloid, while the seeds containing 8.11%. The alkaloids are mainly cytisine, matrine, sophoramine, sophocarpine, aloperine, saccharides and proteins. The anticancer substance is sophocarpine.

ANTICANCER PHARMACOLOGICAL FUNCTIONS

1. Sophocarpine has a remarkable inhibition on sarcoma-180, sarcoma-37, cervical carcinoma-14, Ehrlich's ascites carcinoma and lymphosarcoma-1, with a rate of 30-60%.

2. Sophocarpine can strongly inhibit metabolism of nucleic acid and terminate division of cancer cells.

3. No inhibition of the bone marrow was fond in clinical administration of the drug.

4. The injection of the herb is a broad spectrum anticancer drug and was found inhibiting many types of cancers in animal experiment.

EXPERIMENTAL FORMULAS

For cancer of the rectum:

News Bulletin of Chinese Medicinal Herbs (Vol. 9, 1979) reported retention-enema once daily with 25ml of the preparations from 200 grams of Herba et Semen Sophorae Alopecuroiditis and 10 grams of starch after being mixed with normal saline to the total amount of 1000ml.

For stomach cancer and cervical cancer:

News Bulletin of Chinese Medicinal Herbs (Vol. 10, 1979) reported 20 grams of total alkaloids of the herb and 20ml of dilated HCl are mixed with injection water to the amount of 1000ml for intravenous drip or local injection into the tumor mass once daily. For intravenous injection, 4 to 6ml of the preparation is added to 5% glucose, but for local injection, 2ml is given.

For metastasis of choriocarcinoma:

New Journal of Traditional Chinese Medicine reported the injection of 200mg of sophocarpine once daily or once every other day. The needle is inserted at the juncture between the normal tissues and the tumor mass, to the base of the tumor and the drug is injected radially.

For leukemia:

New Journal of Traditional Chinese Medicine (Vol. 5, 1978) reported the oral administration of the powder of the herb 2 or 3 times daily, each time, 1.5 to 3 grams if it is the powder of the root or the herb and 1 gram if it is the powder of the seed.

For stomach cancer:

Handbook of Medicinal Herbs in Xinjiang reported the oral administration of the following herbs:

Herba et Semen Sophorae Alopecuroiditis 5g
Rhizoma Zingiberis 3g
Herba Taraxaci 6g

HISTORICAL COMMENTS

Handbook of Medicinal Herbs in Xinjiang reported that: "External application of the oil preparation of Herba et Semen Sophorae Alopecuroiditis is effective for eczema and tinea."

Medicinal Herbs Growing in the Deserts in China reported that: "Oral administration of the seeds of the plant, 5 to 7 seeds each time, once daily, cures leukorrhagia. The seeds should be swallowed and not to be chewed. Once chewed, it may cause dizziness and headache."

Journal of Medicinal Herbs in Inner Mongolia reported: "Administration of the decoction of 6 grams of the root of the plant relieves toothache."

THE AUTHOR'S NOTE

The drug is a newly discovered anticancer herb and the aloperine injection was first used to treat chronic epithelioma and malignant hydatidiform mole in 1972 in Jianxi Province. The drug is used alone without the combination of chemotherapy and radiotherapy. The clinical effect was 87.6% for malignant hydatidiform mole and 50% for chronic epithelioma. It has also been noted that sophocarpine of the herb has a better effect than its total alkaloids.

RADIX TINOSPORAE

On *Properties of Drugs* says: "The drug is bitter in taste and very cold in nature with detoxifying function."

It is the root of *Tinospora Sagittata (Oliv) Gagnep* of the family *Menispermaceae*. In the past it was used as Radix Tinosporae Capillipis, mainly containing palmatine, flavonoid glycoside, amino acid and saccharides.

ANTICANCER PHARMACOLOGICAL FUNCTIONS
According a report in Hainan Province on the scanning of anticancer drugs from 1973 to 1975, experiments in vitro with the herb showed an inhibition on tumor cells.

EXPERIMENTAL FORMULAS
For angioma:

Dictionary of Traditional Chinese Medicinal Herbs recorded: 1. The external application three to four times daily of the fresh root of the herb when ground into paste and mixed with wine; 2. Grind the root of the herb into paste and mixed it with *Gauliang* wine for application three to four times a day. It is also good for lipoma.

HISTORICAL COMMENTS
Chinese Pharmacopeia wrote: "The drug has a detoxifying function and is used orally or externally for sore-throat, aphthae, conjunctivitis, distending pain of the ear, cough due to pathogenic heat, cellulitis, carbuncle, snake and insect bite and scorpion sting."

Gan Yuan Xiao Zhi commented: "When sliced and kept in the mouth, the herb is indicative for internal and external stagnancy of pathogenic heat, general poisoning, malaria, sore-throat and toothache. When ground into paste and applied externally, it is effective for furuncles and swelling".

Tianjing Journal of Medicine (Vol. 12, 1971) reported that Radix Tinosporae does not contain colchicine.

HERBA ARTEMISIAE ANNUAE

Essentials of Materia Medica recorded that: "Herba Artemisiae Annuae is bitter in taste and cold in nature and relieves fever and overstrain."

It is the herb of *Artemisia Annua L.* of the family *Compositae*, which is found growing all over China and contains bitter principle, volatile oils, qinghaosu and vitamin A.

ANTICANCER PHARMACOLOGICAL FUNCTIONS
The dried herb, mixed with 60 times of water, is decocted and filtered when hot. The dried filtrate is found inhibiting JTC-26 with a rate of 70 to 90% under the dose of $500\mu g/ml$.

EXPERIMENTAL FORMULAS
For various cancers:

Research Data of Traditional Chinese Medicine (Vol. 6, 1978) reported long-term administration of the following formula: 10 to 15 grams of Herba Artemisiae Annuae, in 300ml of water, is decocted and the broth is divided into three portions taken in three times, daily.

For low fever caused by cancer:

Shanghai Journal of Traditional Chinese Medicine (Vol. 3, 1979) reported the administration of the decoction of the following herbs daily:

Herba Artemisiae Annuae 15g
Radix Cynanchi Atrati 15g
Cortex Lycii Radicis 15g
Radix Scutellariae 15g
Herba Oldenlandiae Diffusae 30 to 60g

For lung cancer, liver cancer, breast cancer and stomach cancer:

Anticancer Preparations of Medicinal Herbs reported the following formula:

Herba Artemisiae Annuae 300g
Radix Actinidiae Chinensis 250g
Radix Vitidis Romanetis 250g
Herba Lobeliae Chinensis 250g
Radix Salviae Miltiorrhizae 250g
Herba Oldenlandiae Diffusae 250g
Fructus Macleayae 100g
Radix et Rhizoma Rhei 100g
Fructus Citri Sarcodactylis 100g
Radix Sanguisorbae 100g

First smash Radix et Rhizoma Rhei and Fructus Citri Sarcodactylis into powder and extract volatile oil from Herba Artemisiae Annuae with distillation method. The rest herbs are decocted into extract to be crushed and mixed with the volatile oil and finally made into tablets with a weight of 0.5g each. The tablets are taken orally, three times a day, each time four tablets.

HISTORICAL COMMENTS

Materia Medica in Tang Dynasty commented: "When applied to incised wound, it can stop bleeding, help the growth of new muscle and relieves pain."

Canon of Materia Medica reported: "The herb is contraindicative for deficiency of blood after birth, diarrhea due to endogenous cold and retention of food in the stomach, and can not be used together with Radix Rehmanniae and Radix Angelicae Sinensis for patients with weak spleen and stomach after birth."

Abstruseness of Materia Medica recorded: "The drug is absolutely contraindicative for deficiency of the stomach."

INDIGO NATURALIS

Kei Bao Materia Medica recorded: "The drug is slightly cold in nature and nonpoisonous and is good at detoxifying drug poison."

The drug is the dried phytochrome extracted from the leaves of *Strobilanthes cusia (Nees) Brenek* of the family *Acanthaceae*, *Indigofera fortunei Craid* of the family *Leguminosae* and *Polygonum tinctorium Ait.* of the family *Polygonaceae*. The leaves and branches of the above plants are collected either in summer or in autumn and immersed in water for two or three days before processing. Then 0.5kg of lime is added to every 5 kilos of leaves and the leaves are stirred until the extract becomes purplish red. The dried extract is the drug, which mainly contains indican, indirubin and ß-sitosterol. Indirubin is the effective anticancer agent, which can be artificially synthesized from potassium indolol and indolone that are used for the production of dye.

ANTICANCER PHARMACOLOGICAL FUNCTIONS

1. Experiments showed that indirubin can prolong the survival period of animals with lymphoma-7212.

2. Subcutaneous and intraperitoneal injections of indirubin with a dosage of 200mg per kilo of body weight, inhibits Walker's carcinoma-256 with a rate of 47-58%.

3. Indirubin promotes the phagocytic function of mononuclear macrophage in both normal animals and animals with tumor, and this suggests that it combats cancer through promoting the immune functions.

4. Indigo Naturalis can reduce the time required for the maturity of the granulocytes and cure chronic granulocytic leukemia through relieving the burden of bone marrow.

EXPERIMENTAL FORMULAS

For sharp pain of liver cancer and pancreatic cancer:

Hilongjiang Journal of Traditional Chinese Medicine (Vol. 4, 1984) reported the external application of the following herbs:

> Indigo Naturalis 60g
> Realgar 60g
> Alumen 60g
> Natrii Sulfas 60g
> Olibanum 60g
> Myrrha 60g
> Borneol 10g
> Sanguis Draconis 30g

Put all the above herbs together and grind them into powder. Each time 30 to 60 grams of the powder is mixed with equal portions of vinegar and pig bile into a paste for external application once daily, each time eight hours.

For cervical cancer:

Research Data of Medicine (Vol. 5 and 6. 1973) recommends the following formula:

> Indigo Naturalis 9g
> Realgar 9g
> Fructus Bruceae 4.5g
> Semen Strychni 4.5g
> Radix Aconiti Lateralis Preparata 4.5g
> Calomelas 4.5g
> Arsenicum 3g
> Salmiacum 3g
> Fructus Mume Carbonisatus 15g
> Borneol 1.5g
> Moschus 3g

All the above herbs are ground into fine powders to be applied to the lesion of the cancer. This can damage the growth and division of the cancer cells and thus leads to the gradual scaling of the tumor mass.

For cancer of the esophagus:

Zhejiang Tumor Bulletin (Vol. 4, 1972) reported the following formula, the herbs of which are ground into fine powder to be melted in the mouth daily, each time 0.9 to 1.5 grams.

> Indigo Naturalis 4.5g
> Gecko 30g
> Mannosum Kaki 15g
> Salmiacum 6g
> Borax 9g
> Sugar 60g

For granulocytic leukemia:

Handbook of Common Anticancer Drugs reported the oral administration of 0.9 to 1.5 grams of Indigo Naturalis three times a day.

HISTORICAL COMMENTS
Origin of Materia Medica commented that: "The drug is indicative for dysphagia and the stale stuff has a better effect".

Simplified Prescriptions commented: "For unperforated scrofula, Indigo Naturalis and Herba Portulacae are smashed and applied to the lesion daily."

Prescriptions of Essential Drugs reported: "In addition to eliminating pathogenic heat and detoxification, the drug removes heat from the blood."

THE AUTHOR'S NOTE
Indigo Naturalis really has anticancer effect. The daily dose is 2 to 4 grams usually, but sometimes can be increased to 6 to 10 grams. The author prescribed 30 grams of Indigo Naturalis and 15 grams of Realgar and had them capsulized to treat chronic granulocytic leukemia together with the volatile oil of Flos Lonicerae. Satisfactory result was achieved.

THALLUS LAMINARIAE SEU ECKLONIAE

Dictionary of Chinese Medicinal Herbs recorded: "The drug, being salty in taste and cold in nature, can soften hard lumps and promote the circulation of body water and is indicative for scrofula, goiter and dysphagia."

The drug is the thallus of *Laminaria japonica A.*, *L. angustata*, *L angustata Var. I*, *L. japonica Var. O.*, of the family *Laminariaceae* and of *Ecklonia kurome O.* and *Undaria pinnatifida cHS.*.

ANTICANCER PHARMACOLOGICAL FUNCTIONS
1. The hot water extract of the above plants, when injected subcutaneously into rats with transplanted sarcoma-180 for five days, showed that *Laminaria angustata* has an inhibitory rate of 94.8%, *Laminaria angustata Var. I.* 92.3%, Laminaria japonica A. 13.6%. Tests verified that the hot water extract mainly contains polysaccharides composed of neutral sugar and acid sugar.

2. Experiments in vitro did not prove the anticancer activity of the drug, hence, it is inferred that indirect anticancer function of polysaccharides is carried out by the host.

3. The dialysate of *Laminaria angustata*, when administered before the transplantation of the tumor cells, has an inhibitory rate of 68.6-80.4%, but given after transplantation, it is 92%.

4. *Laminaria angustata Var. I.* can prolong the survival period of rats with lymphocytic leukemia-1210 with a rate of 125% and the further extract of the sea tangle shows a rate of 141%.

5. The separated substances from *Laminaria angustata Var. I.* are very effective for Meth-A tumor and ß-16 melanoma and sarcoma-180, but not for Lewis' cancer and Walker's ascites carcinoma.

6. *Ecklonia Kurome O.* inhibits the growth hormone of tumors.

EXPERIMENTAL FORMULAS
For thyroma:

1>. *Journal of Zhejiang Traditional Chinese Medical College* reported the administration of the decoction of the following formula a dose daily:

> Thallus Laminariae seu Eckloniae 10g
> Sargassum 10g
> Bulbus Bolbostemmae 10g
> Radix Semiaquilegiae 10g

Radix Angelicae Sinensis 6g
Rhizoma Chuanxiong 6g
Radix Linderae 6g
Fructus Akebiae 9g
Radix Scrophulariae 12g
Lopis Pumicis 12g

2>. *Holy Prescriptions* recorded that 30 grams of the dried Thallus Laminariae seu Eckloniae is collected, washed off salt, ground into powder, rapped in a piece of cloth and soaked in fine vinegar for a while, and finally 3 grams is kept in mouth for melting each time.

For cancer of the esophagus:

General Collection of Holy Relief recorded the following:
Thallus Lminariae seu Eckloniae (washed, baked and ground into powders) 30g
Fine hust of rice 100g
Saliva of old cow 100ml
Juice of Bulbus Lilii 100ml

All the above are stewed into paste, then added with honey and starch and finally made into pills. Each time one pill.

For various cancers:

Research Data of Traditional Chinese Medicine (Vol. 6, 1978) reported that 40 grams of Thallus Laminariae seu Eckloniae is decocted with 1000 grams of wheat for oral administration several times a day.

For malignant lymphoma:

Rhymed Discourse on External Therapy reported the following formula:
Thallus Laminariae seu Eckloniae 30g
Sargassum 30g
Rhizoma Arisaematis 90g
Rhizoma Pinelliae 90g
Moschus 6g
Borneol 6g
Flos Carthami 60g
Concha Ostreae 60g
Halitum 18g

All the above are ground into powder to be mixed with the decoction of 250 grams of Rhizoma Bletillae for external application to the lesion.

HISTORICAL COMMENTS

Canon of Materia Medica commented: "The bitterness of the herb can soften hard masses and its cold nature removes pathogenic heat and disperses lumps, hence the drug is indicative for twelve kinds of edema, goiter and fistula. Dong Tan said that the bitterness of the drug was good for softening hard mass and goiter as hard as a rock can only be cured with this herb."

Collection of Medicinal Herbs recorded: "Thallus Laminariae seu Eckloniae is stronger that Sargassum and long-term administration cures dysphagia."

Chinese Oceanic Medicinal Herbs reported: "Compound Preparation of Thallus Laminariae seu Eckloniae inhibits experimental cancer."

THE AUTHOR'S NOTE

According to the report of *Japanese Chemical and Drug Laboratory* (71) in 1981, the hot water extract of *L. angustata* and *L. angustat Var. I*, dried through lyophilization and given to rats though feeding with a dosage of 100mg/kg of body weight and 50mg/kg of body weight daily, showed an inhibitory rate of 76.3% and 83.6% respectively for sarcoma-180. From this we can see that as a anticancer drug, Thallus Laminariae seu Eckloniae is really a valuable drug for the management of cancer.

FLOS LONICERAE

Origin of Medicinal Herbs commented: "The drug is sweet in flavor and slightly cold in nature and is good for detoxification."

This is the dried flower-buds of *Lonicera japonica, L. hypoglauca, L. confusa* or *L. Similis* of the family *Caprifoliaceae*, which contain flavones, luteolin, luteolin-7-glucoside, inositol and saponins.

ANTICANCER PHARMACOLOGICAL FUNCTIONS

1. Scanning tests in vitro with spread plate method showed that the drug inhibits cells of ascites carcinoma.

2. Scanning tests with bacteriophagic method demonstrated that the drug combats bacteriophage, thus suggesting it has anticancer activities.

3. Experiments in vivo showed that the ether extract of the plant has an inhibitory rate of 22.2% on sarcoma-180 in rats.

4. The mixture of Flos Lonicerae, Polyporus, Poria, Radix Ginseng, Semen Eurgales and Margarita does not have direct effect on cancer cells, but can reduce the activity of catalase and cholinesterase in the liver.

EXPERIMENTAL FORMULAS

For cancer of the nasal cavity:

Fujian Journal of Traditional Chinese Medicine (Vol. 6, 1959) reported the inhalation of the powder of the herb once every two hours.

For breast cancer:

Prevention and Treatment of Tumors reported the following formula:

      Flos Lonicerae 60g
      Semen Vaccariae 30g
      Herba Euphorbiae Lunulatae 30g
      Zijin Ding 12g
      Borneol 6g

Boil the first three drugs into extract, add in the last two drugs, and then grind them into fine powder. Each time 1.5 to 3 grams, four times daily.

For cervical cancer:

New Journal of Traditional Chinese Medicine (Vol. 3, 1980) reported the following herbs:

      Syngnathus 1 piece
      Bungarus Minimus 3
      Hirudo 6g
      Tabanus 6g
      Unguis Hominis 6g
      Rhizoma Coptidis 6g
      Olibanum 6g
      Myrrha 6g
      Scorpio 9g
      Nidus Vespae 9g
      Cortex Phellodendri 9g

Cortex Moutan 12g

herba Conyzae 15g

Grind all the above herbs into powders to be pilled with thick decoction of Flos Lonicerae. The pills are swallowed two or three times daily, each time 6 to 9 grams.

For metastasis of cervical cancer:

Medical Journal of Beijing Traditional Medical College (Vol. 3, 1983) reported the following herbs:

Flos Lonicerae 20g

Herba Taraxaxi 20g

Semen Benincasae 20g

Radix Astragali 20g

Herba Oldenlandiae Diffusae 15g

Flos Sophorae Immaturus 15g

Olibanum 10g

Myrrha 10g

Rhizoma Cyperi Carbonisatus 10g

Massa Medicate Fermentata 10g

Radix Angelicae Sinensis 12g

Herba Violae Yedoensis 12g

Radix Rehmanniae 12g

Radix Ginseng 2g

Sanguis Draconis 1g

Lignum Aquilariae Resinatum 1g

HISTORICAL COMMENTS

Compendium of Materia Medica says: "The drug is indicative for fatal summer fever in children, fulminant and violent diseases with unknown causes, rheumatism, pyogenic infection, carbuncle, cellulitis, tinea, malignant boil and syphilitic skin lesions. It also relieves fever and poisoning."

Abstruseness of Materia Medica recorded: "Flos Lonicerae is good for relieving abdominal fullness with diarrhea, subduing swelling through detoxication and restoring *qi* to treat diseases caused by pathogenic wind. Its detoxication is well-known and it is found very effective for the above diseases."

Tong Tian Mysterious Decree recorded: "To treat carbuncle and cellulitis, 250 grams of Flos Lonicerae is decocted in ten bowls of water to the amount of two and then added 60 grams of Radix Angelicae Sinensis for further decoction unit the broth is about one bowlful for oral administration while it is warm."

HERBA SENECIO INTEGRIFOLII

Lu Chan Yan Materia Medica commented: "The drug is cold in nature and nonpoisonous, and is mainly indicative for carbuncle, ulcers, furuncle and abscess".

The drug is the whole plant of *Senecio integrifolum Turcz.* of the family *Compositae*. *Materia Medica in Tang Dynasty* described that: "The leaf of the plant, which looks like that of *Plantago asiatica L.*, has no veins, and the stem has thin, yellow and while flowers. The plant is found growing thickly in the damp land near water channels."

ANTICANCER PHARMACOLOGICAL FUNCTIONS

Experiments in vitro showed that the administration of three grams of Herba Senecio Integrifolii per milliliter inhibits leukemia remarkably.

EXPERIMENTAL FORMULAS

For leukemia:

1>. *Oncology of Traditional Chinese Medicine* reported the administration of the decoction of the following herbs:

> Herba Senecio Integrifolii 30g
> Radix Rumicis 30g
> Herba Oldenlandiae Diffusae 30g

2>. *Handbook of Common Anticancer Drugs* reported the administration of the following formula a dose daily:

> Herba Senecio Integrifolii 30g
> Herba Galii Aprinis 60g

3>. *Zhejiang Bulletin of Cancer* (Vol. 2, 1976) reported the administration of the following herbs in decoction a dose daily:

> Herba Senecio Integrifolii 30g
> Herba Oldenlandiae Diffusae 30g
> Herba Solani Nigri 30g
> Herba Agrimoniae 30g
> Radix Glehniae 30g
> Flos Lonicerae 18g
> Radix Salviae Miltiorrhizae 18g
> Rhizoma Atractylodis Macrocephalae 15g
> Radix Astragali 12g
> Radix Angelicae Sinensis 12g
> Fructus Psoraleae 12g

HISTORICAL COMMENTS

Kai Bao Materia Medica commented that: "For scabies, rubella and other skin diseases caused by worms, Herba Senecio Integrifolli is ground into fine powder, mixed with water and applied to the lesion."

Dictionary of Chinese Medicinal Herbs wrote: "The drug relieves fever, removes excessive body fluid and kills worms."

THE AUTHOR'S NOTE

The First People's Hospital of Wei County in Zhejiang Province tried the following herbs on acute granulocytic leukemia, acute lymphatic leukemia and monocytic leukemia and found the effective rate was 57.9%:

> Herba Senecio Integrifolii 20g
> Radix Arnebiae 20g
> Herba Galii Aprinis 20g
> Radix Rumicis 15g
> Radix Rehmanniae 15g
> Rhizoma Polygonati 15g
> Radix Paeoniae Lactiflorae 6g
> Rhizoma Chuanxiong 6g
> Radix Glycyrrhizae 6g
> Radix Angelicae Sinensis 6g
> Radix Salviae Miltiorrhizae 6g

HERBA HOUTTUYNIAE

Compiled Essence of All Medical Works commented: "The drug is sweat, acrid and salty in flavor and induces diuresis, cures malaria and diseases caused by summer-heat."

It is the whole plant of *Houttuynia Cordata Thunb.* of the family *Saururaceae*, which contains volatile oil, cordarine, potassium chloride, decanoylacetaldehyde, quercitrin and potassium sulfate.

ANTICANCER PHARMACOLOGICAL FUNCTIONS

1. Bacteriophagic tests in vitro showed that the drug combats bacteriophages and hence suggests that it has an anticancer function.

2. The needle-like crystals, extracted from the herb with a melting point of 140 degrees centigrade, were found effective for stomach cancer.

EXPERIMENTAL FORMULAS

For tumor of the appendix:

Diagnosis, Prevention and Treatment of Tumors reported the following herbs taken in decoction a dose a day:

> Herba Houttuyniae 30g
> Herba Oldenlandiae Diffusae 30g
> Herba Violae yedoensis 30g
> Semen Coicis 15g

For lung cancer:

1 >. *Exchange of Medical Information* (Vol. 9, 1974) reported the decoction of the following herbs:

> Herba Houttuyniae 30g
> Herba Scutellariae Barbatae 30g
> Radix Scrophulariae 30g
> Radix Rehmanniae 30g
> Rhizoma Phragmitis 30g
> Flos Lonicerae 15g
> Radix Trichosanthis 15g
> Rhizoma Bletillae 15g
> Caulis Sargentodoxae 15g
> Radix Pseudostellariae Heterophyllae 15g
> Radix Adenophorae 15g
> Crinis Carbonisatus 15g
> Herba Patriniae Scabiosaefoliae 15g
> Bufo 9g
> Scolopendra 9g
> Rhizoma Arisaematis 9g

2 >. *Shanghai Journal of Traditional Chinese Medicine* (Vol. 3, 1979) reported the following decoction:

> Herba Houttuyniae 30g
> Foliun. Cordylini Fruticosae 30g
> Fructus Akebiae 15g
> Poria 15g
> Polyporus 15g
> Semen Coicis 15g
> Radix Codonopsis Pilosulae 9g

Radix Astragali 9g

Rhizoma Atractylodis Macrocephalae 9g

Pericarpium Citri Reticulatae 9g

Herba Oldenlandiae Diffusae 20g

For Chorionic epithelioma and hydatidiform mole:

Exhibition on Chinese Medicinal Herbs in Wuhan reported the decoction of the following herbs:

Herba Houttuyniae 30g

Semen Coicis 30g

Semen Phaseoli 30g

Semen Benincasae 30g

Herba Patriniae Scabiosaefoliae 15g

Colla Corii Asini 9g

Radix Rubiae 9g

Radix Angelicae Sinensis 9g

Radix Glycyrrhizae 6g

For cancer of the anus:

Shanghai Common Medicinal Herbs reported bath with the decoction of Herba Houttuyniae.

For cancerous edema of the chest and the abdomen:

Diagnosis, Prevention and Treatment of Tumors reported the administration of the following herbs in decoction one dose daily:

Herba Houttuyniae 30g

Semen Phaseoli 90g

For various types of cancers:

Research Data of Traditional Chinese Medicine (Vol. 6, 1978) reported long-term drink of the herb tea prepared with 20 to 30 grams of Herba Houttuyniae and 400ml of water through boiling.

HISTORICAL COMMENTS

Compendium of Materia Medica said: "The drug is effective for carbuncle due to noxious heat, boils, hemorrhoid, malaria and poisoning of Sal Ammoniaci."

Classical Prescription commented: "The drug is especially effective for carbuncle of the lung when smashed and decocted with seasoned Herba Brassicae Junceae." (Carbuncle of the lung means cancer of the lung)

Chinese Pharmacopeia wrote: "The herb is indicative for boils on the back when the fresh herb is smashed and the juice is applied to the swelling."

Prescription from Lu's Philanthropic Clinic recorded: "The fresh drug, when smashed and applied to the nail-like boils, can relieve pain and cure the boils in one or two days."

Simplified Prescription commented: "For decay of the tooth, equal portions of Herba Houttuyniae, Pericarpium Zanthoxyli Bungeani and rape seed oil and a little mud are mixed, made into pills about the size of beans and plugged in the antrum auris on the same side of the decayed tooth."

Dietetic Materia Medica said: "Long-term administration of the herb causes asthenic fever, damages the vitality and weakens bone marrow."

Practical Common Medicinal Herbs: "The fresh leaves of the plant, applied after being made hot at fire, is effective for scabies and boils. Washing with the decoction of the herb is good for swelling caused by the scabies and boils. Chewing the root of the plant prevents the attack of angina pectoris."

THE AUTHOR'S NOTE

As an anticancer drug, Herba Houttuyniae is often used together with other drugs. The Tumor Research Institute of Zhejiang Traditional Chinese Medical College tried Herba Houttuyniae and Herba Sedi in 33 cases of lung cancer and systematic follow-up showed that 24 cases survived for over a year.

Other data reported that the decoction of Herba Houttuyniae could improve the condition and prolong the survival period of patients with lung cancer. Large dose of Herba Houttuyniae is very effective for the complicated infections of lung cancer.

HERBA PATRINIAE SCABIOSAEFOLIAE

Li Shizhen said: "The herb is slightly bitter and sweat and is good at discharging pus and removing blood stasis."

The drug is the whole plant of *Patrinia Scabiosaefolia Fisch.* of the family *Valerianaceae.* Its similar plants such as *P. Villosa Fuss.*, *P. angustifolia hemsl.* and *P. rupestris Juss.* can be used to substitute the herb which contains volatile oil, saponins, tannins and alkaloids.

ANTICANCER PHARMACOLOGICAL FUNCTIONS

1. The hot water extract of Herba Patriniae Scabiesaefoliae showed an inhibitory rate of 50-70% on JTC-26.

2. The hot water extract from the root of the herb inhibits JTC-26 with a rate of 98.2%, but does not damage the normal cells at all, particularly the fibrocytes. It has been regarded as an "anticancer sword with single blade".

3. The hot water extract of the root of the plant showed an inhibitory rate of 57.4% on cancer cells when injected into the abdominal cavity of rats.

EXPERIMENTAL FORMULAS

For cancer of the appendix:

Diagnosis, Prevention and Treatment of Tumors reported the following decoction:

> Herba Patriniae Scabiosaefoliae 30g
> Flos Lonicerae 30g
> Semen Coicis 30g
> Herba Violae Yedoensis 30g
> Herba Scutellariae Barbatae 15g
> Rhizoma Zedoariae 9g
> Rhizoma Scirpi 9g

For Chorionic epithelioma and malignant hydatidiform mole:

Clinical Handbook of Oncology reported the following decoction:

> Herba Patriniae Scabiosaefoliae 30g
> Herba Houttuyniae 30g
> Semen Coicis 30g
> Semen Phaseoli 30g
> Radix Astragali 15g
> Rhizoma Bletillae 15g
> Radix Angelicae Sinensis 9g
> Radix Codonopsis Pilosulae 9g
> Radix Glycyrrhizae 9g

For relapse of carcinoma of the uterine body:

Journal of Beijing Traditional Chinese Medical College (Vol. 3, 1983) reported oral administration of 6 pills of *Xiaojin Dan* together with the following formula:

> Herba Patriniae Scabiosaefoliae 20g
> Caulis Lonicerae 20g
> Flos Lonicerae 20g

Herba Taraxaci 30g

Herba Taxilli 30g

Semen Coicis 15g

Radix Paeoniae Alba 15g

Herba Polygoni Avicularis 12g

Scorpio 3g

Sargassum 10g

Cortex Acanthopanacis 10g

Thallus Laminariae seu Eckloniae 10g

Fructus Forsythiae 10g

For cancer of the esophagus:

Anticancer Herbal Preparations reported the following:

Herba Patriniae Scabiosaefoliae 120g

Cortex Dictamni 120g

Spica Prunellae 120g

Radix Sophorae Tonkinensis 120g

Rhizoma Dioscoreae Bulbiferae 60g

Rhizoma Paridis 60g

All the above herbs are ground into fine powders to be pilled with honey. Each pill is 6 grams and one or two pills are taken each time, three times a day.

For cervical cancer at early stage:

Shanghai Journal of Traditional Chinese Medicine (Vol. 9, 1984) reported the following herbs taken in decoction:

Herba Patriniae Scabiosaefoliae 30g

Herba Scutellariae Barbatae 30g

Spica Prunellae 30g

Semen Coicis 30g

Bulbus Bolbostemmae 15g

Fructus Meliae Toosendan 15g

Rhizoma Smilacis Glabrae 20g

Flos Lonicerae 20g

Pericarpium Citri Reticulatae Viride 15g

Flos Sophorae Immaturus 15g

Radix Glycyrrhizae 3g

HISTORICAL COMMENTS

Records of Famous Physicians commented: "The drug is indicative for carbuncle, general edema, diseases caused by stasis of pathogenic heat, paralysis due to pathogenic wind and after-pain."

Herbs of Medicinal Property reported: "The drug is effective for stubborn illness caused by pathogenic wind and removes chronic stasis of blood."

Materia Medica in Ming Dynasty wrote: "The drug is effective for diseases of the blood and *qi*, cardiac and abdominal pain and lumps."

Prescription of Golden Chamber commented: "To treat abdominal pain with fullness, 100 grams of Semen Coicis, 20 grams of Radix Aconiti Lateralis Preparata and 50 grams of Herba Patriniae Scabiosaefoliae are smashed into powder and each time three to five grams is decocted in 80ml of water to a broth of 40ml for oral administration."

Quang Ji Prescription recommended the decoction of the following herbs for severe postpartum lumbago with hemorrhage and pain in the lumbus and legs:

Herba Patriniae Scabiosaefoliae 30g

Radix Angelica Sinensis 2.4g
Rhizoma Chuanxiong 1.8g
Radix Paeniae Alba 1.8g
Semen Longan 1.8g
The above herbs are decocted in 80ml of water to a broth of 30ml for oral administration.

RHIZOMA POLYGONI CUSPIDATI

Compiled Essence of All Medical Works commented: "The drug, sweat, bitter and acrid in flavor and warm in nature, tonifies the
muscles and bones and increases strength."

The drug is the root of a plant in the family *Polygonaceae*, which mainly activates blood circulation, and is found growing in Northwest China, Central China and Southeast China. It contains emodin, chrysophanol, tannins and polysaccharides. Emodin and chrysophanol are active against cancer.

ANTICANCER PHARMACOLOGICAL FUNCTIONS
1. The hot water extract of Rhizoma Polygoni Cuspidati showed an inhibiting rate of 68% on ascites sarcoma-180 in rats, but the ether extract showed no inhibition at all.
2. Experiments in vitro showed that the hot water extract of the herb inhibited JTC-26 with a rate of 90%.

EXPERIMENTAL FORMULAS
For stomach cancer:
30 grams of Rhizoma Polygoni Cuspidati is prepared into a syrup for oral administration 20 to 30ml each time, 2 to 3 times a day. (*Practical Oncology*)
For leukopenia due to radiotherapy:
Rhizoma Polygoni Cuspidati 30g
Caulis Millettiae 30g
Radix Angelicae Sinensis 30g
Radix Glycyrrhizae 9g
The above herbs are decocted and taken twice daily. (*New Data on Medicine*)

HISTORICAL COMMENTS
Records of Famous Doctors said: "The drug is mainly indicated for abdominal mass and regulates monthly period."
Supplement to Compendium of Materia Medica recorded: "The decoction of the herb is effective for diseases of the bone joints and blood stasis."
Prescriptions Worth a Thousand Gold mentioned: "Mixture of the decoction of the herb with old wine is effective for abdominal mass, tinnitus, heaviness of the limbs, irregular menstruation and impotence, when 600g of Semen Dolichoris Album is sliced and decocted in 2000ml of water to a broth of 200ml to be mixed with 200ml of wine for oral administration 5ml each time."
Zhou Hou's Prescriptions said: "Washing hands or feet with the decoction of the root of the herb cures swelling and pain of the hand and the foot."

SEMEN DOLICHORIS ALBUM

It is defined in *Properties of Medicinal Herbs* that: "The drug, sweet in taste and slightly warm in nature, removes toxic materials of all herbs and plants and is administered through chewing the raw drug or in decoction."

It is the seed of *Dolichos lablab* of *Leguminosae* family, cultivated all over China and also known as Semen Dolichoris Album. Its seeds contain starch, fats, protein, vitamin A, B and C, tartaric acid and two kinds of non-specific plant hemagglutinin.

ANTICANCER PHARMACOLOGICAL FUNCTIONS

1. Tests in vitro showed that Semen Dolichoris is effective in inhibiting oncocytic growth.

2. Tests in vitro with plant hemagglutinin showed that the drug can enable the malignant carcinocytes to take agglutinative reaction and oncocytic superficial structure to alter, eventually bringing cellular toxin into action.

3. Plant hemagglutinin promotes the function of lymphocytes hence, reinforcing the immunity to tumor.

EXPERIMENTAL FORMULAS

For carcinodropsy:

1kg of Semen Dolichoris is fried and then ground into powder to be taken three times a day before meals with Medulla Junci broth. 9 grams of the powder for adults and 3 grams for children each time. (Reported in *Prescriptions for Dropsy in Commentary Anthology of Materia Medica*)

Gastrocancer and other tumors can be treated with the juice extracted from 750 grams of leaves of the herb. The juice is taken frequently without dosage restriction. It is also reported in some foreign countries that the juice has been clinically used to treat other malignant tumors. (Reported in *Journal of Northeast Economic Botany*)

For cancer of the thoracic cavity:

The leaves of the herb, roasted in vinegar and ground into powder, is taken orally. (Reported in *Dietetic Materia Medica*)

HISTORICAL COMMENTS

It is said in *Materia Medica of All Schools in Great Ming Dynasty* that: "Snake bite can be cured with external application of the smashed fresh leaves of the herb."

It is reported in *Newly Edited Materia Medica* that: "The leaves of herb can be used to treat spasm which occurs after vomiting and diarrhea. Add a little vinegar to a handful of fresh leaves of the herb and then smash it. Finally squeeze out the juice and rub it on the affected part of the body."

It is recorded in *Zhen Nan Materia Medica* that: "The drug cures gastrosplenodeficiency, nausea, regurgitation, chronic diarrhea, dyspepsia, mass in the abdomen and infantile malnutrition."

It is suggested in *Popular Materia Medica* that: "White Flos Dolichoris Album can radiate its effect to the *qi* phase to promote the circulation of *qi*, while red Flos Dalichoris Album can penetrate the hemophase to melt away stagnation."

THE AUTHOR'S NOTE

It was reported that Hua Shan Hospital affiliated to Shanghai Medical College had tested the IgG and IgA in 100 patients with malignant tumor and found out that the decoction of Radix Rehmaniae, Radix Codonopsis Pilosulae, Radix Astragali, Plastrum Testudinis and Semen Dalichoris can increase the patient's cellular immunity. The Decoction had been used to treat 56 cases of malignant tumor and the effective rate was found to be 53.6%. It was also reported that Semen Dalichoris alone could increase lymphocytic inversion rate in patients with nasopharyngeal cancer and invigorate vital energy to expel pathogenic factors. In abroad, the seeds of *Vicia faba L.* and *Vicia sativa* pertaining to other bean family are processed into decoction and preparation for external application to treat cancer. Hard testicular tumor can be treated with pounded pea through application to the affected part once a day. Also in abroad, *Phaseolus Vulgarisy L.* is used as an anticancer drug. *Phaseolus Vulgarisy L.*, known as kidney beans and evergreen beans, is one of the most popular kind of vegetables cultivated in Northeast China, the seed and the pod of which are now used as an anticancer and anti-wart drugs.

SQUAMA MANITIS

It is reported in *Zhen Nan Materia Medica* that: "The drug is cold in nature, salty in taste and effective in treating scabies and leprosy, and promotes blood circulation by diminishing *qi* stagnation."

The drug is the scale and the shell of *Manis pentadactyla L.* of *Mandae* family, obtained by killing the pangolin, stripping the flesh and drying the shell in the sunshine. The scales on the shell will come off when put into boiling water, and the shell can be used medically when dried.

ANTICANCER PHARMACOLOGICAL FUNCTIONS

1. Maniticine found in the drug possesses an anti-leukemia function and it is effective when used clinically.

2. *Yinjia* Pills (with ingredients such as Flos Lomicerae, Squiama Manitis and Herba Taraxaci) possess the function of anti-papillocarcinocytic activation.

EXPERIMENTAL FORMULAS

For eczematoid papillary cancer:

> Squama Manitis 9g
> Pericarpium Citri Reticuloutae Viride 9g
> Pericarpium Citri Reticulatae 9g
> Radix Glycyrrhizae 9g
> Radix Astragali seu Hedysari 30g
> Flos Lonicerae 30g
> Radix Angelicae Sinensis 30g
> Fructus Trichosanthis 50g
> Radix Bupleuri 20g

The prescription is taken one dosage and three times a day in decoction. Modifications is made in accordance with the conditions of the patients. (Reported in *Traditional Chinese Medicine Journal*, Vol. 4, 1980)

For malignant lymphoma:

21 sheets of the drug are calcined, ground and applied to the affected part. (Reported in *Yiao Zhengheng's Experienced Prescriptions for Scrofula and Ulceration*)

For cervical cancer:

15g of the drug is calcined yellow and ground into powder to be taken 6 grams a time with millet wine. (Reported in *Miraculous Recipes for Uterosclerosis*)

For hepatocarcinoma:

> Squama Manitis 15g
> Concha Ostreae 30g
> Fructus Meliae Toosendan 9g
> Radix Curcumae 9g
> Semen Persicae 9g
> Flos Carthami 9g
> Cortex Moutan 6g
> Rhizoma Dioscoreae Nipponicae 6g

Lumbricus 12g

The prescription is taken one dosage a day with water. (Reported in *Brief Introduction to Tumor*)

For mammocarcinoma:

1>.   Squama Manitis 12g

Semen Vaccariae 12g

Spica Prunellae 9g

Rhizoma Dioscoreae Bulbiferae 30g

The prescription is taken one dosage a day in decoction. (Reported in *Practical Handbook on Anticancer Drugs*)

2>. Squama Manitis and Spina Gleditsiae of the same amount are ground for external application to ulcerous tumor. (Reported in *Practical Handbook on Anticancer Drugs*)

For haemorrhagia caused by osteoma:

Squama Manitis is roasted in vegetable oil till its turning yellow, then ground into powder to be packed up separately and sterilized for use. Clean away the bleeding and sprinkle the powder immediately on the affected part and finally dress the lesion with pressure. Bleeding stops one to five minutes after the application. (Reported in *Dictionary of Chinese Medicinal Herbs*)

HISTORICAL COMMENTS

It is recorded in *Records of Integrated Chinese and Western Medicine* that: "The drug, with a stinking smell which enables it to scurry actively through the whole human body, can activate viscera, penetrate channels and collaterals, reach joints and apertures, and clear away blood stasis and stagnation. The drug can be used at will to treat furuncle and carbuncle with instant result. The drug is also effective in treating abdominal mass, paralysis, difficult urination and defecation and abdominalgia. It should be borne in mind that the drug is not only effective in curing sores but also in treating many other diseases. I often use the prescription (composed of Squama Manitis 12g, Spina Gleditsiae 12g, Pollen 18g, Rhizoma Anemarrhenae 18g, Olibanum 9g, Myrrha 9g and three Scolopendrae) to cure furuncles and sore at early stage without pus and to treat bubo with satisfactory result. If the sores or furuncles swollen with pus formed, the drug can subside the swelling and release the pus easily. Squama Manitis can be added as a guiding medicine to the prescription for abdominal mass, painful paralysis and difficult urination and defecation."

In *Reference Materia Medica* there was a tale saying that: "Once upon a time, there was a woman who suddenly had a swelling on the nape and it gradually extended to the neck. The swelling was accidentally stabbed one day and a bowel of liquid running out of it. But the wound remained unhealed for a long time. Someone said that the woman was suffering from a so called ant-dripping syndrome caused by swallowing the ants dropped into her food. Squama Manitis, calcined and then ground into powder, was applied to the lesion and it worked instantly. But the drug is forbidden in the treatment of ulcerous carbuncles. The tail part of the drug, short as that of an alligator and quick in movement as that of a carp, is especially strong in action and popularly used in many prescriptions in the raw or the calcined form. It is also roasted with butter, vinegar, oil, soil, or young boy's urine."

It is recorded in *Materia Medica* that: "A proverb goes like this: Administered together with Semen Vacariae, the drug can promote lactation and the mother's milk will run out quickly without stop. This means that the drug is very quick in action and should be ceased once it works. It can not be administered for a long time."

HERBA ANDROGRAPHITIS

In *Quan Zhou Materia Medica*, it is said that: "The drug, bitter in taste and cold and non-toxic in nature, is effective in clearing away pathogenic heat, removes toxic material, diminishes inflammation and subsides swelling."

The drug, also locally known as *Yi Jian Xi* (which means happiness at first sight), Snake Killer, Bitter Herb, is the *Andrographis* of *Acanthaceae* family. The whole plant can be used medically. The herb is cultivated all over China, containing andrographalide, neoandrographolide, Deoxyandrographolide and multi-flavoneous chemical compounds.

ANTICANCER PHARMACOLOGICAL FUNCTIONS

1. Experiments in vivo indicate that the drug can inhibit oncopoiesis in animals.

2. Tests in vitro with bacteriophagic method show that the drug has anti-bacteriophagic function and this suggests that it is of resisting carcino-activation.

3. For trophoblastic tumor, the drug can solidify its cytoplasm and nucleus and induce retrograde variations such as breaking down and dissolving.

4. The drug is low in toxicity, bearing little affection on the heart, the liver and the kidney. The drug also kills bacteria and virus.

5. The decoction of the drug has the function of delaying the degeneration of human embryorenocyte caused by $ECHO_{11}$.

EXPERIMENTAL FORMULAS

For chorioepithelioma and malignant hydatidiform mole:

60 grams of the drug is decocted and taken daily. (Reported in *Anticancer Preparations of Traditional Chinese Medicine*)

Or 50-100ml of Herba Andrographitis Injection (with 5-10% water) and 500ml glucose are administrated intravenously once a day. With vaginal metastasis, the injection is administrated at the metastatic node, 5-10ml a time and once or twice a day. (Reported in *New Traditional Chinese Medicine Journal*, Vol. 5, 1978)

HISTORICAL COMMENTS

It is reported in *Records of Herbs Collected in Lingnan* that: "The drug is effective in removing snake poison and curing cough caused by visceral impairment."

It is said in *Jiangxi Materia Medica* that: "The drug can clear away heat, cool blood, subside swelling, relieve pain and cure cystitis, bronchitis, hypertension and pertussis."

THE AUTHOR'S NOTE

It was reported that seven cases with malignant vesicular mole, chorioepithelioma and massive metastatic vaginonode were treated with Herba Andrographitis through intravenous injection in Meixian Hospital, Guangdong Province, with 5 cured, one improved and one dead. Experiments showed that Herba Andrographis was significantly effective in treating malignant vascular mole and choriovaginoma. The curative effect is reached with 30ml of intravenous injection daily. Chronic application, due to its cold nature, may cause nausea, diarrhea and poor appetite, which can be cured with other medicinal herbs used together with the drug."

HERBA BIDENI BIPINNATA

In *Quan Zhou Materia Medica*, it is defined that: "The drug, warm and non-toxic in nature and bitter in taste, is effective in treating incised wound, expelling stasis and easing pain."

The drug is the whole herb of *Bidens* of *Compositae* family, and it is called A Bundle of Needles and Ghost Fork etc.. Other herbs of the same family such as *Bidens pilosa L.* and *Bidens pilosa L. var. minor* also share the same function with Herba Bideni Bipinnata.

ANTICANCER PHARMACOLOGICAL FUNCTIONS

It is proved by anticancer experiment done with bacteriophagic method that this drug has anti-bacteriophagic function.

EXPERIMENTAL FORMULAS

For esophageal carcinoma:

15-30g of the drug is decocted and taken orally. (Reported in *Treatment Based on the Differentiation of Symptoms and Signs*)

For gastric carcinoma:

> Herba Bideni Bipinnata 30g
> Haematitum 30g
> Rhizoma Dioscoreae 30g
> Flos Inulae 10g
> Pollen Typhae 10g
> Faeces Trogopterorl 10g
> Rhizoma Scirpi 10g
> Fructus Citri Aurantii 10g
> Rhizoma Anemarrhenae 15g
> Rhizoma Dioscoreae Bulbiferae 15g
> Radix Achyranthis Bidentatae 15g
> Poria 20g
> Fructus Crataegi 24g
> Herba Cistanchis Deserticolae 24g

All the above herbs are put together and decocted into thick broth to be taken through sipping frequently, one dosage for two days. (Reported in *Hubei Traditional Chinese Medicine Journal*, Vol. 4, 1984)

HISTORICAL COMMENTS

It is reported in *Materia Medica* that: "Scorpion sting can be cured by external application of the drug."

It is said in *Prescriptions Worth a Thousand Gold* that: "External application of Bipinnota plant pounded with Fructus Arctii and blended with pig fat can cure finger cut."

It is recorded in *Dictionary of Chinese Materia Medica* that: "The drug, bitter in taste, mild in nature and non-toxic, mainly cures spider and fly bites through internal administration and external application."

It is recorded in *Handbook of Chinese Medicinal Herbs* that: "The decoction of the drug cures dysentery, laryngalgia, dysphagia, vomiting, cardiac spasm and esophageal dilatation, and is effective in removing toxic materials, stopping diarrhea and clearing away heat. The drug has been used to treat cecitis in the recent years."

SEMEN IMPATIENTIS

In *Materia Medica*, it is defined that: "The drug, being slightly bitter in taste and warm and slightly toxic in nature, cures abdominal mass and dysphagia."

The drug is the seeds of *Impatiens balsamina L.* of *Balsaminaceae* family, containing balsaminasterol, Parinaric acid, saponins, quercetin glycoside and flavoneous chemical compounds.

ANTICANCER PHARMACOLOGICAL FUNCTIONS
1. Experiments in vivo show that the drug is effective in inhibiting the activation of transplanted tumor-37 in mice.
2. The pharmacologic sensitive test shows that the drug is sensitive to gastrolymphosarcoma.

EXPERIMENTAL FORMULAS
For esophagocarcinoma:

1>. Steep the drug in wine for three days, grind it into powder and then roll the powder with wine into pills of mung bean size. 8 pills are taken each time with warm boiled water. If the patient has difficulty in swallowing, 6 pills are decocted into broth and taken orally. This drug is violent in action, therefore large dosage is forbidden. The prescription should be stopped once the effect has been gained.

2>. Semen Impatientis 30g and Herba Salviae Chinensis 30g are decocted into a thick broth to be blended with 1 or 2 grams of Salmiacum for sipping. (Reported in *Zhejiang Traditional Chinese Medicine Journal*, Vol 3, 1980)

3>. Semen Impatientis 30g, Rhizoma Dioscoreae Bulbiferae 30g, Ocherum Rubrum 30g and Herba Scutellariae Barbatae 30g are decocted and taken daily. (Reported in *Practical Handbook on Anticancer Drugs*)

> For cardiac cancer:
> Semen Impatientis 9g
> Lapis Pumicis 9g
> Dolomitum 9g
> Os Sepiae 30g
> Ocherum Rubrum 6g

All the above herbs are put together and ground into fine powder for rolling with water into pills of the size of mung bean. 16 pills are taken each time in the morning and evening. (Reported in *Collection of Experienced Prescriptions*)

HISTORICAL COMMENTS
It is reported in *Origin of Herbal Canon* that: "The external application of the drug pounded with garlic can cure swelling or tumor mass. The curative effect will be reached quickly if Moschus and Resina Ferulae added."

It is said in *Practical Folk Prescriptions* that: "Dysphagia can be cured effectively with the drug roasted yellow and ground into fine powder, with a dosage of 3 to 9 grams each time, taken orally with old wine."

It is suggested in *Materia Medica* that: "The drug can penetrate bone and soften hard mass with its swift moving nature. When cooking fish, cooks usually put several of its seeds into the boiler to help boiling the hard meat."

ARSENICUM

Li Shicai in the Ming Dynasty said that: "The drug, being sweet and sour in taste, very hot and toxic in nature, cures lingering phlegm-syndrome and all kinds of malaria."

The drug is the natural Arsenolite and classified into the red and the white types. The red one is called red arsenicum, characterized with irregular shape, different size, yellowish or reddish color, crystal or non-crystal property and radiance or non-radiance. The drug is brittle, easily to be broken, and free of stinking smell, but is very toxic. Therefore oral administration is forbidden. The white one is known as white arsenicum and it is similar to red arsenicum in function. The drug is mainly produced in Guangdong, Beijing, Pingshi and Lechang regions and it can also be artificially made from Arsenopyrite or Realgar, mainly containing arsenic trioxide and some impure elements such as sulphur and iron which make it appear red.

ANTICANCER PHARMACOLOGICAL FUNCTIONS

Arsenicum is the protoplasmic toxin, which functions to collapse and deteriorate ulcerous biocytes and kill malignant oncocytes.

EXPERIMENTAL FORMULAS

For dermatocarcinoma:

3 grams of Arsenicum, 1.5 gram of Ungnis Hominis, 1.5 gram of Crinis, 1 gram of Fructus Ziziphi Inermis without core, and 50 grams of Wheat flour fermented with alkali. Ground Arsenicum is mixed with Ungnis Hominis, Crinis and Fructus Ziziphi Inermis, and then wrapped in dough, to be roasted over mulberry charcoal. The burnt dough is ground into powder for sprinkling on the affected lesion. The powder also can be blended with sesame oil into 5% paste for application to the lesion. This prescription is applied once a day or once every other day. The prescription is also effective in treating breast cancer, labial cancer and penis cancer.

For cervical cancer

The flesh of Fructus Ziziphi Inermis and a little of Bormeol are put together and made into powder by sublimation, to which is then added starch and made into tablets as thick as a coin or suppository (each weighs 0.15g and contains 0.1-0.12g of the crude drug). The tablets are applied to the cervical tumor, while the suppository to the cervical canal once every 24 hours with one day interval. The treatment should be stopped during menstruation or metrorrhagia. This prescription is also effective for cervical erosion. (Reported in *Journal of Hubei Medical and Medicinal Industry*, Vol 2, 1974)

For nasopharyngeal cancer, esophageal cancer, rectocancer, cystocancer and cervical cancer:

Arsenicum 15g
Fructus Crotonis (peeled and ground) 7
Fructus Ziziphi 7
Bulbus Allii Fistulosi (steamed and pounded) 7

The four ingredients are mixed up and put into two small sacks for patients to hold one in each hand for 12 hours a time, every other day. (Reported in *Diagnosis and Treatment of Tumor*)

For liposarcoma:

Arsenicum 30g
Sulfur 30g

The two ingredients are melted by heating, and ground into powder when it becomes cold. For treatment, the skin of the tumor is pricked and a little of the powder is applied. The pricked region is dressed with plaster. If ulceration develops, the powder is sprinkled on the ulcer and it will heal very quickly. (Reported in *Handbook on Medicinal Herbs*)

For malignant rete disease:

Arsenicum 1.5g
Melanteritum 30g

The two ingredients are ground into powder and divided into 50 packets. Each packet is steamed with some Fructus Lycii and brown sugar and taken daily. (Reported in *Medical Research Data*, Vol 8, 1974)

HISTORICAL COMMENTS

It is said in *Materia Medica* that: "The drug corrodes carbuncle, deep-rooted carbuncle and slough, and is poisonous to insects, human beings and animals."

It is reported in *Ling Yuan's Prescriptions* that: "Arsenicum is effective for scrofula, when ground into powder and rolled into pills of the size of Semen Firmianae with thick Chinese ink and roasted in pan and kept in a bamboo wear for storage. Puncture the scrofula and apply half a pill to it. The method is repeated till the scrofula fully disappear."

It is recommended in *Prescriptions for Emergencies* that: "Any kind of anal fistula can be treated with Arsenicum that is fried on a new tile and then ground into powder to be wrapped in thin paper and inserted into the anus. If there are several fistulas, do not treat them simultaneously."

THE AUTHOR'S NOTE

The drug, due to its violent toxicity, is usually not administrated orally. If taken orally, it must be decocted with mung bean or beancurd before administration and the dosage and the period of administration should be limited to safe range. Combined with other therapies, 55 cases of acute granulocytic leukemia were given No. 1 Cancer Killer Injection intramuscularly 2 to 4 milliliter each time (each milliliter contains 1 milligram of arsenic trioxide), 1 to 2 times a day. The curative rate was found to be 70% with 12 cases completely alleviated."

RADIX CUDRANIAE

It is defined in *Commonly Used Folk Prescriptions in Zhejiang* that: "The drug, mild in nature and bitter in taste, is effective in clearing away pathogenic heat and cooling blood."

The drug is obtained from of *Cudrania tricuspidata (Carr.) Bur.* of *Moraceae* family, its wood, root, bark, stalk and fruit are for medical use. The root contains flavonoid glycosides, phenol, amino acid, organic acid, stachydrine and morin.

ANTICANCER PHARMACOLOGICAL FUNCTIONS

1. The flavones and the alcohol-steeped paste extracted from the root, stalk and wood of Radix Cudraniae can inhibit mice sarcoma-180 and uterocancer-27 with a steady rate of 30-40%.

2. Screening tests in vitro showed that the drug has a cytotoxic function against cancer cells of the esophagus.

3. Pain-relieving test with hot plate method on mice showed that the drug has a significant pain relieving effect, and this indicates that the drug, to some extent, can alleviate pain caused by cancer.

EXPERIMENTAL FORMULAS

For malignant tumors of the digestive system:

60 to 120 grams of the drug is decocted and taken daily with a dose a day. This prescription also can be administered to treat uterocancer and advanced ovarian cancer. (Reported in *Handbook of Practical Anticancer Drugs*)

HISTORICAL COMMENTS

In *Pharmaceutical Records of Nanning*, it is said that: "The drug can promote menstrual flow through removing blood stasis and cure stranguria with turbid urine, chronic stagnation and calculus."

In *True Materia Medica*, it is suggested that: "The drug nourishes tendons and bones, and activates blood circulation."

In *Ri Hua Zhi Materia Medica*, it is said that: "The drug cures blood stasis caused by metrorrhagia."

THE AUTHOR'S NOTE

It was reported that 266 cases with esophagus cancer were treated with Radix Cudraniae and the total curative rate was found to be 71.28%. (Reported in *Journal of Pharmacology*, Vol.4, 1990) Radix Cudraniae is also effective in treating liver cancer, pulmonary cancer, nasolaryngeal cancer, gastrocancer and enterocancer.

RADIX SALIX BABYLONICAE

It is defined in *Zhennan Materia Medica* that: "The drug is bitter in taste and cold in nature, curing five kinds of stranguria and whitish turbid urine."

The drug is the root of *Salix* of *Salicaceae* family. Its leaves, flowers and branches also can be used medically. Its leaf, stalk-bark and root-bark contain a kind of glucoside called salicin which, bitter in taste, dissolves in water, but not in ethanol. 1kg of the fresh leaves contains 10mg of iodine, being thousand times higher than that contained in general food.

ANTICANCER PHARMACOLOGICAL FUNCTIONS

The main curative effect of the drug is to restore the regenerating capacity of the bone marrow damaged by chemical therapy and to prolong the patient's survival. It has been clinically proved that the drug, combined with chemical therapy, can treat malignant leukemia and proliferate erythrocytic system and macronucleocytes so as to prolong the patient's life.

EXPERIMENTAL FORMULAS

For malignant leukemia:

1>. 30 to 60 grams of fresh willow twigs growing near a valley is cut and decocted for oral taking. The prescription is continued without any intervals.

2>. Equal portions of the fresh roots of the willow, pear, peach, and mulberry trees are decocted and taken by month daily.

HISTORICAL COMMENTS

In *Proved Prescriptions Collected by Yao Zheng*, it is said that: "Goiter can be cured with a wine brewed with 15kg of Radix Salix Babylonicae and 90g of rice in 800ml of water to a broth of 400ml. The wine is taken three times, 40ml a day."

In *Materia Medica*, it is recorded that: "The decoction of willow branch and Cortex Salix Babylonicae cures jaundice and whitish turbid urine. When decocted in wine, the drug cures various pain and swelling, with the functions to dispel pathogenic wind and relieve pain and swelling."

In *Handbook of Prescriptions for Emergencies*, it is reported that: "The drug cures boils and deep-rooted carbuncle. Willow branch and Cortex Salix Babylonicae are often prescribed for breast cancer."

THE AUTHOR'S NOTE

Even in the ancient times, the drug was used to treat tumor. For instance, in the chapter, Application of Heated Drugs, *Medical Rhythmical Essays* Compiled by Wu Shangxian in the Qing Dynasty has reported a therapy known as application of heated Radix Salix Babylonicae, focusing on curing chronic, hard and bluish mammary abscess by applying to the breast the willow root with its bark struck, heated and kept in a bag. Everlasting Paste recorded in the book for curing abdominal mass also contains willow twig. The ingredients in the formula are Ramnlus Salix Babylonicae, Ramulus Mori, Ramulus Sophorace Immatunis (2kg each) and 2kg of sesame oil, which are decocted into paste with the addition of Minium. The paste is then blended with Radix et Rhizoma Rhei and Radix Angelicae

Duhuricae. When applied to the affected lesion, the paste has satisfactory result. In Bai Fu Hospital in Huanggang, Hubei Province, an anticancer paste was developed on the basis of modified "Everlasting Paste" with Ramnlus Salix Babylonicae, Ramulus Sophorae Immatunis, Ramnlus Pruni Persicae, Radix et Rhizoma Rhei, Radix Angelicae Duhuricae and Olibanum and Myrrha. The paste was applied to the tumor lesion of 16 cases with esophageal cancer, changed once daily and accompanied with other oral drugs. The total curative effect 62.5%.

SEMEN ABRI

In *Supplement to Materia Medica*, it is defined that: "The drug, being hot in taste and slightly toxic in nature, activates the nine apertures and curing abdominal distension."

The drug is the dried seed of *Abrus precatorius L.* of the family *Leguminosae*, cultivated mainly in Yunnan, Guangxi and Guangdong. Its seed, also known as Red Bean and Beauty Bean, has an aperture in the middle and is in oval shape with one end black and the other red, containing abrin, abrissic acid, hemolioprotein, lipase, urea enzyme and glycyrrhizin.

ANTICANCER PHARMACOLOGICAL FUNCTIONS

1. Thoracic injection of abrin into mice one or three days after the inoculation of ascites cancer can completely inhibit oncocytoplasia. But it will lose its effect when heated under 100 degrees centigrade for 30 minutes before injection.

2. Abrin extracted from the drug by NaCl can inhibit MFS fabriosarcoma in mice.

3. The mechanism of the drug's function lies in the fact that it can strongly inhibits the synthesis of protein and decomposition of polyribose in cells.

4. The protein crystal extracted from the drug, contains 4.5% neutral protein and 9.3% gluosamine which are found inhibiting the activation of tumors.

5. The abrin extracted from the drug, undergone DEAE fibrocolum chromatography and polyacrylamide electrophoresis, can be divided into two parts with electrophoresis done with 0.05M potassium phosphate buffer solution containing 0.1 MNaCl. The two parts of the protein are found resisting tumors and Yoshida's sarcoma.

6. The experimental animals, having been cured of Yoshida's sarcoma with abrin, acquire immunity to the illness.

7. The dissolvable protein in the seed is found resisting tumor (Yoshida's sarcoma and fibrosarcoma in mice) both in vivo and in vitro.

EXPERIMENTAL FORMULAS
For dermatocancer:
Semen Abri is pounded and applied to the lesion. (*Natural Drug Magazine*, Vol. 11, 1971)

HISTORICAL COMMENTS
Chen Zangqi said that: "The drug cures gastralgia, headache caused by heat accumulation and phlegm syndrome due to pathogenic wind, and kills all kinds of parasites and ascarides."

In *Materia Medica*, it is said that: "The drug keeps borneol odor from dispersing."

In *Major Poisonous Plants in the North*, it is reported that: "The leaf, root and seed of Abri are poisonous, especially the seed."

THE AUTHOR'S NOTE
The poison of the drug comes from its abrin, the function of which, similar to that of ricin in the seed of castor-oil plant, is to cause hemagglutination, hemolysis and histionecrosis. If swallowed with

its hard shell, the seed will not exert any poisonous effect. But if chewed, even half a seed will cause poisoning. So oral administration of the drug is forbidden lest it will cause poisoning.

SEMEN JUGLANDIS

It is defined in *Handbook of Chinese Medicinal Herbs in Shandong* that: "The drug is bitter in taste, astringent and mild in nature, and removes toxic materials and subsiding swelling."

The drug is obtained from *Juglans regia L.* of *Juglandaceae* family, the kernel, septum, green shell and leaf of which are for medical use. The outer shell contains juglone, hydrojuglone ß-glucoside, tannins and gallic acid; the fruit and leaves contain flavone; the kernel contains fatty oil, protein, saccharides; the leaves contain inositol, caffeic acid and gallic acid; the leaves and the unripe fruit contain vitamin C, alkaloids, juglone, anthraquinone and tannins in large quantity. The leaves and fruit also contain volatile oils.

ANTICANCER PHARMACOLOGICAL FUNCTIONS

1. The unripe walnut steeped in wine can inhibit ascites cancer and sarcoma-180 and sarcoma-37 in mice. It is thought that this is because of the vitamin C it contains, which can remarkably stop the synthesis of ammonium nitrite in the body.

2. Black Semen Juglandis inhibits spontaneous mammocancer and ascites cancer of mice.

3. Juglone and polysaccharides inhibits the cytonucleofission of sarcoma-180 and the solid ascites cancer of mice.

4. LD50 was measured to be 214g/kg (raw herb) after thoracic injection of the substance extracted from green walnut to mice, and this indicates low toxicity.

EXPERIMENTAL FORMULAS

For gastrocancer:

Steep the unripe walnuts in wine for a month, during which it may be exposed to sunshine in the afternoon. The wine is condensed to 60% when prepared and it is called *Qing Long Yi Jiu* for oral administration three times a day, 10ml each time. Radix Acanthopanacis Senticosi Tablet (each tablet contains 1.5g of the crude drug) is prescribed for the patient at the same time with a dose of three times a day, three tablets each time. (Reported in *Traditional Chinese Pharmacology*, Vol. 7, 1980)

For esophageal cancer and gastrocancer:

Ten fresh twigs, each being 0.3 meter long and a finger thick, are boiled together with 3 eggs for 4 hours. Only the eggs are taken for treatment. (Reported in *Differentiation of Symptoms and Signs*)

For leukemia:

In abroad, the kernel of *Juglans nigaa* is blended with milk and apple for oral administration. It is reported to be very effective. In China, 7421 Injection is prepared with the same herb.

For hepatocancer:

Ramulus Juglandis 30g
Herba Scutellariae Barbatae 30g
Radix Sophorae Tonkinensis 30g
Fructus Trichosanthis 30g
Herba Oldenlandiae Diffusae 30g
Radix Astragali 30g
Herba Taraxaci 60g
Radix Codonopsis Pilosulae 15g
Flos Lonicerae 15g

Squama Manitis 15g

Radix Glycyrrhizae 12g

The prescription is taken one dosage a day. (Reported in *Erxi Journal of Science and Technology*, Vol. 4, 1979)

For gastrolymphosarcoma:

Three eggs are boiled with 120-150 grams of walnut twig (fresh or dried). The eggs are simmered for four hours and taken with some of the decoction. The remaining decoction is taken later. (Reported in *Jiangsu Journal of Traditional Chinese Medicine*, Vol. 2, 1980)

For malignant granulocytic leukemia:

1>.   Cortex juglandis 90g

Radix Codonopsis Pilosulae 15g

Radix Angelicae Sinensis 15g

Radix Paconiae Alba 12g

Radix Astragali 12g

The prescription is taken in decoction one dose a day. (Reported in *Anticancer Preparation in Traditional Chinese Medicine*)

2>.   Semen Juglandis 30g

Radix Codonopsis Pilosulae 30g

Radix Astragali 18g

Radix Angelicae Sinensis 15g

Colla Cornus Cervi 9g

Fructus lycii 15g

Radix Rehmanniae 24g

Radix Polygoni Multiflori 30g

Fructus Rubi 18g

Rhizoma Polygonati 24g

Rhizoma Atractylodis Macrocephalae 18g

Poria 15g

Radix Glycyrrhizae 7.5g

(Reported in *New Traditional Chinese Medicine*, Vol. 4, 1977)

For mammocancer:

Semen Julandis 100g

Cortex Juglandis 9g

Bulbus Fritillariae Cirrhosae 9g

Flos Loniarae 9g

Fructus Forsythiae 9g

The prescription is decocted in liquid composed of wine and water for oral administration. (Reported in *Mei's Experienced Prescriptions for Breast Cancer*)

For other cancers:

Semen Juglandis 100

Rhizoma Zedoariae 120g

Radix Angelicae Sinensis 120g

Semen Impatientis 120g

Natrii Sulfas 250g

Oviductus Notarchi 250g

The ingredients are decocted for one day and one night. 3-9 Semen Juglandis are taken each day. (Reported in *Anticancer Consultation*)

HISTORICAL COMMENTS

In *Materia Medica*, it is said that: "The drug supplements *qi* to invigorate blood, moistures dryness to eliminate phlegm, nourishes the kidney, dredges *sanjiao*, warms the lung to smoothen the intestines, cures cough due to deficient cold attack, painful and swollen waist and feet, abdominal hernial pain, fistula, swelling, pustule, and removes copper poison."

In *Guide to Drug Administration*, it said that: "The drug cures fistula and scrofula."

In *Popular Prescriptions*, it is said that: "Heart burn due to food can be relieved with one walnut chewed with ginger broth."

In *Zhao's Experienced Prescriptions*, it is said that: "Abdominal flatulence can be cured definitely with one walnut and one date (with the shell and core removed) wrapped in paper and calcined for oral administration before chewing with a cup of ginger broth."

In *Collection of Simple Prescriptions*, it is said that: "Scabies can be cured quickly with Realgar (3g) and Folium Artemisiae Argyi (3g) pounded, wrapped in cotton and tied to scrotum."

In *Miraculously Effective Prescriptions*, it is said that: "Intestine pain due to *qi* can be cured with one walnut fried, ground and taken with wine."

THE AUTHOR'S NOTE

Injections made from walnut tree branches and twigs are popularly used to treat various tumors, being effective in alleviating esophageal cancer and cardiac cancer, promoting appetite, easing pain, invigorating blood, supplementing liver, decreasing and eradicating some tumors. The General Hospital affiliated to Beijing Military Headquarter has prepared a series of injections from walnut tree branches and twigs, such as 12130 (with Cortex Juglandis added), 12131 (with Radix Semiaquilegiae added), 12132 (with Radix Rumicis Obtusifolii added), 12133 (with Radix Actinidiae Chinensis added) and 12134 (with Radix Gossampinis added). In *Mei's Newly Compiled Recipes*, there is a prescription for treating mammocancer, saying that: "Mammary hyperplasia causes no pain at earlier stage but conceals great danger, for it may gradually develop into mammocancer. This disease can be cured with 3 grams of Cormus Iphigeniae pounded together with three walnuts and taken with wine every day. The hyperplasia needs prompt treatment lest it may develop into cancer."

RADIX DAUCIS CAROTAE

It is defined in *Daily Used Materia Medica* that: "The drug is hot and sweet in taste and non-toxic in nature, regulating intestines to promote *qi* circulation and expelling pathogenic materials detained in the stomach."

The drug is the root of *Drancus* of *Umbelliferae* family with two years of growth. The major root of the plant is thick and fleshy, about one *chi* (0.3m) in length and one *cun* (0.033m) in diameter. The leaf is large and tetrapterous. The stalk grows to 1-1.3m high in the early summer with little white flowers arranged in compound umbel and the fruits are thorny. The plant, cultivated all over China, contains volatile oil, while its root containing carotene, fats, proteins, saccharides, vitamin A, B, C, G, malic acid, mucilage, choline, folic acid and lignans.

ANTICANCER PHARMACOLOGICAL FUNCTIONS

1. Deficiency of vitamin A increases the risk of cancer in both animals and human beings. Clinical pharmacological observation of the American Cancer Academy for 20 years suggests that people who often eat carrot have 40% less chance to develop cancer than those who eat no carrot.

2. The folic acid contained in carrot resists tumor in experimental animals, and its derivative amethopterin has certain curative effect on infantile leukemia.

3. Animal experiment in Japan indicated that the lignin in carrot can increase biological immune capacity by 2-3 times, indirectly inhibiting or eradicating internal cancer cells.

4. The injection of lignin extracted from carrot into mice with sarcoma-180 has prolonged the life of the mice (60 days), while the mice in the control group all died. Biopsy indicated that cancer cells in the treated group had all disappeared .

EXPERIMENTAL FORMULAS
For leukemia:
Certain quantity of fresh carrots is squeezed to get juice for oral administration 50-100ml each time with a little sugar. Other anticancer herbs may also be given at the dame time. (*Traditional Chinese Medical and Pharmaceutical Correspondence*, Vol. 6, 1974)

HISTORICAL COMMENTS
In *True Materia Medica*, it is said that: "The drug smooths chest disorder and disperses pathogenic materials accumulated in the intestines and the stomach."
In *Dictionary of Chinese Materia Medica*, it is reported that: "The drug regulates the diaphragm, the intestines and the stomach, calms the viscera, and promotes appetite with no side effect."
In *Introduction to Medicine*, it is defined that: "The drug is sweet and hot, favorable for the supplementation and moisturization of body organs and effective in reinforcing the kidney, with the same functions as Fructus Cnidii."

THE AUTHOR'S NOTE
Carrot is rich in carotene which turns into vitamin A when absorbed. So correct absorption of carotene is essential to the resistance against cancer. Carotene is dissolvable in fat, therefore only after being dissolved in fat can it be turned into vitamin A and absorbed with the efforts of the mucous membrane of small intestine. So dietetic carrot must be cooked with cooking oil in order that carotene can be fully dissolved and absorbed. When cooked together with beef and mutton, it is not only highly nutritional, but also tasty. A little vinegar is supposed to be used in cooking carrot, otherwise the carotene will be destroyed. From the point of view of nutrition, it is improper to eat carrot in raw because only 15% of carotene can be absorbed.

It was reported by *Daily News in Japan* in November 30, 1981, that a professor in Chicago University concluded, after observing 2107 males aging from 40 to 55 for 15 years since 1975, that a fairly amount of carotene in daily food could reduce the risk of cancer. At the 15th Symposium on Chinese Pharmacology held in Japan in 1982, Japanese scholars reported a prescription called SA, which is widely used in Korea to resist cancer. The SA contains traditional Chinese medicinal herbs, such as Poria, Cortex Cinnamomi, Radix Ophiopogonis, Rhizoma Atrctyleodis Macrocephalae, Rhizoma Atractylodis Lanceae, Rhizoma Dioscoreae, Radix Glycyrrhizae, Cortex Magnoliae and Fructus Ziziphi Inermis, and the preparation made from the fresh and natural juice of carrot and cucumber. Experiments have proved that the drug significantly inhibits nephrocytic canceration in rats. The SA of low concentration (35-105μg/ml) works well in inhibiting the growth of carcinocytes without inhibiting the multiplication of the normal cells.

FRUCTUS BRUCEAE

In *Records of Integrated Chinese and Western Medicine*, it is defined that: "The drug, being extremely bitter in taste and cool in nature, cools blood and removes toxic materials."
The drug is obtained from *Brucea* of *Simarubaceae* family cultivated in the southern provinces of China. The seed, in the shape of an egg, is lightly yellow, greasy and extremely bitter. The fruit contains bruceoside, a kind of phenol and fatty acid, brusatol and bruceine A, B, C, and G.

ANTICANCER PHARMACOLOGICAL FUNCTIONS

1. The oil preparation, the water preparation and the kernel of Fructus Bruceae can lead to oncohistocytic retrograde variation and necrosis of the experimental papilloma in mice, and a similar effect is found when administered to the normal skin tissues and the cancer tissue. But the oil preparation has a weaker effect.

2. Animal experiment shows that the drug can inhibit mice sarcoma-180 and Walker's cancer-256 and spermospore.

3. The external experiment shows that its hot water extract inhibits JTC-26 with a rate of 90%.

4. Injection of the milk preparation of Fructus Bruceae to mice evidently inhibits carcinocytes of ascites hepatoma and also increases the leukocytes reduced by cyclophosphamide. The CAMP in carcinocytes becomes evidently increased after seven days' continual administration of the drug.

EXPERIMENTAL FORMULAS

For Rectocancer:

Intramuscular injection is made from a proper amount of Fructus Bruceae and administrated every other or third day with 2ml each time and 15 days as a course of treatment. (*Diagnosis, Prevention and Treatment of Cancer*)

For esophageal cancer:

> Semen Persicae 120g
> Hirudo 60g
> Haematitum 150g
> Fructus Bruceae 60g

The herbs are ground into powder and blended with lotus root starch for oral administration with 9 to 12 grams each time, 3 to 4 times a day. Patients with deficient symptoms should take this prescription with great caution. (*Newly Compiled Introduction to Traditional Chinese Medicine*)

For squamous epithelial carcinoma of the external auditory meatus:

1>. Semen Fructus Bruceae is wrapped in dried longan pulp and is taken three times a day with the following dosage: 9 grains, each time for the first week; 10 grain, each time for the second week; 11 for the third week; 12 for the fourth week; and 15 for the fifth week.

2>. The drug is pounded with vaseline and applied to the affected part once a day. (*Guangxi Traditional Chinese Medicine*)

For colocancer:

The drug is pounded and decocted for enema. (*Zhejiang Journal of Traditional Chinese Medicine*, Vol. 2, 1980)

For cervical cancer:

> Fructus Bruceae 4.5g
> Semen Strychni 4.5g
> Radix Aconiti Lateralis Preparatae 4.5g
> Calomelas 4.5g
> Realgar 9g
> Arsenium 6g
> Indigo Naturalis 9g
> Salmiacum 6g
> Fructus Mume Carbonisatus 15g
> Borneol 1.5g
> Moschus 3g

This prescription is for external application to the lesion.

For papillary tumor of the external auditory meatus:

Drop the ether extract of Fructus Bruceae into the ear or apply the oil to the lesion. (*Chinese Medical Journal*, Vol. 3, 1950)

HISTORICAL COMMENTS

It is reported in *Chinese Medical Dictionary* that: "The drug is effective in cooling blood to stop haemorrhagia, expelling stagnation to promote blood generation and curing dysentery caused by evil heat with instant effect, especially dysentery with fresh blood."

It is said in *Magic Prescriptions for Dysentery* that: "Burned Pericarpium Punicae (3g), Sliced Opium (6g), Fructus Bruceae (with oil squeezed, 90g), Radix Ginseng (0.9g), Alumen (0.6g), and Lignum Aquilariae Resinatum (0.9g) are pounded into fine powder and rolled with rice porridge into pills of 0.03-0.06g each. For curing dysentery, 1-2 pills are taken each time."

THE AUTHOR'S NOTE

Experiment in vivo with Methyl alcohol extract from the part of Fructus Bruceae above ground according to the standard set by International Tumor academy, shows that the drug evidently inhibits the activation of lymphocytic leukemia-338 (*Journal of Foreign Pharmacology*, Vol. 5, 1982). Five monomers have been further separated out from the ethanol extract of degreased Semen Bruceae, among which four are quassinoids, resisting cancer when used externally (*Traditional Chinese Pharmacological News*, Vol. 11, 1979). The butanol extract of the herb inhibits ascites cancer, Walker's sarcoma-256 and lymphatic leukemia-388 with evident effect.

PORIA

It is defined in *Secret Recipes* that: "The drug, warm in nature and bland in taste, opens atriae and promotes the production of body liquid."

The drug is obtained from the fungus on *Poria Cocos (schw.) Wolf* of *Polyporaceae* family, also known as Cloudy Poria and Pine Poria. The outer peel, the reddish part beneath the peel (red Poria), and the white part round the pine root in the middle (Poria god) of the fungus are for medical use. The fungus parasitizes on the root of *Pinus tabulacformis carr.* or the root of *Pinus massomiana lamb.. Records of Renowned Doctors* says that: "Poria grows under large pine trees in mountains and valleys, containing ß-pachyman (about 93% of the weight of the dried Poria), pachgmic acid, choline, adenine and other substances. *Shen Nung's Materia Medica* ranks Poria as a top-grade medicine.

ANTICANCER PHARMACOLOGICAL FUNCTIONS

1. The dissolvable dextran in Poria evidently inhibits mice sarcoma-180 with an effective rate of 96.88%.

2. The ethanol extract of the drug inhibits sarcoma-180 of ascites type in rats with an effective rate of 6.5%.

3. The drug increases the phagofunction of macrophagocyte and promote the formation of immunoglobulin.

EXPERIMENTAL FORMULAS

For uteromusculoma:
> Radix Salviae Miltiorrhizae 15g
> Poria 15g
> Rhizoma Scirpi 5g
> Rhizoma Zedoariae 5g
> Cortex Cinnamomi 10g

Cortex Moutan 10g

Semen Persicae 10g

Squama Manitis 10g

Concha Ostreae 10g

The prescription is taken one dosage a day in decoction. (*Journal of Zhejiang Traditional Chinese Medicine College*, Vol. 1, 1984)

For cystocancer:

Poria 30g

Polyporus 30g

Herba Scutellariae Barbatae 30g

Herba seu Radix Cirsii Japonici 30g

Herba Cephalanoploris 30g

Herba Oldenlandiae Diffusae 30g

Pollen Typhae Carbonisatus 30g

Rhizoma Dryopteris Crassirhizomae Carbonisatus 30g

Flos Sophorae Immaturus Carbonisatus 30g

Rhizoma Anemarrhenae 12g

Cortex Phellodendri 12g

Radix Rehmanniae 12g

The prescription is taken in decoction. (*Exchange of Medical Information*, Vol. 9, 1974)

For breast cancer:

Poria 9g,

Radix Astragali 4.5g,

Pericarpium Citri Reticulatae Viride 4.5g,

Radix Ginseng 3g

Rhizoma Chuanxiong 3g

Radix Bupleuri 3g

Radix Glycyrrhizae 3g

Semen Gleditsiae Sinensis 3g

Radix Angelicae Sinensis 3g

Radix Paeoniae Alba 3g

Radix Rehmanniae 3g

Fructus Chaenomelis 6g

The prescription is taken in decoction. (*Journal of Jiangsu Traditional Chinese Medicine*, Vol. 1, 1962)

For gastrocancer:

Poria 4g

Radix Ginseng 4g

Rhizoma Atractylodis Macrophalae 4g

Rhizoma Pinelliae 4g

Pericarpium Citri Reticulatae 2g

Fructus Ziziphi Inermis 2g

Radix Glycyrrhizae 1g

The above herbs are ground into powder to be taken 1g a time and three times a day. (*Elucidation on Clinical Application of Prescriptions in the Han Dynasty*)

For other cancers:

15g of Poria is decocted in 300ml of water and taken orally in three times. This prescription is taken one dosage a day. (*Traditional Chinese Medical And Pharmaceutical Research Data*, Vol. 6, 1978)

HISTORICAL COMMENTS

In the book *On Pharmaceutical Properties*, it is said that: "The drug increases appetite, stops hiccup, tranquilizes the mind and cures pulmonary flaccidity syndrome."

In *Ri Hua Zhi Materia Medica*, it is said that: "The drug cures five kinds of impairments and seven kinds of damage, wakes up the mind and benefits intelligence."

In *Records of Integrated Traditional Chinese and Western Medicine*, it is reported that: "Poria has to be cut into thin pieces or pounded before decocting, otherwise, it can not be fully decocted."

THE AUTHOR'S NOTE

One hundred cases of uteromusculoma were treated with modified Poria-Rambles Cinnamomi Decoction (Ramulus Cinnamomi, Poria, Cortex Moutan, Semen Persicae, and Radix Paeoniae, 4 grams each) with 36 to 200 doses of the decoction in general. The tumor mass disappeared in 46 cases and reduced to half of its original size in 34 cases.

HERBA ARTEMISIAE CAPILLARIS

In *Modified Materia Medica*, it is defined that: "The drug is bland in taste and apt to drainage, ranked as number one medicine for treating the impairment of the spleen and the stomach due to pathogenic wet heat."

The drug is obtained from the seedling of *Artemsia Capillaris Thunb.* of *Compositae* family, mainly containing scoparone, chlorogenic acid, caffeic acid and volatile oils. Many herbs of this family bear anticancer function. In Japan, for instance, the decoction of *Folium Artemisia princeps. p.* is used for treating various cancers.

ANTICANCER PHARMACOLOGICAL FUNCTIONS:

1. The drug intensely resists carcinogenic model and its carcinogenic virus, inhibiting Aspergillus flavus and aflatoxin B with 100% effective rate.

2. The hot water extract inhibits ascites sarcoma-180 with an effective rate of 21.6%, while the ethanol extract works with a rate of 18.5%.

EXPERIMENTAL FORMULAS

For cheilocarcinoma:

Herba Artemisiae Capillaris 3g
Radix Stellariae 3g
Cornu Rhinoceri 3g
Herba Dendrobii 3g
Fructus Citri Aurantii 3g
Radix Ophiopogoni 3g
Radix Glycyrrhizae 3g
Radix Rehmanniae 3g
Radix Scutellariae 3g
Rhizoma Anemarrhenae 3g
Folium Eriobotryae 3g
Folium Lophatheri 20g
Medulla Junci 20g

The prescription is taken in decoction after meal. (*Orthodox Surgery*)

For primary liver cancer:

Herba Artemisiae Capillaris 12g

Fructus Gardeniae 9g
Rhizoma Scirpi 9g
Rhizoma Zedoariae 9g
Squama Manitis 9g
Radix Curcumae 9g
Fructus Citri Aurantii 9g
Concha Osteae 30g
Herba Scutellariae Barbatae 30g
Rhizoma Paridis 30g
Herba Oldenlandiae Diffusae 30g
Nidus Vespae 15g.

The prescription can be modified in accordance with the patient's condition. (*Shanghai Journal of Traditional Chinese Medicine*, Vol. 9, 1979)

HISTORICAL COMMENTS

Records of Renowned Doctors says that: "The drug cures jaundice, difficult urination, headache due to pathogenic heat, and abdominal mass."

Ri Hua Zhi Materia Medica suggests that: "The drug cure pestilence, mania due to pathogenic heat, headache and dizziness, pain caused by wind, miasma, female abdominal mass, and extreme renal deficiency."

Screened Materia Medica holds that: "The drug diminishes stasis, stops pain, activates diaphragm and expels phlegm."

HERBA SAGINAE JAPONICAE

It is defined in *Dictionary of Chinese Materia Medica* that: "The drug, bitter and hot in taste and cool in nature, cures scrofula and carbuncle."

The drug is obtained from a herb of *Caryophyllaceae* family, the whole plant is for medical use. In Materia Medica, Herba Aristolochiae Mollissimae was mistaken as Herba Saginae Faponicae. Long time ago, Chen Cangqi pointed out that Herba Aristollochiae Mollissimae was characterized by its large and thick size (not as thin as silk). Herba Saginae Japonicae is cultivated in the Changjiang River Basin, the Huanghe River Basin and the south of Northeast China, containing saponins, volatile oils and flavonoid glycosides.

ANTICANCER PHARMACOLOGICAL FUNCTIONS

1. The water extract of the drug is evidently resistant against sarcoma-180, sarcoma-77, cervical cancer-14 and lymphatic leukemia-615 in rats.

2. The water extract of the drug also bears curative effect on multiple malignant leukemia and chronicle granulocytic leukemia.

3. The drug inhibits cervical cancer-14 with an effective rate of 53.35% and 57.9% respectively.

4. Its saponin and volatile oil inhibits sarcoma-180 of mice with 11% and 14.8% effective rate. These low rates suggest that flavoglycoside is its effective anticancer element.

EXPERIMENTAL FORMULAS

For lymphodenoma:

15-30 grams of the drug is decocted for oral administration. The fresh herb is pounded and applied to the lesion. (*Handbook of Commonly Used Chinese Medicinal Herbs*)

HISTORICAL COMMENTS

In *Supplementation to Materia Medica*, it is reported that: "The drug, growing in shady places with the size of a rat paw, is extremely hot in taste, curing dermatitis rhuis when crushed and applied to the lesion."

In *Collection of Folk Recipes in Guizhou*, it is reported that: "The drug cures carbuncle and suppurative dermatitis when applied externally, carious tooth when sucked, and epistaxis when filled into the nose."

In *Newly Compiled Materia Medica in Zhejiang*, it is said that: "The drug cures hemoptysis and hematemesis when dried, ground and blended with Gypsum Fibrosum which has been saturated in young boy's urine. The pulvis is taken 3 to 9 grams each time and once or twice daily. This formula removes hemostasis while in the process of stopping hemorrhage."

RADIX RUBIAE

It is defined in *Materia Medica* that: "The drug diminishes stagnation with its warm nature, penetrates liver with its sour taste and enters blood with its salty taste, especially effective in promoting blood circulation and invigorating blood."

The drug is obtained from a herb of *Rubiaceae* family. The root is for medical use, mainly containing purpurin, alizarin and pseudopurpurin.

ANTICANCER PHARMACOLOGICAL FUNCTIONS

1. The acetyl chemical compound of the two kinds of cyclic hexapeptide extracted from Radix Rubicae evidently inhibits lymphocytic leukemia-388 with a higher curative value.

2. These two kinds of peptide also evidently inhibit the activation of lymphocytic leukemia-1210, monoactone-38, Lewis pulmonary cancer and solid tumor.

3. The external experiment shows that the liquid, in which Radix Rubicae was soaked, inhibits JTC-26 with an effective rate of 90%.

4. The internal experiment shows that the extract from the drug by methanol inhibits sarcoma-180 of ascites type in rats with an effective rate of 80% and the liquid, in which the drug was soaked, inhibits with an effective rate of 13%.

EXPERIMENTAL FORMULAS

For esophageal cancer:

1>.   Radix Rubiae 10g
       Bulbus Allii Macrostemi 10g
       Cormus Iphigeniae 10g
       Fructus Trichosanthis 25g
       Semen Persicae 6g
       Semen Armeniacae Amarum 6g
       Rhizoma Pinelliae 6g
       Fructus Arctii 6g
       Radix Cyathulae 6g
       Flos Mume 6g
       Flos Inulae 6g
       Cortex magnoliae 5g
       Radix Salviae Miltiorrhizae 15g
       Ocherum Rubrum 15g

The prescription is taken in decoction one dosage a day. (*Collection of Shi Jinmen's Experienced Prescriptions*)

2>.　　Radix Rubiae 9g

　　　　Calyx Kaki 9g

　　　　Fructus Aesculus Wilsonii 9g

　　　　Rhizoma Pinelliae 9g

　　　　Flos Inulae 9g

　　　　Herba Lobeliae Chinensis 24g

　　　　Pericarpium Zanthoxyli Bungeani 2.5g

　　　　Flos Rosae 1.5g

　　　　Semen Canavaliae Gladiatae 15g

The prescription is taken in decoction one dosage a day. (*Prescriptions for Tumors*)

For uteromusculoma:

　　　　Radix Rubiae 10g

　　　　Ramulus Cinnamomi 10g

　　　　Poria 10g

　　　　Semen Persicae 10g

　　　　Cortex Moutan 10g

　　　　Radix Paeoniae Latiflorae 10g

　　　　Olibanum 10g

　　　　Myrrha 10g

　　　　Radix Salviae Miltiorrhizae 15g

　　　　Os Sepiae 15g

　　　　Concha Ostreae 30g

The above ingredients are pounded into powder and rolled with honey into pills. (*Journal of Zhejiang Traditional Chinese Medicine*, Vol. 1, 1985)

For cancers with blood vomiting:

　　　　Radix Rubiae 4.5g

　　　　Radix Notoginseng 3g

　　　　Extractum Spatholobi 6g

The prescription is taken in decoction one dosage a day. (*Supplementation to Medicine*)

HISTORICAL COMMENTS

In *Collection of Comments on Materia Medica*, it is said that: "The drug promotes blood circulation when used with wine, stops hemorrhage when roasted. The drug also can invigorate blood, activate channels, cure hemostasis and arthralgia due to blood deficiency without any side effect on blood. The drug benefits women when combined with Radix Angelicae Sinensis and Radix paeoniae Alba."

In *Pearl Bag*, it is said that: "The drug diminishes various symptoms caused by stagnant blood."

In *Ri Hua Zhi Materia Medica*, it is suggested that: "The drug stops epistaxis and cures leukorrhagia, puerperal faintness, no lactation milk, menoxenia, stool with blood, anal fistula and hemorrhoid."

In *Ge Zhu Prescriptions*, it is mentioned that: "The drug relieves pain caused by wind, promotes menstruation, induces abortion and cures jaundice and abdominal mass."

In *Elucidation on Materia Medica*, it is said that: "The drug promotes blood circulation. Patients suffering from hemopathy complicated with diarrhea and poor appetite are excluded from using this drug."

GLOSSOGYNE

It is defined in *Elicitation on Materia Medica* that: "The drug, being sweet in taste and cold in nature, draws out smallpox virus."

This drug is obtained from *Lentinus Pleurotaceae* of *Agaricales Basidiomycetes* family, mainly growing on the branches of *Castanea mollissima Bl.*, *Lithocarpus glaber (Thunb.) Nakai*, and *Quercus dentata Thunb.*. The whole fungi can be used medically. The fungus is produced all over China and edible when fresh or dried with caution, containing multi-carbohydrates, protein, vitamin A, B2 and a great quantity of ergosterol which turns into vitamin D when exposed to ultraviolet ray.

ANTICANCER PHARMACOLOGICAL FUNCTIONS

1. Lentinan resists carcinogenic materials effectively and inhibits tumor with an effective rate of 70%. In abroad, Lentinan extracted from Letnus edodes was used to inhibit sarcoma-180 in mice with an effective rate of 70-100%. Two carcinogenic material found in the juice of Glossogyne pertains to carbohydrate.

2. Animal experiment shows that the carbohydrate in *Tricholoma ionides (Bull. ex Fri.) Quel.*, *Agaricus bisporus (Lange) sing.*, and *Pleurotus ostreatus (Jaeq. ex Fr.) Quel.* of the same family of Glossogyne inhibits tumor with rates of 91.3%, 12.7% and 75.3.%, respectively.

3. It is still unclear about the anticancer mechanism of carbohydrate. Some people have suggested that carbohydrate can stimulate reticuloendothelial system nonspecifically, increasing the immune reaction capacity of the host against specific carcinocytic antigen.

EXPERIMENTAL FORMULAS

For various cancers:

Glossogyne is taken as a food or decoction. (*Traditional Chinese Medical and Pharmacological Research Data*, Vol. 6, 1978)

HISTORICAL COMMENTS

In *Rest and Diet Recipes*, it is reported that: "The drug, sweet in taste and moderate in nature, increases appetite and cures turbid urine and incontinence."

In *Dictionary of Chinese Materia Medica*, it is said that: "The drug nourishes *qi* to increase appetite, eases diseases caused by pathogenic wind and promote blood circulation."

In *True Materia Medica*, it is suggested that: "Glossogyne is the best food. All mushrooms and fungi are affected by heat radiated from earth, but only Glossogyne is sweet in taste and moderate in nature, increasing appetite, curing urine incontinence and improving middle *jiao* deficiency. The top grade Glossogyne is produced in winter which is fleshy and as large as a copper coin."

THE AUTHOR'S NOTE

Nearly all the carbohydrates extracted from various edible mushrooms have anticancer function.

HERBA ISODI

In *Handbook of Ningxia Medicinal Herbs*, it is said that: "The drug, bitter in taste and cold in nature, clears away heat to remove toxic materials and invigorates spleen to promote blood circulation."

The drug is obtained from *Isodon glaucocalyx (Maxim.) kudo* of *Labiatae* family, cultivated over the northeast and the northwest of China, also known as *She Zong Guan*. The whole herb is for medical use. Its stalk and leaf contain volatile oil and the whole herb reacts with alkaloid, lactone and flavone. The anticancer element in Japanese Herba Isodi is found to be enmein.

ANTICANCER PHARMACOLOGICAL FUNCTIONS

1. Isodon glaucocalyx kudo has evident cytotoxicity over esophageal carcinocytic strain.

2. The ethanol extract of Japanese Herba Isodi inhibits sarcoma-180 in rats with an effective rate of 90.7% and the hot water extract with an effective rate of 20%.

3. Enmein bears anticancer function, prolonging the survival of mice after ascites cancer having been inoculated. Bi-ethylenmein shows even greater effect in resisting cancer.

4. The exposure of colon bacillus to ultraviolet rays proved that Japanese Herba Isodi resists the activation of mutation, the effective ingredient being Enmein.

5. Isodon glancocalyx kudo inhibits various tumors when transplanted to animals, and Enmein is thought to be the effective element.

6. Isodon glancocalyx kudo inhibits the activation of ascites cancer.

7. The herb has cytotoxicity over Hela cells no matter in what season it is collected. But those collected in May have the highest effect, the lowest effective concentration being 1:3200.

8. Ponicidin extracted from the herb has evident cytotoxicity over ascites carcinocytes cultured externally, and inhibits metastasis of tumor with positive effect without involving the normal functions of the bone marrow, the liver and the kidney.

EXPERIMENTAL FORMULAS

For esophagocancer and gastrocancer at earlier or meddle stage:

1>. 90 to 120 grams of the fresh drug is decocted for oral taking as tea.

2>. 5kg of the whole herb is boiled in 15kg of water for an hour, then the residue of the first boiling is decocted again in 10kg of water for another hour. The two decoctions are filtered and condensed into 3000ml, with each milliliter containing 5g of the crude drug. The broth is taken three times a day, 10ml each time. (*Medical Research Correspondence*, Vol. 5, 1974)

For various cancers:

10g of the drug's leaves and stalk is decocted in 150ml of water for oral administration three times daily. (*Traditional Chinese Medical and Pharmaceutical Research Data*, Vol. 6, 1978)

For cancer of the breast:

Herba Isodi 30g
Herba Aristolochiae Mollissimae 30g
Herba Taraxaci 30g
Herba Pyrolae 15g
Herba Pteridis Multifidae 15g

The prescription is taken in decoction one dosage a day. (*Surgery in Traditional Chinese Medicine*)

HISTORICAL COMMENTS

In *Jilin Medicinal Herbs*, it is said that: "The drug invigorates the stomach and regulates the intestine, curing poor appetite and digestion."

In *Handbook of Ningxia Medicinal Herbs*, it is reported that: "The drug clears away heat to remove toxic materials, invigorates the stomach to activate blood, curing gastritis, acute hepatitis and cold with fever."

In *Newly Compiled Materia Medica in Zhennan*, it is suggested that: "The drug has been used to treat cancer and tumor."

THE AUTHOR'S NOTE

Nanjing Pharmaceutical Academy has separated out 11 substances from the drug, among which 9 were tested for the anticancer function, and 5 were found evidently prolonging the survival of mice with ascites cancer and killing QGY7702 cells of liver cancer in human. Two new diterpene compounds were found to have high activation, prolonging the life of rats suffering from ascites cancer with effective rates of 111.8% and 171.8% respectively. (*Jiangsu Medicine and Pharmacology*, Vol. 10, 1984)

Sugar Coated Ginseng and Herbal Isodi Tablet developed in Zhejiang Province was used to treat 101 cases of gastrocancer who had undergone an operation. The survival rate for a year was found to be 82.2%, while that of the control group with only chemotherapy was 64.1%. The former is obviously higher than the latter. The Tumor Department of the First Teaching Hospital of Henan Medical College has used the tablets for years and their experience indicates that the tablet is one of the best drugs for breast cancer.

HERBA GELSEMII

It is defined in *Canon of Materia Medica* that: "The drug, hot in taste and warm in nature, cures incised wound and lactostasis."

The drug is obtained from Gelsemium elegans Benth. of Loganiaceae family, growing in Zhejiang, Fujian, Guangdong, Guangxi, Guizhou, and Yunnan provinces, containing koumine, kouminidine, gelsemine, sempervine and kounidine. Kouminicine is very poisonous. The whole herb is for medical use.

ANTICANCER PHARMACOLOGICAL FUNCTIONS

1. All the biological alkali contained in the drug inhibits sarcoma-180 transplanted to mice.
2. Gelsemine is effective to relieve pain and carcinalgia in rats. The recommended dosage is 0.5-2mg.

EXPERIMENTAL FORMULAS

For gastrocancer:

30 grams of the drug is decocted for oral taking as tea. (*Reference for Clinical Treatment of Tumor*)

For tumors of the abdominal cavity:

      Herba Gelsemii 15g
      Folium Artemisiae Argyi 15g
      Radix Sanguisorbae 15g
      Radix Arnebiae 15g
      Rhizoma Zedoariae 15g
      Radix Salviae Miltiorrhizae 30g
      Hirudo 10g

The prescription is used with care if the patient has hypermenorrhea or metrorrhagia. (*Reference for Clinical Treatment of Tumor*)

HISTORICAL COMMENTS

In *Records of Renowned Doctors*, it is said that: "The drug diminishes hemostasis."

In *Origin of Materia Medica*, it is reported that: "The herb with purple color eliminates hemostasis and that with green color expels phlegm stagnation."

In *Atlas of Guangxi Medicinal Plants*, it is suggested that: "Paste made from the drug reduces tumor."

In *Records of Lingnan Medicinal Herbs*, it is pointed out that: "To cure scrofula, certain amount of Herba Gelsemii and Rhizoma Dioscoreae Cirrhosae are pounded, decocted in vinegar for an hour and applied to the lesion for three days after cooling down."

Thirty-eight cases of liver cancer were treated in Guangxi Medical College with 125mg of the powder of the drug for oral administration. The herb was especially effective in one case, moderately effective in 3 cases and effective in 19 cases. The drug contains dead poison and the dosage recommended in *Clinical Guide for Tumor Diagnosis* seems to be too large.

RHIZOMA TYPHONII

It is defined in *Sichuan Chinese Pharmacological History* that: "The drug, very warm in nature and hot-sweet in taste, contains toxin and cures gastralgia and arthralgia due to blood disorder."

The drug is obtained from *Typhonium giganteum Engl.* of *Araceae* family, containing Mucilage, Calcii Oxalas, Sucrose, Saponins, ß-sitosterol, Inositol and alkaloids. The commercial plant is divided into Rhizoma Typhonii and Radix Aconiti Coreani, which differ in actions.

ANTICANCER PHARMACOLOGICAL FUNCTIONS
External screening test shows that the drug is active against cancer.

EXPERIMENTAL FORMULAS
For reticulocytic sarcoma:
Collect a single-rooted fresh lotus and pound it into paste for application to the lesion; or apply the paste made by blending the powder of the herb with warm water to the lesion. (*Journal of Hubei Traditional Chinese Medicine*, Vol. 6, 1980)
For lymphoma:
The drug is pounded for external application to the lesion. (*Traditional Chinese Pharmacology*)

HISTORICAL COMMENTS
It is reported in *History of Medicinal Plants in China* that: "The drug cures lymphotuberculosis."
It is recommended in *Chinese Pharmacology* that: "The drug relieves pain, removes toxic material and promotes *qi* or the circulation of vital energy."
It is pointed out in *Folk Herbal Medicine in Jiangxi* that: "Scrofula can be treated with fresh single-rooted lotus which is pounded with a little egg white and applied to the lesion once daily."

THE AUTHOR'S NOTE
The commercial drug is often used as Rhizoma Typhonii. Actually the two drugs are quite different in actions. Rhizoma Typhonii is the root of *Aconitum Coreanum (Levl.) Rap.* of *Ranunculaceae* family, containing aconitines. It is pointed out in Origin of Materia Medica that: "The drug penetrates stomach *yin* to reach the *yang* phase, leads the effect of medicine upwards to activate the heart and the lung, clears away heat accumulated by cryoplasia due to *yang* deficiency with drugs expelling pathogenic wind as adjuvant. But Rhizoma Typhonii itself does not function to dominate pathogenic wind." It has been proved that A. Kusnezoffii Reichb. of the same family also resists cancer, but there is still no report on whether Radix Aconiti has this function.

RHIZOMA PARIDIS

Su Jing in the Tang Dynasty said that: "The drug, bitter in and slightly cold and toxic in nature, cures convulsion due to pathogenic heat accumulated in the abdomen."

The drug is obtained from *Paris* of *Liliaceae* family, which is a perennial herb with short and oval radix and stalk. Its section is powderish in texture and whitish in color. The single stalk on the earth is erect and about 1 meter high, the top is covered with palmately compound leaves arranged in one layer in most and two layers in a few. The whorled leaves usually appear to be 6 to 8. The flower is either yellow or green, under which protrudes a bract. The fruit is purple black with an opening along the dorsal suture. The root is for medical use. The drug is produced all over China. Plants of the same family such as *P. polyphylla Sm. var. yunnanensis (Franch) Hand. Mazz.*, *P. polyphylla var. stenophylla Franch.*, and *P. polyphylla var. appendiculata Hara* are also used as the substitutes for the drug.

ANTICANCER PHARMACOLOGICAL FUNCTIONS

1. Screening test in vitro shows that the drug inhibits oncocytes.

2. Experiment in vivo indicates that the butanol extract of the drug inhibits animal tumor. Saponin I and VI have a cytotoxicity over leukemia-338 and leukemia-1210.

3. The drug has been proved to have a cytotoxicity by bean sprout screening method.

4. Bacteriophagic screening test shows that the drug is anti- bacteriophagic, and this suggests that the drug has active functions against cancer.

5. The drug has been proved to inhibit mice sarcoma-180 , sarcoma-37 and solid hepatocancer.

6. Experiment in vitro proved that the hot water extract of the herb inhibits JTC-26 with an effective rate of 50-70%.

EXPERIMENTAL FORMULAS

For encephaloma:

1>.   Rhizoma Paridis 30g
        Radix Clematidis 30g
        Fructus Chaenomelis 9g

The prescription is taken, one dosage a day, in decoction with 3g of Radix Notoginseng powder. (*Handbook of Practical Anticancer Drugs*)

2>. 30 grams of Rhizoma Paridis and 10 pieces of Bellamya are pounded with 1 gram of Borneol for application to the liver region once a day, totally for three days. (*Journal of Zhejiang Traditional Chinese Medicine*, Vol. 10, 1984)

For nasopharyngocancer:

        Rhizoma Paridis 50-100g
        Ramulus Uncariae cum uncis 15g
        Rhizoma Arisaematis 50-150g
        Herba Conyzae 15g
        Radix Pseudostellariae Heterophyllae 15g
        Spica Prunellae 15g
        Rhizoma Alismatis 50g
        Radix Rubi Parvifolii 100g

The prescription is taken one dosage a day. (*Practical Oncology*)

For esophagocancer:

        Rhizoma Paridis 12g
        Radix et Rhizoma Rhei 9g
        Semen Momordicae 9g
        Mirabilite 12g
        Rhizoma Pinelliae 0.3g

The ingredients are ground into powder and rolled with honey into pills of 3 grams each. 3 to 4 pills are sucked daily. (*Prevention and Treatment of Common Tumors*)

For liposarcoma:

Rhizoma Paridis (6g) and Radix Polygoni Multiflori (240g) are pounded in a stone pot into paste for application to the tumor and covered with oil paper, twice a day. (*Journal of New Traditional Chinese Medicine*, Vol. 2, 1977)

HISTORICAL COMMENTS

It is said in *Materia Medica* that: "The drug cures convulsion, epilepsy with shaking of the head, mania, carbuncle, vulvitis, infantile twitch of the hands and feet, scrofula, sore throat, snake bite, ascariasis, teniasis, oxyuriasis and edema." A proverb says that: "I am Rhizoma Paridis, living deep in the mountains; Once carbuncle is caught in my sight, I cure it easily."

In *Properties of Medicinal Herbs*, it is said that: "The drug invigorates blood to promote the circulation of *qi*, reinforces essence to supplement the kidney and cures various diseases."

In *Collection of Pin Hu Simple Prescription*, it is pointed out that: "Pyogenic scrofula can be cured with the liquid squeezed out of the drug and Rhizoma Paridis."

HERBA LEONURI

It is defined in *Elicitation on Materia Medica* that: "The drug, hot and sweet in taste, and slightly warm and nontoxic in nature, diminishes hematostasis and promotes hematopoiesis."

The drug is obtained from a plant of *Labiatae* family. The whole plant is for medical use. The plant is cultivated in most part of China, mainly containing leonurine, stachydrine, V_a and rutin.

ANTICANCER PHARMACOLOGICAL FUNCTIONS

The hot water extract of the herb inhibits sarcoma-180 in rats with an effective rate of 78%. It was found to resist cancer activation with a higher effect and increases the body weight of the mice, with anticancer and nutritional functions. Radix Catharanthi, tested simultaneously, inhibits tumor with a higher rate (95.9%), but the body weight of the mice become reduced.

EXPERIMENTAL FORMULAS

For celiac tumor with hemostasis:

300 grams of the drug is decocted in half water and half wine for oral administration. (*Min Dong Materia Medica*)

For breast cancer:

2.5kg of the drug is cut into small pieces and decocted into thick broth for oral administration frequently. (*Prescriptions-worth a Thousand Gold*)

For uterocancer:

15g of the drug is decocted in 300ml of water for oral administration three times a day. (*Traditional Chinese Medical and Pharmaceutical Research Data*, Vol. 6, 1978)

HISTORICAL COMMENTS

It is said in *Collection of Comments on Materia Medica* that: "The drug promotes blood circulation without affecting the new blood and nourishes blood without inducing any hematostasis, and deserves to be ranked as a holy medicine for curing hemopathy."

It is reported in *Materia Medica*: "The whole herb is for medical use. When treating hematophase syndrome (caused by the invasion of heat-wind into the hematophase in the *Jueyin* Channel of the hand and the foot), ophthalmopathy and menoxenia, the seed is preferred; while when treating swelling, ulcer, carbuncle, edema and puerperal diseases, the whole herb is preferred. This is because the root, the stalk, the flower and the leaf of the herb are effective in promoting circulation of body fluid, and its seed is good at nourishing."

It is pointed out in *Corrigendum to Materia Medica* that: "The drug, though not very warm or hot, is classified into drugs of warm and dry nature due to its strong smell and bitter taste, fit for treating cryopathy in winter, but not for pyropathy in summer."

RHIZOMA ALPINIAE

It is defined in *Corrigendum to Materia Medica* that: "The drug, extremely hot in taste and warm in nature, pertains purely to *yang* and cures cold syndrome of the middle-*jiao*."

The drug is obtained from a herb of the *Zingiberaceae* family. Its radix is for medical use, containing 0.5-1.5% of volatile oils, flavonids, kaempferol, quercetin and galangol. Its decoction resists a variety of bacteria such as anthrax bacillus and pneumococcus.

ANTICANCER PHARMACOLOGICAL FUNCTIONS

1. Experiment in vivo with the hot water extract of the drug on sarcoma-180 of ascites type in rats shows that the drug inhibits tumor with an effective rate of 51.8% and evidently resists cancer activation.

2. The drug inhibits aflatoxin B_1 with 100% effective rate.

EXPERIMENTAL FORMULAS

For various cancers of the body surface:

An appropriate amount of the drug is pounded into powder, blended with vaseline and applied to the lesion. (*Traditional Chinese Pharmacological Correspondence*, Vol. 6, 1974)

For hepatocarcinoma:

   Rhizoma Alpiniae 10g
   Flos Caryophylli 10g
   Fructus Amomi 10g
   Rhizoma Zingiberis 15g
   Bulbus Allii 8g
   Salt 5g

The above ingredients are pounded and applied to the acupoints of Zhongwan and Zu Shan Li (on both feet) once a day. (*Journal of Zhejiang Traditional Chinese Medicine*, Vol. 10, 1984)

For gastralgia caused by stomach cancer:

Equal portions of Rhizoma Alpiniae and Semen Arecae are roasted into powder and taken 6 grams each time with millet porridge. (*Selected Prescriptions*)

HISTORICAL COMMENTS

It is pointed out in *Corrigendum to Materia Medica* that: "The drug cures frequent regurgitation accompanied with watery diarrhea and undigested food in the stool."

It is reported in *Newly Compiled Materia Medica* that: "To cure gastrodynia, the drug has to be combined with Rhizoma Atractyloidis Lanceae, otherwise the curative effect is not stable because Rhizoma Alpiniae itself can not diminish wetness."

It is said in *Annotation on Materia Medica* that: "The drug, contraindicating to salt, is effective in treating nausea caused by gastrothermosis, acute gastroenteritis due to sunstroke, diarrhea induced by enterothermosis and gastrodynia caused by gastrasthenia."

SARGASSUM

It is defined in *Canon of Materia Medica* that: "The drug, bitter in taste and cold in nature, cures tumor, goiter, scrofula, stasis, carbuncle and abdominal mass."

The drug is obtained from the thallus of *S. fusiforme (Herv.) Setch.* and *S. pallidum (Jurn.) C. Ag.* of *Sargassaceae* family. The former contains alginic acid and mannitol, while the latter sargassan and polypeptide. However, both pertains to phaeophyta, which usually contains phenols of sargassan.

ANTICANCER PHARMACOLOGICAL FUNCTIONS

1. The crude extract of the drug has certain inhibiting effect on uterocancer-14, sarcoma-180 and lymphoma-I of ascites type (L_1) transplanted to animals.

2. The hot water extract of Sargassum Kiellanianum inhibits sarcoma-180 transplanted subcutaneously to rats with an effective rate of 93.7% after the drug being administrated celiacally for ten days in succession. Statistical analysis showed that its main substance is polysaccharides and the total amount of carbohydrate it contains is about 60%.

EXPERIMENTAL FORMULAS

For breast cancer:
>Sargassum 30g
>Thallus Laminariae 30g
>Semen Cassiae 30g
>Fructus Ligustri Lucidi 15g
>Flos Lonicerae 15g
>Radix Salviae Miltiorrhizae 15g
>Pericarpium Citri Reticulatae 15g
>Radix Rehmanniae 15g
>Radix Pseudostellariae Heterophyllae 18g
>Poria 12g
>Fructus Lycii 12g
>Herba Dendrobii 12g

The prescription is taken one dosage a day. (*Exchange of Medical Information*, Vol. 6, 1974)

For osteoangioma:
>Sargassum 60g
>Rhizoma Drynariae 60g
>Fossillia Ossis Mastodi 60g
>Concha Ostreae 60g
>Radix Dipsaci 60g
>Rhizoma Polygonati 60g
>Rhizoma Cibotii 60g
>Herba Taxilli 60g
>Caulis Lonicerae 60g
>Vascular Aurantii 60g
>Cortex Eucommiae 90g
>Spica Prunellae 90g
>Rhizoma Scirpi 30g
>Radix Zedoariae 30g
>Radix Salviae Miltiorrhizae 30g
>Tabanus 30g
>Olibanum 30g
>Myrrha 30g
>Herba Dendrobii 120g

Scolopendra 15g

Rhizoma Curcumae Longae 30g

Radix Achyranthis Bidentatae 30g

Cornu Cervi 90g

The above ingredients are decocted in an appropriate amount of water and then added with 500g of honey to make a paste for oral administration with 2 to 3 spoonful each time, 4 times a day. (*Prevention and Treatment of Tumor*)

For osteoangioendthelioma:

Sargassum 30g

Thallus Laminariae seu Eckloniae 30g

Concha Ostreae 30g

Rhizoma Drynariae 30g

Spica Prunellae 30g

Herba Dendrobii 15g

The prescription is taken one dosage a day in decoction. (*Prevention and Treatment of Tumors*)

For lung cancer:

Sargassum 15g

Carapax Eretmochelytis 15g

Plastrum Testudinis 15g

Fructus Bruceae 7.5g

Bufo 6g

The first four ingredients are put between two new tiles, calcined over coal fire till turning yellow, ground into powder and blended with Bufo powder. The prepared powder is packaged in capsules and taken 6g a time with boiled water, twice a day. (*Newly Compiled Traditional Chinese Medicine*)

For uteromusculoma:

Sargassum 40g

Thallus Laminariae seu Eckloniae 20g

Concha Ostreae 40g

Rhizoma Arisaematis 15g

Bulbus Fritillariae Cirrhosae 15g

Fructus Trichosanthis 15g

Radix Paeoniae Latiflorae 15g

Radix Angelicae Sinensis 15g

Pollen Typhae 15g

Faeces Trogopterore 15g

Rhizoma Zedoariae 10g

Rhizoma Scirpi 10g

Radix Salviae Miltiorrhizae 40g

Spica Prunellae 20g

The prescription is taken in decoction. (*Jilin Chinese Herbal Medicine*, Vol. 3, 1983)

For carcinoma of the parotid gland:

Sargassum 30g

Concha Ostreae 30g

Rhizoma Dioscoreae Bulbiferae 30g

Thallus Laminariae seu Eckloniae 15g

Radix Ranunculi Ternati 15g

The prescription is taken one dosage a day in decoction. (*Handbook of Practical Anticancer Drugs*)

HISTORICAL COMMENTS

It is reported in *Newly Compiled Materia Medica* that: "The drug is specific for hard mass and sclerosis with its salty taste. However the drug alone cannot exert such a remarkable effect, it is frequently used with other medicines to guide it to enter into the channels. A man asked me to treat his mother suffering from goiter during my visit to the Yan and the Zhao Kingdom. I wrote out a prescription containing Sargassum (15g), Poria (15g), Radix Platycodi (3g), Rhizoma Arisaematis (3g), Rhizoma Atractylodis Macrocephalae (15g), Radix Glycyrhizae (3g), Pericarpium Citri Reticulatae (4.5g), Semen Sinapis (6g). The prescription was taken in decoction. The first four doses reduced the goiter by half and the last four diminished it completely."

It is recorded in *Doctor's Panacea* that: "Scrofula with macrocervix can be cured with the drug (torrefied in buckwheat flour) and Bombyx Batryticatus (roasted), decocted in Albamyrice broth and made into pills of the size of a Chinese parasol seed for oral administration with millet gruel. The dosage for each is 60 pills."

It is suggested in *Handbook of Prescriptions for Emergencies* that: "To treat hypomaxilloscrofula, 300 grams of Sargassum is immersed in 500ml of wine for several days and taken frequently with a little each time."

It is said in *Prescriptions According to Three Categories of Pathogenic Factors of Diseases* that: "For all kinds of goiters caused by the disorder of *qi*, overstrain, deficiency of the spleen, and psychotension, Sargassum, Radix Gentianae, Gecko, Medulla Tetrapanacis, Thallus Laminariae seu Eckloniae, Alumen, Usnea and Massa Medicata Fermentata are ground into powder and taken three times a day with 1 gram of wine. During the administration of the formula, no crucian carp, pork, hot and crude vegetables are taken."

THE AUTHOR'S NOTE

A case of opthalmoma was cured in Ophthalmology Dept. of Beijing Hospital with 223 doses of a prescription composed of Sargassum, Spica Prunellae, Thallus Laminariae seu Eckloniae, Rhizoma Smilacis Glabrace and Folium Pyrrosiae. The prescription was taken one dose daily without any other medication.

It is said that Sargassum antagonizes Radix Glycyrrnizae, but Li Shizhen said: "Li Donghuan treated scrofula with Scirrhomalacia Prescription, using Sargassum and Radix Glycyrrnizae simultaneously. That is because the hard mass is so stubborn that mild medicine cannot subdue it, therefore antagonistic ones must be applied." The combination of these two drugs for treating goiter is also recorded in *Principles for Treatment* and *Golden Mirror of Medicine*. It was reported in *Journal of Zhejiang Traditional Chinese Medicine* (Vol. 3, 1980) that a case (female, 59 years old) of osteoma with osteolytic fracture was treated with Sargassum, Radix Glycyrrnizae and Thallus Laminariae seu Eckloniae (15 grams each). The symptoms were, after several months, greatly improved with no further progression of the tumor. This is an example of using "antagonistic medicine".

RADIX STEPHANIAE TETRANDRAE

It is defined in *True Materia Medica* that: "The drug, bitter in taste and extremely cold in nature, seems to be dangerous but swift to subdue diseases."

The drug is obtained from a herb of *Menispermaceae* family, the root of which is for medical use. Besides, *Cocculus trilobus (Thunb.) DC.* of *Menispermaceae* family and *Aristalochia fangchi Y.C. Wu et L.D, Chow et S.W. Hwang* of the *Aristolochiaceae* family, are also used as the substitutes for the drug. The family of the herb is very complex, the one with anticancer function is *Stephania tetrandra S.M.*, mainly containing tetrandrine and fangchinoline.

ANTICANCER PHARMACOLOGICAL FUNCTIONS

1. Experiments in vitro showed that with a concentration of 1:4000, tetrandrine kills cancer cells with a rate of 100%; with a concentration of 1:6000, it kills only 25%. This indicates that the efficacy of the drug is closely related to its quantity.

2. Experiments in vivo with animals showed that abdominal injection of tetrandrine 50mg/kg or oral administration of 100mg/kg was effective as a therapy.

3. Tetrandrine inhibits ascites carcinocytes and liver carcinocytes of ascites type in mice.

EXPERIMENTAL FORMULAS

For obstruction of esophageal cancer and cardia cancer:

Radix Stephaniae Tetrandrae 12g
Rhizoma Arisaematis 12g
Herba Eupatorii Fortunei 12g
Lignum Acronychiae 24g
Fructus Mume 15g
Pericarpium Citri Reticulatae 9g
Squama Manitis 4.5g
Radix Euphorbiae Ebracteolatae 0.6-1.5g

The prescription can be taken continuously without course restriction. (*Medical Research Correspondance*, Vol. 12, 1973)

For nasopharyngeal cancer:

Radix Stephaniae Tetrandrae 30g
Rhizoma Fagopyri Cymosi 30g
Radix Achyranthis Bidentatae 30g

The above herbs are decocted for oral administration. Medulla Junci is pounded for sucking and Herba Sedi Sarmentosi is pounded for external application. (*Selection of Data on New Medicine from a National Exhibition*)

HISTORICAL COMMENTS

It is said in *Renewed Materia Medica* that: "The drug clears away heat and expels hematostasis."

It is reported in *On Properties of Medicinal Herbs* that: "The drug cures buccal distortion, and chiralgia, expels phlegm detention and stops cough and asthma due to deficiency of the lung."

SPICA PRUNELLAE

It is defined in *Canon of Materia Medica* that: "The drug, bitter and hot in taste and cold in nature, cures carbuncle and goiter."

The drug is obtained from a herb of *Labiatae* family, and its spica is for medical use. The whole herb contains triterpenoidal saponins, vitamin B_1, C, and K, and carotene, while the spica contains delphinidin, cyanidin and ursolic acid.

ANTICANCER PHARMACOLOGICAL FUNCTIONS

1. The condensed decoction of the drug inhibits JTC-26 with an effective rate of 50-70%.

2. It was reported that the ordinary decoction of the drug inhibits the growth of sarcoma-180 and ascites cancer in rats, but the mortality was the same as that of the control group. So it is suspected that the inhibiting effect was exerted by its toxin.

EXPERIMENTAL FORMULAS

For multiple osteoangioma:

        Spica Prunellae 15g

        Herba Pteridis Multifidae 24g

        Radix Bupleuri 9g

        Radix Gentianae 9g

        Carapax Trionycis 24g

        Cortex Lycii Radicis 12g

        Bombyx Batryticatus 12g

        Periostracum Cicadae 12g

        Lumbricus 12g

        Radix Isatidis 15g

        Radix Rhapontici Uniflori 6g

        Rhizoma Zingiberis 2g

The prescription is taken one dosage a day in decoction. (*Journal of Shanghai Traditional Chinese Medicine*, Vol. 7, 1984)

For thyroid adenocarcinoma:

        Spica Prunellae 20g

        Caulis Polygoni Multiflori 20g

        Concha Ostreae 30g

        Rhizoma Dioscoreae Bulbiferae 9g

        Radix Curcumae 15g

        Rhizoma Acori Graminei 15g

        Radix Adenophorae 15g

        Radix Bupleuri 10g

        Rhizoma Scirpi 10g

        Rhizoma Zedoariae 10g

The prescription is taken one dosage a day. (*Journal of Traditional Chinese Medicine*, Vol. 9, 1983)

For thyroid cyst:

1>.   Spica Prunellae 60g

        Radix Salviae Miltiorrhizae 24g

        Pericarpium Trichosanthis 24

        Thallus Laminariae seu Eckloniae 24g

        Sargassum 24g

        Rhizoma Cyperi 24g

        Cormus Iphigeniae 24g

        Radix Bupleuri 15g

        Radix Paeoniae Lactiflorae 18g

        Radix Paeoniae Albae 18g

The prescription is taken in decoction one dose a day.

2>.   Spice Prunellae 60g and lean pork 60g are simmered and taken every other day to reinforce the curative effect. (*Hunan Medical and Pharmaceutical Journal*, Vol. 3, 1980)

HISTORICAL COMMENTS

It is reported in *Recompiled Materia Medica* that: "The drug cures scrofula, goiter, carbuncle, mammoabscess and mammocancer."

It is pointed out in *Prescriptions of Materia Medica* that: "The drug is contraindicative for those suffering from *qi* deficiency."

FRUCTUS LAGENARIA

It is defined in *Zhennan Materia Medica* that: "The drug, slightly sweet in taste and cold in nature, promotes circulation of body fluid."

The drug is obtained from a herb of *Cucurbitaceae* family, and the shell of its fruit is for medical use. The dried drug contains 20% of glucose and pentosan. Besides, it also contains cucurbitacin B, which is a terpene compound effective against cancer.

ANTICANCER PHARMACOLOGICAL FUNCTIONS

1. Cucurbitacin inhibits the respiration and aoxygen fermentation of Ehrlich's ascites carcinocytes.

2. The drug inhibits sarcoma-180 and Ehrlich's ascites carcinoma-256.

EXPERIMENTAL FORMULAS

For nasopharyngeal carcinoma:

The old drug is calcined and ground into powder with a little Moschus and Borneol, to be blown into the nose several times a day, each time a little bit. (*Hunan Scientific and Technological Information*, Vol. 2, 1974)

For Lymphosarcoma:

The drug with long stem is calcined and ground into powder to be applied to the lesion, or blended with sesame oil and applied to the lesion. (*Medical Secrets of Hua Tuo*)

HISTORICAL COMMENTS

It is reported in *Essential Prescriptions Worth a Thousand Gold* that: "The drug cures diabetes, pyogenic sore and nasolaryngeal cancer."

It is recorded in *Imperial Prescriptions* that: "Gingivitis and gingivalgia can be treated with Fructus Lagenaria (240g) and Radix Achyranthis Bidentatae (120g), when ground into powder for oral administration 13 grams each time. The herbs can also be decocted for gargling 3 to 4 times a day."

It is said in *Zhennan Materia Medica* that: "The drug is used in low dosage to treat rubella."

THE AUTHOR'S NOTE

In the early 50s, plants of *Cucurbitaceae* family were found to have powerful anticancer effect, with an efficacious chemical compound, tetracyclic triterpenes, generally known as cucurbitacin. Cucurbitacin B inhibits sarcoma-180 in mice with 21-55% effective rate, cucurbitacin D with 50-56%, cucurbitacin E with 40-42%, cucurbitacin I with 5-44% and others, more or less, also have anticancer actions. The application of cucurbitacin was restricted in the past because of its strong toxicity. But pharmaceutical experiment done by Yunnan Provincial Pharmaceutical Research Institute proved that NaAc significantly reduces the toxicity of cucurbitacin B and E compound on white rats, and this has greatly enhanced its application. Besides, cucurbitacin has also been separated out from plants pertaining to *Cruciferae* and *Scrophulariaceae* family.

RHIZOMA HELEOCHARIDIS

It is defined in *Guide to Materia Medica* that: "The drug, sweet in taste, slightly cold and slippery in nature, invigorates *qi* and regulates the functions of the stomach and the intestines, curing five kinds of dysphagia."

The drug is obtained from a herb of *Cyperaceae* family, its root for medical use. A part from protein and sugar, it also contains puchiin which inhibits Staphylococcus aureus, Bacillus coli and Bacillus gasoformans, and is not liable to be absorbed by activated carbon.

ANTICANCER PHARMACOLOGICAL FUNCTIONS
It was found by a cooperative research group on the prevention and treatment of tumors in Shanghai that screening tests proved that all the preparations of the drug inhibits animal tumors when administrated externally.

EXPERIMENTAL FORMULAS
For malignant encephoastrocytoma:

      Rhizoma Heleocharidis 60g

      Radix Semiaquilegiae 30g

      Herba Scutellariae Barbatae 30g

      Herba Oldenlandiae Diffusae 30g

      Concha Haliotidis 30g

      Rhizoma Paridis 15g

      Rhizoma Pinelliae 15g

      Rhizoma Atractylodis Macrocephalae 15g

      Radix Notoginseng 10g

      Bombyx Batryticatus 10g

      Rhizoma Gastrodiae 10g

      Scorpio 3g

The prescription is taken one dosage a day in decoction. (*Journal of Integrated Chinese and Western Medicine*, Vol. 2, 1985)

For esophageal carcinoma:

Ten pieces of the drug are boiled in a copper pot and taken very day. (*Popular Knowledge of Medicine and Hygiene*)

HISTORICAL COMMENTS
It is said in *Newly Compiled Materia Medica* that: "The drug, when sliced and dried, is specifically effective for abdominal mass, and would be more effective if used together with Carapax Tronycis, with no damage to the vitality."

It is reported in *True Materia Medica* that: "The drug is sweet in taste and cold in nature, clearing away asthenic heat accumulated in the chest, diminishing celioblotion and curing dysentery with blood."

It is recorded in *Daily Diet* that: "The drug is contraindicative for cold syndrome due to *qi* deficiency."

THE AUTHOR'S NOTE
General verruca can be cured with the drug when broken into pieces for rubbing the lesion with its white pulp till the callus becoming soft and coming off with slight pain and punctate bleeding. The therapy is repeated three to four times a day and totally for 7-10 days.

RHIZOMA ZEDOARIAE

It is defined in *Origin of Medicine* that: "The drug, bitter in taste and mild in nature, relieves diaphragm pain."

The drug is obtained from *Curcuma* of *Zingiberaceae* family, and its radix is for medical use. *C. Wenyujin Y.H. Chen et C. Ling* is used as the substitute for the drug. The drug mainly contains volatile oil, fats, stigmasterol, ß-elemene, triterpenic acid, resin, mucilage and flavonoid glycosides.

ANTICANCER PHARMACOLOGICAL FUNCTIONS

1. 0.3ml of 100% *C. Wenyujin Y.H. Chen et C. Ling* injection was administrated celiacally to mice with experimental sarcoma and the inhibiting rate was 53%.

2. Local injection of its volatile oil causes necrosis of the tumor tissue and makes the tumor comes off eventually without evident affect on the normal surrounding tissues.

3. Oral administration of the drug has no effect on ascites cancer of mice, but can inhibit mice sarcoma-180.

4, The hot water extract of the drug inhibits mice sarcoma-180 with 80% effective rate when celiacally injected with total cellular volumetric method. The hot water extract from the leftovers of the ethanol extract has an inhibiting rate of 77.1%. This means that the active part of the herb is not soluble in ethanol and can not be destroyed by ethanol liquid. It is inferred that the effective elements are polysaccharide, organic acid, amino acid and polypeptide.

5. This drug can increase the total number of lymphocytes and reinforce body immune capacity.

6. The substance, ß-elemene, evidently prolongs the survival of mice with ascites cancer and ARS, showing no evident inhibition on hematopoiesis. The external culture bears higher phagohepatocytic function.

EXPERIMENTAL FORMULAS
For cervical cancer:

      Rhizoma Zedoariae 15g
      Radix Angelicae Sinensis 9g
      Radix Paeoniae Latiflorae 9g
      Semen Arecae 9g
      Thallus Laminariae seu Eckloniae 9g
      Semen Persicae 9g
      Carapax Trionycis 9g
      Radix et Rhizoma Rhei 9g
      Semen Longan 2.4g
      Succinum 1.2g
      Fructus Citri Aurantii 4.5g
      Radix Aucklandiae 6g

The prescription is taken one dosage a day in decoction. (*Compendium for Nourishing Yin*)
For cystocarcinoma:

      Rhizoma Zedoariae 9g
      Rhizoma Scirpi 9g
      Pericarpium Citri Reticulatae Viride 6g
      Pericarpium Citti Reticulatae 6g
      Herba Pogostemonis 6g
      Rhizoma Cyperi 6g
      Radix Glycyrrhizae 6g
      Rhizoma Zingiberis 3g
      Fructus Ziziphi Inermis 2

The prescription is taken one dosage a day in decoction. (*Diagnosis and Treatment of Tumors*)
For Celiac tumor:

Same amount of Rhizoma Zedoariae, Cortex Cinnamomi and Fructus Foeniculi are ground into powder and taken orally. (*Collection of Comments on Materia Medica*)

For spermatocytoma:

20ml of 1% Rhizoma Zedoariae oil is added to 500ml of 5% glucose saline for intravenous injection, and Gossypol is taken orally 10ml a time and three times a day. (*Journal of Shandong Traditional Chinese Medical College*, Vol. 1, 1980)

HISTORICAL COMMENTS

It is reported in *Materia Medica of All Schools in the Ming Dynasty* that: "The drug diminishes all kinds of stagnation due to the disorder of *qi*, increases appetite to digest food, promotes menstruation, expels hematostasis, relieves pain caused by trauma and cures dysentery with blood or celiorrhagia due to visceral disorder."

It is said in *Atlas of Materia Medica* that: "The drug expels blood stasis, removes phlegm and cures globus hystericus."

It is suggested in *Origin of Canon* that: "The drug is torrefied for diseases of the Liver Channel, simmered for diseases of the Heart-spleen Channel and roasted with goat or chicken blood for regulating menstruation with *Siwu Tang*.

THE AUTHOR'S NOTE

In 1979, scholars at Tokyo Pharmacologic University, selected 112 kinds of medicinal herbs, through screening tests in vivo with sarcoma-180, finding that plants of ginger family have a higher anticancer effect. Among the 112 selected herbs, 13 pertain to ginger family and among the 13, 12 are active against cancer with a rate of 92%. Rhizoma Zedoariae is one of the 12 plants. (*Journal of Crude Drugs*, Vol. 2, 1979 and Vol. 2, 1982) The experiments show that the application of radiotherapy or chemotherapy after a period of clinical administration of Rhizoma Zedoariae not only increases the curative effect of the therapies, but also prevents leukocytic reduction. (*Journal of Chinese Pharmacology*, Vol. 2, 1981) In 1976, it was reported in Liaoning Province that 173 cases of cervical cancer received treatment with only Rhizoma Zedoariae and 28.9% of the patients were cured and 71.68% were found effective. In 1976, a national summary on the drug showed that among the 173 tumor cases (a majority in the advanced stage) of 29 different types of cancer, excluding cervical cancer, Rhizoma Zedoariae cured 11 cases and were effective in 56 cases.

RADIX ET RHIZOMA PODOPHYLLI

It is defined in *Commonly Used Chinese Medicinal Herbs* In Tibet that: "The drug, being bitter and slightly hot in taste, warm and slightly toxic in nature, is good at harmonizing blood, stopping hematorrhagia, removing toxic materials and subsiding swelling."

The drug is obtained from *Podophyllum emodi Wall.* of *Berberidaceae* family. Its radix contains podophyllotoxin, quercetin and delphinidin. The herbs of this family, such as *Dysosma Pleiantha (Hce.) Woods.*, *Diphylleia sinensis Li* and *Berberis soulieana Schneid.*, are also active against cancer.

ANTICANCER PHARMACOLOGICAL FUNCTIONS

1. Podophyllotoxin inhibits the division of cells at the middle phase and suppresses the growth of animal tumor.

2. Its derivative VM-26, with low toxin, inhibits the combination of thymine with DNA in low concentration, and is also effective for reticulocytoma at the advanced stage. But it is found also inhibiting the bone marrow.

EXPERIMENTAL FORMULAS

For cervical cancer in the form of cauliflower:

The liposoluble substance extracted from the drug's radix is dissolved in 75% alcohol to make 10-20% solution to be saturate on a cotton ball for dressing on the entire tumor lesion for 24 hours. This treatment is given every day or every other day or every third day according to the patient's conditions. (*Tumor Prevention and Treatment in Qinghai*, Vol. 1, 1972)

HISTORICAL COMMENTS

It is said in *Chinese Medicinal Herbs in Shaanxi* that: "The drug promotes the circulation of blood and *qi* and relieves pain."

It is reported in *Chinese Herbal Medicine* that: "All the substances (pertaining to podophyllotoxin category) bear certain anti-oncocytic effect, but are only used as external drugs clinically because of its toxin."

THE AUTHOR'S NOTE

Podophyllum peltatum of the same family also has activities against cancer. The artificial etoposide from the extract of the root and the stalk of the drug by ethanol is similar to colchicine in action and is difficult to be dissolved in water. If incubated with Hela cells, it will break single-chained DAN. This drug can delay and kill G2 lymphatic maternal cells. The drug has been clinically employed since 1973 and proved to be effective for microcytic bronchocancer, testocancer, acute non-lymphocytic leukemia and malignant lymphoma. It has been confirmed from the clinical treatment of 250 cases that the drug is effective in treating mononucleocytic leukemia, acute granulocytic leukemia, Hodgkin's disease, malignant lymphosarcoma and mammocancer. But 50 cases treated with its oral capsules showed no effect. Its toxin usually affects hematopoietic system with occasional loss of hair and vomiting.

FRUCTUS AKEBIAE

Wang Ang in the Qing Dynasty said that: "Its seed is similar to that of the Chinese honey locust, brown and lustrous, biter in taste, cold and non-toxic in nature."

The drug is obtained from *Akebia* of *Ladrizabalaceae* family, produced in the central and northern regions of China. The drug is generally divided into three kinds: *A. trifaliata (Thunb.) Koidz. var. australis (Diels) Rehd.*, *A. trifoliata (Thunb.) Koidz.*, and *A. quinata (Thunb.) Decne.*.

ANTICANCER PHARMACOLOGICAL FUNCTIONS

1. Experiments in vitro with JTC-26 showed that the drug decocted has an inhibiting rate of 50-70%.

2. The drug inhibits mice sarcoma-180 and sarcoma-37.

EXPERIMENTAL FORMULAS

For uterine and ovarian tumor:

15 pills of the drug are taken orally every day or the decoction of the drug is taken daily for a long period of time. (*Materia Medica of All Schools In Great Ming Dynasty*)

For liver cancer:

       Fructus Akebiae 30g

       Fossilia Spiriferis 30g

       Herba Verbenae Officinalae 30g

The herbs are decocted and taken daily. (*Handbook of Practical Anticancer Drugs*)

For chorioepithelioma and malignant hydatidiform mole:

1>.   Fructus Akebiae 60g
          Semen Livistonae 60g
          Herba Scutellariae Barbatae 60g
          Radix Cudraniae 60g

The above herbs are taken in decoction daily.

2>.   Fructus Akebiae 60g
          Radix Rhodomyrtis Tomentosae 60g
          Herba Oldenlandiae Diffusae 60g

The herbs are taken in decoction daily. (*Anticancer Prescriptions of Traditional Chinese Medicine*)

HISTORICAL COMMENTS

It is suggested in *Dietetic Canon* compiled by Cui Yuxi that: "The drug taken in diet expels phlegm and cures dysentery with blood and mucus."

It is said in *Materia Medica of All Schools in Ming Dynasty* that: "The drug cures all syndromes induced by pathogenic wind, visceral impairment, all kinds of injury, loss of hair, pestilence, snake bite and blindness due to fright, indigestion with detained food, irregular urination and restlessness."

CAULIS MARSDENIAE

It is defined in Dictionary of *Chinese Materia Medica* that: "The drug, bitter and cold, promotes lactation and urination, and resists cancer."

The drug is obtained from *Marsdenia* of *Asclepiadaceae* family, its vine and stalk are for medical use. The drug, cultivated in South China, contains steroidal saponins, saccharides, a little alkaloids, resin and phytochromes.

ANTICANCER PHARMACOLOGICAL FUNCTIONS

1. The drug inhibits mice sarcoma-180. According to the result of analysis and clinical application, its curative effect is exerted through reinforcing the non-specific immunity of the body. It has been found that oral administration is superior to intravenous injection according to the curative effect on cancer of the esophagus. It shows toxic effect during the period of administration with symptoms such as polyuria and polyperspiration.

2. *Marsdenia Condurango* of the same family has already been made into oral liquid for treating gastrocancer in some foreign countries. The biological alkali extracted from *Tylophora Crebriflora* has been proved to inhibit adenocancer-755, rat lymphosarcoma, sarcoma-256, lymphocytic leukemia-388 and leukemia-1210. However, this alkali was found to have irreversible toxicity one the central nerve system and therefore has been stopped in use. The herb growing in China does not contain such toxin and its curative effect may be confirmed by immunology.

EXPERIMENTAL FORMULAS

For cancer of the digestive system:

A 100% water solution, made from the liquid extracted from the drug, is taken 10 drops (3ml) orally every 3 hours. The prescription is continued for several months or half a year. (*Medical Reference*, Vol. 2, 1972)

For cervical cancer, Hodgkin's disease, esophageal and cardia cancer:

9 to 120 grams of the drug is simmered for over 3 hours and the broth is divided into three portions. A portion each time, three times a day. (*Collection of Herbs from All Over China*)

For other cancers:

30 to 45 grams of the drug is decocted with 10 grains of Fructus Piperis for oral administration daily. (*Selected Herbs in Yunnan*)

For lymphosarcoma:

30 grams of the drug is decocted for oral administration daily. (*Treatment Based on Differentiation of Symptoms and Signs*)

HISTORICAL COMMENTS

It is reported in *Catalogue of Medicinal Herbs in Guizhou* that: "The drug invigorates blood to promote myoplegia and lactation, curing cough, trauma, fracture and lactopenia."

It is pointed out in *Simao's Selection of Chinese Medicinal Herbs in Yunnan* that: "The drug clears away heat to remove toxic materials and subsides inflammation to relieve pain."

THE AUTHOR'S NOTE

The drug has already been used clinically to treat cervical cancer, lymphosarcoma, cancer of the digestive system, Hodgkin's disease, osteosarcoma, mandible and lingual squamous epithelial carcinoma. It was reported in *New Medical Information* (Vol. 4, 1972) that 100 cases of cervical cancer were treated in the hospital affiliated to No. 142 Army with the drug and it was found remarkably effective in 32 cases and effective in 46, with a total effective rate of 78%. Another 40 cases of tumor were treated with this drug in a hospital in Wuhan with an effective rate of 62.5%. This drug is different from *Fissistigm Glucescens (Hance) Merr* which, though sharing the same nomenclature, pertains to *Annonaceae* family and has not been reported to resist cancer activation.

CORTEX MORI

Li Dongyuan from the Jin Kingdom said that: "The drug can reinforce pneuma to supplement asthenia with its sweet taste and clear away pulmonary pathogenic heat to stop cough with its hot taste."

The drug is obtained from *Morus alba L.* of *Moraceae* family, its cork is for medical use. The drug contains umbelliferone, scopoletine, mulberrin and tannins. Its extract is effective in tranquilizing mice and promoting their urination, therefore, it is said in *Materia Medica* that: "The drug is good for promoting drainage."

ANTICANCER PHARMACOLOGICAL FUNCTIONS

1. Animal experiments in vivo showed that the hot water extract of the drug inhibits mice sarcoma-180 of ascites type with an effective rate of 51.8%.

2. The experiments in vitro showed that the hot water extract of the drug inhibits JTC-26 with an effective rate of 70-90%.

EXPERIMENTAL FORMULAS

For esophageal cancer and gastrocancer:

30 grams of the drug (with its coarse bark) is decocted with 90 grams of millet vinegar for 1 hour and taken in one time or several times. Glucose powder can be added to the decoction if it is two sour. (*Journal of Fujian Traditional Chinese Medicine*, Vol. 3, 1965)

For other cancers:

15 grams of the drug is decocted in 250 grams of water and taken in three times. (*Research Data of Traditional Chinese Medicine*, Vol. 6, 1978)

For superficial cancer:

The drug is dried in shade, ground, blended with wine and applied to the swelling. (*Prescriptions Worth a Thousand Gold*)

HISTORICAL COMMENTS

It is said in *Explanation to Medicinal Herbs* that: "The drug cures hemoptysis due to pyrophlegm, stuff nose when used together with Flos Chrysanthemi Morifolii and Semen Dolichoris Album, and hemorrhoids when combined with Radix Adenophonne and Radix Astragali."

It is reported in *Yu Qiu's Explanation to Herbs* that: "The juice squeezed from the drug cures black naevus, deteriorated muscle, incised wound and stasis."

THE AUTHOR'S NOTE

It is reported in *Atlas of Materia Medica* compiled by Su Song that: "Incised abdominal wound without the projection of the intestine is sutured with thread made from the drug and then applied with warm chicken blood. An Jincang in the Tang Dynasty used this method to close abdominal cut." Researches carried out at home indicated that wounds of dogs can be sutured with the thread made from the drug, with no need to remove the stitches."

HERBA TAXILLI

It is defined in *Canon of Materia Medica* that: "The drug is bitter and bland, curing lumbago and carbuncle, and nourishing the hair."

The drug is the leaves or branches of *Viscum coloratum (Komar.) Nakai, Taxillus chinensis (DC.) Danser*, and *Prunus mume (Sieb.) Sieb. et Zucc.* of the *Loranthaceae* family. It is said in *Sichan Materia Medica* that: "The herb is often found parasitizing on other trees and its leaves are quite similar to each other." It is said in *Tang Materia Medica* that: "Herba Taxilli is only found parasitizing on *Quercus dentata Thunb., Zelkova Schneideriana Hand. Mazz., Salix babylonica L., Homonoia riparia Lour.*, and *Liquidambar formosana Hance*." But for medical purpose, Herba Taxilli and Herba Viscum are regarded as the most desirable. Herba Viscum mainly contains oleanolic acid, while Herba Taxilli mainly contains quercetin and avicularin.

ANTICANCER PHARMACOLOGICAL FUNCTIONS

1. Experiments in vitro showed that the drug inhibits JTC-26 with a rate of 50-70%.

2. The hot water extract inhibits mice sarcoma-180 with an effective rate of 39.5% and the ethanol extract with an effective rate of 17.5%.

3. The hot water extract from *Taxillus chinensis (DC) Danser* inhibits mice sarcoma-180 with an effective rate of 77.9%.

4. The toxic peptide of the herb has been extracted from Yiscumalbum in some foreign countries, which is an alkaline protein with a molecular weight of 60000, effective in stimulating the enlargement of mice thymus gland. Injection of $0.5\mu g$ of toxic peptide daily before transplantation in the animal experiment, inhibits the growth of sarcoma-180 with a rate of 90%, and it still works well when its concentration several times lower than that of the other anticancer drugs. It was clinically observed that the drug hinders the growth of cancer. The drug is mainly used abroad to treat cancer of the breast and the uterus.

5. Experiments in vivo showed that the herb parasitized on Ramulus Litchi inhibits the growth of cancer cells.

6. Animal experiments with Herba Visci Articulati showed the herb resists the activation of cancer.

EXPERIMENTAL FORMULAS

For cardia cancer:

A small cup of the juice of the crude drug is taken orally. (*Collection of Pin Hu Prescriptions*)

For oophoric cyst:

    Herba Taxilli 15g
    Radix Angelicae Sinensis 15g
    Radix Rehmanniae 15g
    Rhizoma Cyperi 15g
    Radix et Rhizoma Rhei 15g
    Semen Persicae 12g
    Fructus Citri Aurantii 12g
    Corium Stomachichum Galli 12g
    Radix Paeoniae Latiflorae 12g
    Radix Paeoniae Albae 12g
    Rhizoma Scirpi 12g
    Rhizoma Atractylidis Macrocephalae 12g
    Fructus Crataegi 12g
    Radix Curcumae 12g

The above herbs are decocted and taken daily. A dose a day. (*Journal of Zhejiang Traditional Chinese Medicine College*, Vol. 1, 1984)

For nasopharyngeal cancer:

    Herba Taxilli 15g
    Herba Scutellariae Barbatae 15g
    Rhizoma Zedoariae 15g
    Ramulus Uncariae cum Uncis 12g
    Rhizoma Ardisiae 12g
    Cormus Iphigeniae 12g
    Semen Livistonae 30g
    Scolopendra 3
    Nidus Vespae 3g

The above herbs are taken in decoction. (*Oncology of Traditional Chinese Medicine*)

For tumor in the upper part of the neck:

The plant parasitized on pomegranate tree is ground with vinegar for rubbing on the tumor lesion. (*Newly Compiled Experienced Prescriptions*)

For other cancers:

15 grams of the leaf, or stalk or flower of the herb parasitized on *Herba viscum coloratum (komar.) Nakai* is decocted in 300ml of water and the broth is divided into three portions for oral administration three times a day, each time a portion. (*Research Data of Traditional Chinese Medicine*, Vol. 6, 1978)

HISTORICAL COMMENTS

It is said in *True Materia Medica* that: "The drug is specific for invigorating kidney to supplement blood."

It is reported in *Elucidation on Materia Medica* that: "The drug is bitter and sweet in taste, moderate in action, not cold or warm in nature, and nonpoisonous."

It is pointed in *Renewed Materia Medica* that: "The drug cures *yin* deficiency, reinforces renal function, nourishes joints, regulates menstruation, supplements blood, stabilizes embryo and relieves pain."

RADIX EUPHORBIAE EBRACTEOLATAE

It is defined in *Properties of Medicinal Herbs* that: "The drug is bitter, hot and toxic, curing phlegm and abdominal mass."

The drug, though of different varieties, is usually referred to *Euphoria fischeriana S., E. ebiacteolata. H.,* and *Stellera chamaejasme L.* of the *Thymelaeaceae* family. The radix of the herb is for medical use. The drug is produced all over China.

ANTICANCER PHARMACOLOGICAL FUNCTIONS

1. The injection prepared from the drug inhibits solid liver cancer in mice with a rate of 43.85-52.43%, higher than that of the control group treated with Herba Crotalariae, Vinblasline and Hydroxyl catharamine.

2. The liquid extracted from the drug inhibits mice sarcoma-180 with a high effective rate: 41.2-45.29% when administrated intravenously and 37.67-44.0% when administrated celiacally.

3. The decoction of the drug relieves pain. The pain threshold of mice can be increased by 20-50% with 6 grams of the crude drug per kilograms of body weight administered through gastric lavement.

EXPERIMENTAL FORMULAS

For hepatocarcinoma:

      Radix Euphorbiae Ebracteolatae 6g
      Carapax Trionycis 30g
      Radix Salviae Miltiorrhizae 30g
      Bufo 30g
      Fructus Crataegi 30g
      Herba Scutellariae Barbatae 30g
      Scorpis 5g
      Rhizoma Scirpi 15g
      Rhizoma Zedoariae 15g
      Fructus Phyllanthi 15g
      Hirudo 10g

The above herbs are taken in decoction with a dosage a day. (*Journal of Zhejiang Traditional Chinese Medicine College*, Vol. 3, 1980)

For cancer of the stomach, the lung, the liver, the thyroid and the nipple:

3 grams of the drug is decocted in 200ml of water for a while, then the drug is filtered out and two eggs are added for further boiling. Both the broth and the egg are eaten. (*Journal of Yantai Medicine and drugs*, Vol. 3, 1971)

For cancer of the breast:

500 grams of the drug and 500 grams of Fructus Ziziphi Inermis are boiled together. Then take away the drug and eat 5 Fructus Ziziphi Inermis each time and 2-3 times a day. (*Reference for Clinical Treatment of Tumor*)

HISTORICAL COMMENTS

It is said in *Introduction to Materia Medica* that: "The drug cures deep-rooted carbuncle cause by parasites and scrofula."

It is recorded in *Supplementation to Zhou Hou's Prescriptions* that: "Abdominal solid mass and the stagnation of *qi* along the two sides of the rib can be cured with Radix Euphorbiae Ebracteolatae (60g), Flos Inulae (30g) and Radix Aconiti Lateralis Preparata (60g), when pounded, screened and made into honey coated pills for oral administration two or three pills each time."

It is pointed in *Handbook of Highland Medical Herbs* that: "The drug is not indicative for pregnant women and should be used with care for chronic gastroenteric ulcer."

It is reported in *Dictionary of Traditional Chinese Medicinal Herbs* that: "The compound injection, made with Caulis Millettiae, Semen Coicis and Herba Scutellariae Barbatae, is given intravenously once a day with a dose of 20-40ml of the injection mixed with 5% glucose. 20 cases of stomach cancer at the advanced stage received the drug and it was found that the drug alleviated the symptoms when administrated before operation and reinforced the curative effect and stabilized the patient's condition when administrated after operation."

RADIX CYNANCHI PANICULATI

It is defined in *Canon of Materia medica* that: "The drug is hot in taste and warm in nature, relieving severe pain."

The drug is obtained from a herb of the *Asclepiadaceae* family, its radix or the whole plant is for medical use. The drug, cultivated in most areas of China, contains paeonol, sarcostin, deacylcynanchogenin, acetic acid and cinnamic acid, its radix containing flavonoid, saccharides, amino acid and paeonol.

ANTICANCER PHARMACOLOGICAL FUNCTIONS
1. Screening tests with lymphocytic leukemia-615 indicated that the drug inhibits leukemia cells.
2. Bacteriophagic method proved that the drug resists the activation of cancer.

EXPERIMENTAL FORMULAS
For lung cancer:

        Radix Cynanchi Paniculati 30g
        Rhizoma Polygonati Odorati 30g
        Semen Descurainiae 30g
        Radix Codonopsis Lanceolatae 30g
        Bufo 30g
        Gecko Chinensis 5g
        Scolopendra 5g
        Poria 15g
        Fructus Phyllanthi 15g
        Radix Glycyrrhizae 10g
        Gecko 1 pair

The prescription can be modified in accordance with the patient's condition. (*Journal of Zhejiang Traditional Chinese Medicine*, Vol. 3, 1980)

For headache caused by tumor of the sella turcica region:

The injection made from the drug is administered intramuscularly or on the acupoints 50-100mg a time and 200mg a day. The pain will be relieved several hours or half an hour after the injection of the drug. The curative effect can last for 3-12 hours. (*Traditional Medical and Pharmaceutical Correspondance*, Vol. 2, 1973)

HISTORICAL COMMENTS
It is said in *Records of Famous Doctors* that: "The drug invigorates *qi*."

It is reported in *Jilin Chinese Medicinal Herbs* that: "The drug is effective in promoting urination, reinforcing renal function, tranquilizing the mind to relieve pain, expelling cold to diminish stasis, removing snake poison and regulating channels to promote blood circulation."

It is pointed out in *Dictionary of Chinese Materia Medica* that: "The drug relieves pain, stops cough, promotes drainage to subside swelling and invigorates blood to remove toxic materials."

It is suggested in *Nanjing Folk Medicinal Herbs* that: "Toothache can be cured by gargling with the wine in which the seedling of the drug has been steeped."

It is mentioned in *Shanghai Prescriptions* that: "Malignant celialgia caused by visceral disorder can be cured with the drug powder and Benzoinum (steeped in wine, ground into fine powder, screened and simmered into paste which is made into pills as large as Semen Firmianae and taken with vinegar once ten pills with no time restriction).

FRUCTUS CASSIAE OCCIDENTALIS

It is defined in *Dictionary of Chinese Materia Medica* that: "The drug is bitter in taste, cold and toxic in nature, clearing away liver heat to improve eyesight, regulating stomach, promoting defecation and 'removing toxic materials."

The drug is obtained from *Cassia* of the *Leguminosae* family, the fruit and the stalk bark are for medical use. The radix and fruit contain emodin, chrysarobin, tannin, toxoprotein, fats, and mucilage, while the leaves contain cassiollin.

ANTICANCER PHARMACOLOGICAL FUNCTIONS
1. Emodin evidently inhibits cytopnea of ascites cancer.
2. The drug inhibits human pulmonary carcinocytic multiplication.

EXPERIMENTAL FORMULAS
For gastrocancer and liver cancer:
9 to 15 grams of the drug is decocted for oral taking. The prescription is taken one dosage a day. (*Treatment and Diagnosis Based on Differentiation of Symptoms and Signs*)
For lymphocarcinoma:

        Fructus Cassiae Occidentalis 30g
        Herba Oldenlandiae Diffusae 30g
        Spica Prunellae 30g
        Sargassum 30g
        Concha Ostreae 30g
        Flos Chrysanthemi Indici 30g
        Herba Aristolochiae Mollissimae 30g
        Fructus Trichosanthis 30g
        Thallus Laminariae seu Eckloniae 15g
        Rhizoma Dioscoreae 15g
        Semen Persicae 12g
        Radix Adenophorae 12g
        Semen Vaccariae 12g
        Nidus Vospae 12g

The above herbs are taken in decoction one dose a day, and at the same time, *Xiaojin Pian*, 5 tablets each time, twice a day; *Tiannong Pian*, 5 tablets each time, three times a day. (*Anticancer Preparations in Traditional Chinese Medicine*)

HISTORICAL COMMENTS
It is said in *Supplementation to Materia Medica* that: "The drug cures furuncle and carbuncle."
It is reported in *Jiangxi Chinese Herbs* that: "The drug cures gastralgia."

It is pointed out in *Major Toxic Plants in North China* that: "Eating the seeds and the root of the plant by accident will cause diarrhea and nausea, which can be treated by gastric lavement, egg white, active carbon, tannic acid protein and symptomatic therapies."

FRUCTUS GARDENIAE

It is defined in *Guide to Materia Medica* that: "The drug is bitter in taste, cold and light in nature, and red in color, clearing away cardiac and pulmonary pathogenic heat accumulation through promoting urination."

The drug is obtained from *Gardenia jasminoides Ellis* of the *Rubiaceae* family, the flower, the leaves and the radix are for medical use. The drug is produced in Zhejiang, Guangdong, Guangxi, Yunnan and Guizhou. The fruit contains flavones, crocin, ß-sistosterol and geniposide.

ANTICANCER PHARMACOLOGICAL FUNCTIONS

1. The hot water extract slightly inhibits mice sarcoma-180 of ascites type.

2. Screening tests with bacteriophagic method for selecting anticancer drugs showed that this drug inhibits the activation of cancer.

EXPERIMENTAL FORMULAS

For acute lymphocytic leukemia:

28 grains of the calcined Fructus Gardeniae are decocted in water into a broth of 50-100ml for oral taking in the morning and in the evening. The number of the drug is increased to 48 the following day. The prescription is continued with a weak interval after administration for 3 to 4 weeks. (*Oncological Bulletin*, Vol. 4, 1975)

For cheilocarcinoma:

Fructus Gardeniae 9g
Bombyx Batryticatus 9g
Radix Glycyrrhizae 9g
Herba Pogostemonis 9g
Gypsum Fibrosum 12g
Radix Ledebouriellae 12g
Scorpis 3g
Scolopendra 6g

The prescription is taken one dosage a day in decoction. (*Prevention and Treatment of Tumor*)

For other cancers:

10 grams of the drug is decocted in 200ml of water and the broth is taken in several times. (*Traditional Chinese Medical and Pharmaceutical Research*, Vol. 6, 1978)

HISTORICAL COMMENTS

It is said in *Origin of Materia Medica* that: "The drug diminishes hemostasis caused by pathogenic heat and cures celialgia when used together with Rhizoma Corydalis."

It is recorded in *Pu Ji Prescriptions* that: "Difficulty in micturition can be cured by 2-7 Fructus Gardeniae, a little salt and a single-clove garlic, pounded together and pasted on a sheet of paper for application to the navel or the scrotum."

It is reported in *Guide to Materia Medica* that: "The drug clears away heat when used crudely, stops haemorrhagia when torrefied black, cures nausea when roasted in ginger juice, clears intrinsic heat with its pulp and extrinsic heat with its peel."

FRUCTUS TRAPAE BISPINOSAE

It is defined in *Records of Famous Doctors* that: "The drug is sweet in taste, mild and non-toxic in nature, regulating middle *jiao* to supplement the viscera."

The drug is obtained from *Trapa* of *Trapaceae* family. The plants of this family, such as *Trapa bispinosa*, *Trapa quadrispinosa* and the fruit of *Trapa bicornis Osbeck*, are for medical use. The drug is produced in the southern provinces of China, the kernel of the fruit contains ergostatetraen, ß-sitosterol and large quantities of starch. Its stalk, leaf and stem are all for medical use.

ANTICANCER PHARMACOLOGICAL FUNCTIONS
1. The water extract of the seed resists ascites cancer and liver cancer AH-13 in mice.
2. The anticancer activity of the fruit of *Trapa bispinosa* differs greatly from that of *Trapa quadrispinosa*. The hot water extract of the latter inhibits mice sarcoma-180 with an effective rate of 60% and the ethanol extract with an effective rate of 38.8%. Whereas the hot water or the ethanol extract of the former shows no inhibiting effect. Animal experiment done abroad with another herb of the family has proved that it has certain anticancer effect.

EXPERIMENTAL FORMULAS
For gastrocancer:

30 to 60 grams of the shell of the old drug or kernel is ground into powder and taken in raw or with honey 6 grams a time. This prescription also can be used to treat esophageal cancer, uterocancer and mammary cancer. (*Therapy Based on Differentiation of Symptoms and Signs*)

For esophagocancer:

       Fructus Trapae Bispinosae 9g

       Caulis et Folium Wisteriae Sinensis 9g

       Fructus Chebulae 9g

       Semen Coicis 9g

The prescription is taken one dosage a day in decoction for three times. (*Dietetic Herbs and Simple Prescriptions*)

For various cancers:

       Fructus Trapae Bispinosae 60g

       Semen Coicis 30g

       Herba Tetragoniae 30g

       Caulis Wisteriae Sinensis 9g

The prescription is taken one dosage a day in decoction and it has a miraculous curative effect. (*Journal of Jiangsu*, Vol. 1, 1962)

For mammary cancer, uterocancer and esophagocancer:

30 to 60 grams of the leaves, fruit stem or fruit of the drug is decocted with 30 grams of millet. The decoction is taken for several days as a tea. (*National Collection of Medicinal Herbs*)

For cervical cancer:

20 to 30 grains of the crude flesh of the herb is simmered in water into brown decoction and taken in 2 to 3 times. The prescription can be taken for a long time and is also effective in treating gastrocancer. (*Prescriptions of Modern Gynecology*)

HISTORICAL COMMENTS
Atlas of Materia Medica says that: "The drug cures erysipelas."

Materia Medica reports that: "The drug clears away accumulated heat caused by exogenous diseases, cures consumptive disease, dispels alcohol poisoning and removes stubborn poison."

Supplementation to Materia Medica suggests that: "Wart can be cured with the fresh herb when rubbed on the lesion for one or two times a day."

Dictionary of Chinese Materia Medica points out that: "Frequently occurring wart can be cured with the stalk of the herb."

THE AUTHOR'S NOTE

In *Key to Family Care* written by a scholar in Japan it is suggested that about 30 grains of the fresh pulp or dried fruit of the herb is simmered daily in clay pot with bowls of water into a decoction (similar to strong tea in color) for oral administration three or four times a day, or for washing the vagina and the uterus. The decoction, though with a mud smell, has no side effect and works well when used externally and internally. Doctors believe that incurable cancers can be tried with this recipe, which is found effective not only for uterocancer but also for gastrocancer. For lavement, the decoction is diluted 3 to 5 times thinner than that for oral administration. *Research Materials of Chinese Pharmacology* (Vol. 6, 1978) reported that the herb, crushed and decocted, can be used for treating various types of cancer.

RHIZOMA SMILACIS CHINAE

It is defined in *Records of Famous Doctors* that: "The drug is sweet in taste, warm and mild in nature, containing no poison and invigorating the blood and *qi*."

The drug is obtained from *Smilax* of the *Liliaceae* family. The radix contains multiple steroidas saponins, one of which has been proved to be the combination of diosgenin, D-glucose and L-rhamnose.

ANTICANCER PHARMACOLOGICAL FUNCTIONS

1. Bacteriophagic screening tests showed that the drug resists bacteriophagia, indicating that it is active against cancer.

2. The drug inhibits mice sarcoma-180 with an effective rate of 30-50%, prolongs the survival of patients with ascites sarcoma with an effective rate of 50%, and inhibits encephaloma-ß-22 with an effective rate of over 50%.

3. The hot water extract of Japanese Rhizoma Smilacis inhibits 67.1% of mice sarcoma-180 and the ethanol extract inhibits the growth of tumor with an effective rate of 28.9%.

EXPERIMENTAL FORMULAS

For esophageal, gastric, nasopharyngeal, rectal and cervical cancer:

500-625 grams of the dried drug is steeped in 3-3.5kg of water for an hour and then simmered for 3 hours. The decoction, after the residue of the drug being removed, is decocted with 30-60g of fat pork for 1 more hour till it condenses into 500ml. The decoction is taken several times daily. (*Dictionary of Chinese Materia Medica*)

For esophagocancer:

500 grams of the fresh drug is decocted in 1500 grams of water into a condensed broth of 500 grams, which is further decocted after the removal of the residue and the addition of 100g of fat pork. The broth and the fat is divided into three portions for oral administration three times a day, each time a portion. (*Dictionary of Chinese Materia Medica*)

For acute leukemia:

Rhizoma Smilacis Chinae 60g
Radix Astragali 30g
Radix Codonopsis Pilosulae 15g
Radix Rehmanniae 15g
Radix Sophorae Tonkinensis 15g

Radix Angelicae Sinensis 12g
Arillus Longan 12g
Radix Paeoniae Alba 12g
Colla Corii Asini 12g
Herba Oldenlandiae Diffusa 30g

The prescription is taken one dosage a day in decoction. (*Medical Research Correspondance*, Vol. 8, 1974)

HISTORICAL COMMENTS

It is reported in *Complete Record of Holy Prescriptions* that: "Stranguria can be cured with 60 grams of the powder of the drug with a dose of 6 grams each time taken with millet porridge, when combined with washing of the waist and belly with Herba Thymi broth."

THE AUTHOR'S NOTE

The drug is astringent in nature, unfit for patients with intrinsic heat (including those treated by radiotherapy), and should be decocted together with fat pork to neutralize the saponins and foreign matter lest it may irritate the gastroenteric system and cause nausea and vomiting. Cases of esophagocancer were treated in Ri Tang Hospital affiliated to Chinese Medical Academy with Rhizoma Smilacis Pills with a dose of 6-8 pills each time three times a day. The pills were effective to alleviate the symptoms. (*Information of Chinese Herbal Medicine*, Vol. 3, 1972) A case of esophagocancer was treated in Hunan with total of 14.5kg of the crude herb, and his symptoms were relieved and the patient survived for four years without recurrence.

SALMIACUM

Su Jing in the Tang Dynasty said that: "The drug is salty, bitter and hot in taste, warm in nature, diminishing mass formation and hemostasis."

This drug is a white crystallized powder or fiber-like hard crystal. The drug has no smell, remains unchanged in the air, disperses when heated, dissolves in water but not in ethanol. The drug is toxic, mainly containing ammonium chloride. The Halitum Purpureum on sale mainly contains sodium chloride.

ANTICANCER PHARMACOLOGICAL FUNCTIONS

The drug inhibits mice sarcoma-180, rat cancer of ascites type and cancer-256.

EXPERIMENTAL FORMULAS

For esophagocancer:

1>. 30 grams of the drug is ground into powder, decocted and filtrated. The broth is, with the addition of vinegar (1kg of the broth and 1kg vinegar), boiled till it becomes a yellowish crystallized powder. The powder is taken three times a day and 0.6-1g a time. (*Prevention and Treatment of Tumor*)

2>. Salmiacum 3g
Borax 15g
Radix Glycyrrhizae 30g
Borneol 0.9g
Galla Turcica 9g

The above herbs are ground into powder and rolled with honey into pills of peach-stone size, for sucking with a dose of 3 to 4 pills a day. (*Newly Compiled Introduction to Traditional Chinese Medicine*)

3>.　　Salmiacum 3g
　　　　Radix Isatidis 30g
　　　　Herba Euphorbiae Lunulatae 30g
　　　　Calculus Bovis 60g
　　　　Radix Clemadis 60g
　　　　Rhizoma Arisaematis 9g

The above herbs are made into dry extract for oral administration with 1.5g each time, four times a day.

4>.　　Salmiacum 6
　　　　Borax 60g
　　　　Nitrum 30g
　　　　Chalcocitum 15
　　　　Lignum Aquilariae Resinatum 9g
　　　　Borneol 9g

The herbs are ground into powder and taken 0.9g every 30 minutes through sucking. The curative effect is usually observed 6 hours after the administration and the prescription is continued for 2 days. (*Traditional Chinese Medical and Pharmaceutical Correspondance*, Vol. 3, 1972)

5>.　　Salmiacum 30g
　　　　Radix et Rhizoma Rhei 30g
　　　　Rhizoma Coptidis 30g
　　　　Radix Scutellariae 30g
　　　　Radix Glycyrrhizae 10g

The prescription is taken in decoction. (*Anticancer Preparations of Traditional Chinese Medicine*)
For celiac tumor:

　　　　Salmiacum (rinsed in vinegar for one night)　　　15g
　　　　Fragrant Inkstick 0.3g
　　　　Rhizoma Zingiberis 0.3g
　　　　Radix Aconiti Lateralis Preparata 0.3g
　　　　Rhizoma Zedoariae 0.3g
　　　　Lacca Sinica Exsiccata 0.3g
　　　　Pericarpium Citri Reticulatae Viride 0.3g
　　　　Cortex Cinnamomi 0.3g
　　　　Fructus Crotonis (stripped off the peel) 0.3g
　　　　Scirpi 0.3g
　　　　Radix et Rhizoma Rhei 0.3g
　　　　Radix Aucklandiae 0.3g

The above ingredients are processed into pills of mung bean size. 5 pills are taken each time. (*Great Charity Prescriptions*)

For osteosarcoma:

120 grams of Salmiacum and 5 grams of Borneol are steeped in sorghum wine for a week. The wine is used for rubbing the lesion. (*Anticancer Consultation*)

For nasopharyngeal cancer:

Halitum Purpureum is ground into powder in porcelain ware and 500g of Radix Semiaquilegiae is steeped in 5kg of wine for a week. 0.9-1.2g of the powder is taken with 30ml of wine each time, three times a day. (*Explanation on Herbs and Prescriptions*)

HISTORICAL COMMENTS

It is recorded in *Materia Medica* that: "The drug cures dysphagia, celioscirrhi, chronic diarrhea, pharyngoblockage, nevus and warts."

It is reported in *Holy Prescriptions* that: "To cure chronic abdominal mass and celialgia, 60 grams of the drug is torrefied in vinegar, mixed with three pieces of Fructus Chaenomelis (stripped off the pulp), dried in bowl under the sun till it breaks up, and then ground into powder to be mixed with five liters of millet vinegar for further decoction. The decoction is mixed with honey and powdered Rhizoma Cyperi to make pills of Semen Firmiane size. A pill is taken with wine each time."

It is reported in *Effective Prescriptions* that: "Deng Caiqing has treated dysphagia and regurgitation with 6g of the drug wrapped in buckwheat dough for calcining. Then 3 grams of the wet herb is collected from the middle part of dough for further calcining and grinding with 6 grams of Semen Arecae and 2 pieces of Flos Caryophylli. 0.21g of the powder is taken each time with millet wine and three times a day. The prescription should be stopped when rehabilitation has reached. The patient can then take rice porridge for half a month accompanied with stomach invigorating medicine. There is another prescription: 3 grams of Stomach-Calming Powder is ground with 1.5g of the drug and 1.5g of Rhizoma Zingiberis. The powder is taken 6 grams a time in decoction. Vomiting with black and hard substance may occur immediately after the administration of the decoction. (Note: Attention and care should be given to the use of these two prescriptions, particularly the former one. Dysphagia and regurgitation are the symptoms of esophagocancer and gastrocancer which can be tried with this prescription.)

It is pointed out in *Holy Prescriptions* that: "Perineal carbuncle and malignant swelling can be treated with the drug (0.25kg) wrapped in silk and sucked in the mouth.

It is suggested in *Boji Prescriptions* that: " Three Holy Pills (containing Sulfur, Hydrargyrum and Salmiacum) cures chronic abdominal mass with instant result."

HERBA OLDENLANDIAE CHRYSOTRICHAE

It is defined in *Zhejiang Folk Medicinal Herbs* that: "The drug is slightly bitter in taste and mild in nature, containing no poison, dispersing retained blood to heal intrinsic trauma."

The drug belongs to the *Rubiaceae* family, the whole of which is for medical use.

The drug is a folk remedy, not recorded in *Materia Medica*. The one recorded in *Supplementation to Medical Mirror* and *Supplementation to Materia Medica*, according to the description, is not the drug in question but *Agrimonia pilosa Ledeb.* of the *Rosoaceae* family. The drug is mainly produced in South of Changjian River and the southern provinces, containing corymbosin, diterpenoid acids, ß-sitosterol, ursolic acid, oleanolic acid, stearic acid, oleic acid and linoleic acid.

ANTICANCER PHARMACOLOGICAL FUNCTIONS

1. Bacteriophagic screening tests in vivo showed that the drug resists bacteriophagia, indicating an active function against cancer.

2. Experiments in vitro proved that the drug inhibits cervical cancer-14 in mice.

EXPERIMENTAL FORMULAS

For cancer of the nasal cavity and the accessory nasal sinuses:

60 grams of the fresh drug is pounded into juice and taken orally twice a day. (*Prescriptions in Traditional Chinese Medicine*)

For cancer of the stomach:

60 grams of the drug is decocted with 60 grams of Rhizoma Smilacis Chinae for oral taking. (*Basic Knowledge of Traditional Chinese Medicine*)

For vocal ligament tumor:

      Herba Oldenlandiae Chrysotrichae 30g

      Rhizoma Fagopyri Cymosi 30g

Herba Solani Nigri 30g

Herba Solani Lyrati 30g

Herba Duchesneae 24g

Folium Pyrrosiae 15g

Radix Ophiopogonis 12g

The prescription is taken in decoction and 9 grams of Radix Scrophulariae can be added to the formula. (*Basic Knowledge of Traditional Chinese Medicine*)

For various malignant tumors:

30g of the drug is decocted for oral taking. This prescription can be taken for a longer period. (*Therapies Based on Differentiation of Symptoms and Signs*)

HISTORICAL COMMENTS

It is said in *History of Chinese Medicinal Plants* that: "The drug steeped in wine or taken with water cures haemorrhagia due to overstrain, relaxes and activates tendons, and also subsides unidentified swelling and heals sprain when pounded and applied to the lesions."

It is recorded in *History of Hunan Medicinal Herbs* that: "The drug expels hemostasis through activating *qi*, removes toxic materials through clearing away heat, cools blood, reinforces teeth and improves eyesight."

It is pointed out in *Newly Compiled Materia Medica in North Zhenan* that: "The drug stops haemorrhagia when pounded and applied externally. A case of haemorrhagia caused by glossotrauma was cured with the fresh whole herb, when other drugs and pressing method failed to stop bleeding. The decoction of the drug can treat blood stool and hemouria when taken orally."

It is reported in *Anticancer Herbal Preparation* that: "Cases of gastrocancer were treated with *Shelian* Decoction (Herba Oldenalandiae Chrysotrichae, Herba Scutellariae Barbatae, Herba Lobeliae Chinensis, Semen Coicis, Herba Hydrocotyli Sibthorpioditis, and Radix Hostae Plantagineae) with satisfactory result in No. 3 Hospital in Nanchang City, Jianxi Province. The prescriptions are also effective in treating esophageal cancer, liver cancer and rectocancer. A patient, named Wu, male and 42, had cardia cancer and the carcinoma evidently shrunk after the administration of the prescription for 5 months. No recurrence occurred as he continued the drug to reinforce the curative effect."

RADIX ASTRAGALI

It is defined in *Canon of Materia Medica* that: "The drug is sweet in taste and slightly warm in nature, curing carbuncle, subcutaneous ulcer and chronic sore, removing pus to relieve pain and improving deficiency syndrome to cure infantile diseases."

The drug is obtained from the herbs of the *Leguminosae* family, among which *A. membranaceus (Fisch) Bge.* and *A. membranaceus Bge. var. mongholicus (Bge.) Hsiao* are regarded as the qualified ones. Besides, *A. floridus Benth.*, *A. tibetanns Benth ex Bge.*, and *A. yunnanensis Franch* are also used as the substitutes of the drug, which contains saccharose, glucuronic acid, mucilage, bitter principles, choline, folic acid, ß-sitosterol, polysaccharides, trace elements and 0.0092-0.032ppm% iodine. The *A. Scaberimus Bge.* has been used to treat cancer in some foreign countries.

ANTICANCER PHARMACOLOGICAL FUNCTIONS

1. Astragalan bears general biological activation. Experiments in vivo showed that it is against cancer, but fails to kill cancer cells directly in experiment in vitro. This indicates that it works through promoting body immunity.

2. It is proved that the decoction of the drug can effectively induce generation of anticancer interferon in human body.

3. The decoction of the drug can evidently promote the function of the macrophagocytes to engulf SRBC after administrated to mice (25g/kg) orally for 5 days.

4. Experiments in vitro with bean sprout method indicates that the drug bears inhibiting function.

5. Experiments in vivo showed that the hot water extract of the drug inhibits mice sarcoma-180 with a rate of 41.7%, but the alcohol extract showed no effect.

EXPERIMENTAL FORMULAS

For cancer with aphagia due to deficiency syndrome:

Radix Astragali 180g
Radix Glycyrrhizae 30g
Fructus Ziziphi Inermis 1

The ingredients are smashed into small pieces and decocted in a small bowel of water for oral taking without time restriction. (*Local Prescriptions*)

For vomiting blood due to lung cancer:

6 grams of the drug and 15 grams of Herba Spirodela polyrrhizae are ground into powder for oral administration 3 grams each time with ginger-honey broth. (*Holy Prescriptions*)

For cavernous hemangioma:

Radix Astragali 30g
Herba Solani Lyrati 30g
Fructus Fici Pumilae 30g
Rhizoma Smilacis Glabrae 30g
Radix Codonopsis Pilosulae 12g
Radix Paeoniae Alba 12g
Radix Arnebiae 9g
Cortex Moutan 9g

The prescription is taken in decoction and modified in accordance with the patient's condition. (*Journal od Shanghai Traditional Chinese Medicine*, Vol. 6, 1979)

For nasopharyngeal cancer:

Radix Astragali 15-30g
Radix Paeoniae Latiflorae 10g
Rhizoma Chuanxiong 10g
Semen Persicae 10g
Flos Carthami 10g
Rhizoma Acori Graminei 10g
Radix Angelicae Sinensis 10-12g
Caulis Millettiae 15-24g
Radix Salviae Miltiorrhizae 15-24g
Pericarpium Citri Reticulatae 9g

The prescription is taken in decoction and modified in accordance with the patient's conditions. (*Journal of Traditional Chinese Medicine*, Vol. 9, 1983)

For osteoma:

Radix Astragali 30g
Fructus Crataegi 30g
Poria 30g
Semen Coicis 30g
Herba Oldenlandiae Diffusae 30g
Radix Angelicae Sinensis 10g
Fructus Mume 10g
Radix Trichosanthis 10g

Rhizoma Cibotii 12g

Radix Dipsaci 12g

Rhizoma Dioscoreae Bulbiferae 12g

Rhizoma Dioscoreae 15g

The prescription is taken in decoction one dosage a day. (*Journal of Hubei Traditional Chinese Medicine*, Vol. 6, 1980)

HISTORICAL COMMENTS

It is said in *Comments on Materia Medica* that: "The drug nourishes the lung to invigorate the spleen, reinforces and protects *qi* to expel toxic materials, and eradicates pathogenic wind to remove toxic materials."

It is reported in *Well-Compatiblized Materia Medica* that: "The drug cures deficiency syndrome when roasted with honey, stomach disorder when roasted with milk, and gastric deficiency when roasted with millet broth, removes toxic materials when roasted with salty water, warms stomach and heals dysentery when roasted with wine, clears away cardiac and asthenic heat and cures sore and ulcer when used crudely, and disperses stagnated *qi* when combined with Cortex Mori."

It is recorded in *Concord Prescriptions* that: "Furuncle, subcutaneous ulcer, carbuncle in the back, appendicitis, mastitis, unidentified swelling, sudden malignant pain, high fever accompanied with aversion to cold, and exogenous disease can be treated, without the consideration of age, with Herba Lonicerae (150g), Radix Astragali (150g), Radix Angelicae Sinensis (36g), and Radix Glycyrrhizae 30g). The herbs are ground into powder and 6 grams of the powder is decocted in one and a half cup of wine to one cup of broth for oral administration each time. If the disease is on the upper part of the body, the prescription is taken after meal, and if the disease is on the lower part of the body, the prescription is taken before the meal and again a little while after the first administration."

THE AUTHOR'S NOTE

Mr. Yie Juquan said that: "30 grams of the crude drug is decocted into a cup of strong decoction for oral administration 3 times, each time, one third. Preliminary tests indicated that the drug administered after operation reduces recurrence."

RADIX SCUTELLARIAE

Miao Xiyong in the Ming Dynasty said that: "The drug is bitter in taste and mild and non-toxic in nature, clearing away various pathogenic and damp heat."

The drug is obtained from a herb of the *Labiatae* family, the radix is for medical use. The herbs of the same family, such as *S. amoena C.H. Wright* and *S. hypericifolia Lëve.*, can also be used medically. The drug is produced all over China. The effective substances contained in the drug are baicalein, baicalin, wogonin and flavonoides.

ANTICANCER PHARMACOLOGICAL FUNCTIONS

1. Experiments in vivo showed that the hot water extract of the drug inhibits JTC-26 with an effective rate of 100%, but also strongly inhibits normal cells.

2. Experiments in vitro showed that the ethanol extract of the drug inhibits mice sarcoma-180 with an effective rate of 37.7%, and the hot water extract with an rate of 11.5%.

3. Wagonin has been proved to have a strong action against the activity of cancer pharmaceutically and clinically, and to inhibit the cells of leukemia.

EXPERIMENTAL FORMULAS

For nasopharyngeal cancer:

        Radix Scutellariae 12g

        Caulis Aristolochiae Manshuriensis 12g

        Rhizoma Ligustici 12g

        Radix Codonopsis Pilosulae 12g

        Bulbus Fritillariae Thunbergii 9g

        Fructus Forsythemi 9g

        Flos Chrysanthemi 9g

        Radix Paeoniae Alba 15g

The prescription is taken in decoction. (*Diagnosis and Treatment of Tumor*)

For laryngocancer:

        Radix Scutellariae 10g

        Radix Platycodi 10g

        Bulbus Fritillariae Thunberi 10g

        Radix Ophiopogonis 10g

        Fructus Gardeniae 10g

        Radix Sophorae Tonkinensis 10g

        Folium Perillae 6g

        Herba Menthae 6g

        Radix Tinosoprae 6g

        Rhizoma Paridis 15g

        Fructus Arctii 12g

        Radix Isatidis 20g

        Anemarrhena, Phellodendron and Rehamania Pill 1

The prescription is taken in decoction twice a day. (*Oncology in Traditional Chinese Medicine*)

For haemorrhagia caused by colocancer:

9 grams of the drug is ground into powder and decocted in a bowl of water. Both the decoction and the residue are taken orally. (*Materia Medica*)

For external and middle auditory meatus cancer:

        Radix Scutellariae 7.5g

        Realgar 22.5g

        Azurite 15g

The herbs are ground into powder for blowing into the ear. (*Medical Consultation*)

HISTORICAL COMMENTS

It is said in *Herbal Antithetical Couplet* that: "The drug relieves celialgia when combined with Cortex Magnoliae and Rhizoma Coptidis, induces pregnancy with Fructus Schisandrae, Rhizoma Paridis Tetraphyllae and Concha Ostreae, and cures scrofula with Radix Astragali, Radix Ampelopsis and Semen Phaseoli."

It is recorded in *Key Prescriptions* that: "The drug functions in nine ways: 1. To clear away pathogenic heat accumulated in the Lung Channel; 2. To cool down heat accumulation in summer; 3. To clear away wind-heat located in the upper *jiao* and the skin; 4. To clear away all kinds of heat syndromes; 5. To nourish *yin* and reduce *yang* after parturition; 6. To invigorate thoracic *qi*; 7. To diminish phlegm located above the diaphragm; 8. To clear away pathogenic heat accumulated in the upper *jiao* and expel splenodampness; and 9. To calm the fetus."

THE AUTHOR'S NOTE

A renowned Japanese doctor treated a woman, 38 years old, with breast tumor on the right side, as large as a berry and free from the surrounding tissues, with Sixteen Ingredients Decoction which is composed of Radix Angelicae Duhuricae, Radix Aucklandiae, Radix Linderae, Cortex Magnoliae, Fructus Citri Aurantii, Semen Arecae, Radix Ledebouriellae and Radix Glycyrrhizae (2 grams each), and Radix Angelicae Sinensis, Rhizoma Chuanxiong, Radix paeoniae, Ramulus Cinnamomi, Radix Ginseng, Folium Perillae and Radix Platycodi (3 grams each). The patient was advised to continue the prescription if the tumor would have shrunk, and to take operation if there would be no response at all after 15 days of administration. However, after taking only 16 doses, the tumor disappeared completely. This prescription is originally recorded in *Rehabilitation of All Diseases* written by Gong Tingxian in the Ming Dynasty, also known as Two Plus Eight Dispersing Decoction, miraculously effective in curing unidentified stubborn tumors.

RHIZOMA COPTIDIS

It is defined in *Canon of Materia Medica* that: "The drug is bitter in taste and cold in nature, curing ophthalmalgia due to pathogenic heat stimulation."

The drug is obtained from a herb of the *Ranunculaceae* family, the radix is for medical use. The drug has many varieties, among which *Coptis Chinensis Franch.* and *C. deltoidea C.Y. cheng et Hsiao* are regarded as the best. The drug mainly contains berberine (7-9%) and chemical compounds such as obakulactone and obacunone.

ANTICANCER PHARMACOLOGICAL FUNCTIONS

1. It is suggested that berberine belongs to serous toxin or cytodivision toxin. It is found in histoculture that it inhibits cytopnea and oxygen absorption, and induces metacytolipsis. Fluorescent photo shows that it exists in the granules of cells.

2. The drug inhibits cellular respiration and particularly the function of the yellow enzyme which is of low concentration in cancer tissues. Therefore, cancer tissues are more sensitive to berberine than the normal cells.

3. Experiments in vivo with the water extract of the drug showed that it inhibits JTC-26 with a rate of 100% when transplanted to the JTC-26 culture medium with a dose of 500μm/ml. But simultaneously it inhibits the normal fibroembryocytes with the same rate.

EXPERIMENTAL FORMULAS

For cervical cancer:
1>.   Fructus Chebulae 6g
        Borax 6g
        Rhizoma Coptidis 6g
        Fructus Mume 6g
        Moschus 0.12g

The above herbs are ground into fine powder to be blended with Moschus for external application to the lesion once daily after washing the vagina.
2>.   Herba oldenlandiae Diffusae 60g
        Herba Scutellariae Barbatae 60g
        Rhizoma Smilacis Glabrae 30g
        Rhizoma Dryopteris Crassirhizomae 30g
        Semen Coicis 30g
        Rhizoma Dioscoreae 30g
        Flos Lonicerae 15g
        Radix Arnebiae 15g
        Radix Salviae Miltiorrhizae 15g
        Radix Angelicae Sinensis 12g

Pericarpium Citri Reticulatae Viride 9g

The prescription is taken twice daily in decoction.

For rectocancer:

Rhizoma Coptidis 15g

Cortex Phellodendri 15g

Radix Scutellariae 15g

Calculus Bovis 18g

Succinum 30g

Cormus Iphigeniae 30g

Rhizoma Bletillae 30g

Rhizoma Dioscoreae 30g

Radix Notoginseng 60g

Pericarpium Citri Reticulatae 9g

Bulbus Fritillariae Cirrhosae 9g

Radix Curcumae 9g

Fructus Mori 9g

Radix Glycyrrhizae 9g

Flos Lonicerae 9g

Agkistrodon 9g

Cornu Rhinoceri 0.9g

Miniuim

The above herbs are ground into powder to be blended with Minium, rolled into pills for oral administration 1 pill a time and 2 to 3 times a day after meal. A course includes 30 days of administration. (*Anticancer Preparations of Traditional Chinese Medicine*)

For radiant dermatitis caused by radiotherapy:

Rhizoma Coptidis 30g

Cortex Phellodendri 3g

The herbs are decocted and filtrated. The broth is applied to the lesion with a piece of gauze saturate with the decoction. (*Journal of Heilongjiang Traditional Chinese Medicine*, Vol. 4, 1984)

For external and middle auditory meatus cancer:

Rhizoma Coptidis 30g

Alumen 15g

Pig Bile 30g

The herbs are dried in shade before being ground into powder for blowing into the ear 1 to 2 times a day. (*Diagnosis and Treatment of Tumor*)

For esophageal cancer:

Rhizoma Coptidis 6g

Rhizoma Pinelliae 6g

Fructus Amomi Rotundus 6g

Radix Ginseng 6g

Poria 6g

Caulis Bambusae in Taeniam 6g

The herbs are decocted in fresh ginger water before taking. (*General Introduction to Management of Complicated Diseases*)

HISTORICAL COMMENTS

It is said in *Ri Hua Zhi Materia Medica* that: "The drug cures five kinds of impairment and seven kinds of trauma, invigorates *qi*, relieves gastralgia and palpitation with fear and restlessness, moistens the heart and the lung, promotes myopoiesis and stops haemorrhagia."

It is suggested in *Rei Zhai's Key Prescriptions* that: "The drug expels stagnated blood in the tongue."

It is recorded in *Materia Medica* that: "The drug alleviates symptoms of slight poisoning caused by overdosage."

It is reported in *Elucidation on Materia Medica* that: "The drug cures *qi* deficiency, lack of blood, weak spleen and stomach, *yin* deficiency, and restlessness due to the intrinsic heat accumulation. To treat these disorders, the drug is contraindicative to salt, and any violation may endanger the patient's health."

It is advised in *Introduction to Medicine* that: "The drug, roasted after being steeped in wine, works upward to the brain, the eye, the mouth, and the tongue, and roasted with ginger juice, cures pyogenic infection, summer-heat attack, malignant infection, pyogenic swelling, sore and ulcer. The use of ginger is to neutralize pathogenic cold without altering its nature so as not to entrap heat."

CORTEX PHELLODENDRI

It is defined in *Canon of Materia Medica* that: "The drug is bitter in taste and cold in nature, clearing away pathogenic heat accumulated in the viscera and the gastroenteric system."

The drug is obtained from a herb of the *Rutaceae* family, generally divided into two categories, i.e. *Phellodendron amurense Rupr.* and *P. Chinensis Schneid.*. The bark without cork is for medical use. The drug is produced in most parts of China, mainly containing berberine, phellodendrine and ß-sitosterol.

ANTICANCER PHARMACOLOGICAL FUNCTIONS

1. The hot water extract from the drug inhibits mice sarcoma-180 with an effective rate of 82%.

2. The drug inhibits JTC-26 with an effective rate of 90% when administrated externally.

3. Berberine under a dose of 2.5-7.5mg/kg does not activate ascites cancer, but the phosphate of its biological alkali inhibits it.

EXPERIMENTAL FORMULAS

For differential squamous epithelial carcinoma:

    Cortex Phellodendri 10g

    Rhizoma Cimicifugae Foetidae 10g

    Alumen 30g

    Gypsum 20g

The herbs are ground into powder, blended with boiled food oil and applied to the lesion twice a day. (*Journal of Shaanxi Traditional Chinese Medicine*, Vol. 4, 1984)

For cervical cancer:

    Cortex Phellodendri 15g

    Radix Scutellariae 15g

    Rhizoma Coptidis 15g

    Radix Arnebiae 15g

    Alumen 30g

    Borax 30

The herbs are ground into fine powder to be mixed with a little Borneol. (*Medical Research Correspondence*, Vol. 5, 1973)

For angioma:

    Cortex Phellodendri 9g

    Catechu 6g

Bulbus Fritillariae Cirrhosae 1g
Cinnabaris 1g
Camphora 1g
Calomelas 1g
Hydrargyrum 1g
Borneol 0.9g

The herbs are ground into powder for application to the lesion frequently. (*Biography of Hua Tuo*)

For glossocancer:

The drug is applied to the tongue frequently. (*Theoretical Essays of Medicine*)

For labiocancer at the early stage:

The powder of the drug is blended with juice of Radix Rosae Mutiflorae for external application. (*Holy Prescriptions*)

HISTORICAL COMMENTS

It is said in *Elucidation of Drugs* that: "Because its bitter taste works on the bones and moves downwards, the drug, roasted with wine and taken with Four Ingredient Decoction, enters the hemophase, curing vacillating osteoalgia on the four extremities, weakness of the feet and the kneels with sour pain, malignant sores all over the body, serious beriberi, hiccup, nausea, and hemopyrosis due to *yin* deficiency. This is because that the bitter taste is able to disperse the heat gathered in the *yin* phase and eliminate ascarid."

It is reported in *Origin of Materia Medica* that: "The drug is for reducing sthenic heat, controlling flaming heat of the *yin* nature when roasted with wine, extinguishing the lower *jiao* fire when roasted with salt, expelling the phlegm fire when roasted with ginger, eliminating damp heat when roasted black with ginger juice, diminishing the deficiency fire when roasted black with salty wine, and curing the loss of *yang* with reddish complexion due to excessive heat caused by *yin* deficiency when used together with Herba Anaphalidis juice."

It is recorded in *Secret Treatment* that: "The drug cures flaming heat accumulated in the urinary bladder, dysuria, damp swelling of the lower *jiao*, dysentery with blood at the beginning, naval pain and kidney *yin* deficiency."

It is suggested in *Luo's Diagnostic Mirror* that: "The drug cures stomatitis when roasted with honey for gargling. If not effective, Radix Codonopsis Pilosulae, Rhizoma Atractylodis Macrocephalae, Radix Glycyrrhizae, Rhizoma Zingiberis and Radix Aconiti Lateralis Preparata are added to the drug."

RHIZOMA DIOSCOREAE BULBIFERAE

Li Shizhen in the Ming Dynasty said that: "The drug is bitter in taste, mild in nature and nonpoisonous, reducing heat by cooling the blood and curing goiter through removing toxic materials."

The drug is obtained from *Dioscorea bulbifera L.* of the *Dioscoreaceae* family, the radix is for medical use. The drug contains such chemical elements as diosbulbin A, B, and C which are all demethyl-furanditerpenes with bitter taste.

ANTICANCER PHARMACOLOGICAL FUNCTIONS

1. The drug inhibits mice sarcoma-180 and cervical cancer-14.

2. Bacteriophagic experiment proved that the drug is against the activity of bacteria, suggesting that the drug resists cancer.

EXPERIMENTAL FORMULAS

For rectocancer, cardiac cancer and inferior esophageal cancer:

500 grams of the drug is cut into small pieces, rinsed in 1500ml of alcohol, sealed by Gypsum Fibrosum, simmered for 2 hours with millet chaff, steeped in cold water for 7 days, then filtrated and taken a little each time and totally 50-100ml a day. This prescription is also effective in treating gastrocancer, cervical cancer and mammary cancer. (*Classification of Commonly Used Chinese Medicinal Herbs*)

For esophageal cancer and cardiac cancer:

Anticancer Pill II is taken 1 to 2 pills (each weights 6 grams) a time and twice a day with warm boiled water. Anticancer Tablet II is taken 3 to 5 tablets (each weights 0.5 gram) a time and three times a day with warm boiled water. (*Anticancer Prescriptions of Traditional Chinese Medicine*)

For thyroid tumor:

1>. 15 grams of the unprocessed drug is taken daily. (*Yunnan Medical Journal*, Vol. 2, 1965)

2>. The drug is steeped in wine for oral administration 3 to 4 times a day with a total dosage of 100ml. (*National Oncological Research Bulletin*, Vol. 8, 1970)

HISTORICAL COMMENTS

It is recorded in *Materia Medica* that: "The drug eliminates fire by cooling the blood, cures goiter through removing the toxic materials."

It is reported in *Dictionary of Chinese Materia Medica* that: "The drug cures, when ground with water and taken orally or applied externally, various malignant sores, swelling, fistula, pharyngitis, snake and dog bite."

"The wine made with the drug is effective in curing various goiter and *qi* stagnation", recorded in *Materia Medica*.

It is said in *Prescriptions Worth a Thousand Gold* that: "Patients with goiter for one or two years may drink the drug wine frequently so as to keep the fragrant smell vacillating in the body. This therapy is quite effective."

THE AUTHOR'S NOTE

Several cases of esophageal cancer were treated in Hubei Traditional Chinese Medical College with 2% glycerina of the drug dropped into the esophagus, and quick and evident effect was achieved (Reported in *Chinese Pharmaceutical information*, Vol. 3, 1972). A case of rhabdomyoma in Jiangxi was reported to be cured by the wine made with the drug with an oral dose of 60-80ml a day.

LUMBRICUS

It is defined in *Canon of Materia Medica* that: "The drug is salty in taste and cold in nature, curing abdominal mass."

The drug is obtained from *Pheretima aspergillum (Perrier)* of the *Megascolecidae* family or from *Allolobophora caliginosa (Savigny) trapezoides (Ant. Dugés)* of the *Allolobophora* family. All contains lumbrifebrine, lumbritin, various substances containing nitrogen, and a kind of enzyme which automatically dissolves when pH ranges between 8.0 and 8.2.

ANTICANCER PHARMACOLOGICAL FUNCTIONS

1. The extract of the drug is, by methylene blue method, effective in treating colon cancer and liver cancer, and inducing generation of bacteriophage.

2. The hot water extract of the drug inhibits JTC-26 with an effective rate of 50-70%.

EXPERIMENTAL FORMULAS

For gingival hemorrhage:

   Lumbricus (dried) 3g

   Alumen 3g

   Moschus 1.5g

The herbs are ground into powder, sprinkled on wet cloth for application to the lesion. (*Holy Prescriptions*)

For glossocancer:

One Lumbricus is melted in salty water and applied to the lesion. (*Holy Prescriptions*)

For malignant lymphosarcoma:

A handful of Lumbricus is calcined over coal fire into powder. A spoonful of the powder is mixed up with the powders of 1.5 gram of Olibanum, 1.5 gram of Myrrha, 1.5 gram of Calomelas and 9 sheets of Squama Manitis. Then the mixed powder is blended with food oil for application to the lesion. (*Materia Medica*)

For liver cancer:

   Lumbricus 15g

   Squama Manitis 15g

   Concha Ostreae 15g

   Semen Persicae 9g

   Flos Carthami 9g

   Radix Curcumae 9g

   Semen Meliae 9g

   Cortex Moutan 6g

   Rhizoma Dioscorea Nipponicae 6g

The prescription is taken one dosage a day in decoction. (*Brief Introduction to Oncology*)

For celiac tumor:

White-necked Lumbricus is pounded into juice and taken orally. (*Newly Compiled Experienced Prescriptions*)

HISTORICAL COMMENTS

It is said in *Materia Medica* that: "The drug cures swelling and nasal polyp."

It is reported in *Supplementation to Materia Medica* that: "The extremely hot nature of the drug eliminates flaming fire and morbid heat, therefore, the drug cures high fever in patients with exogenous febrile diseases; and the salty taste of the drug comes downwards to promote micturition, therefore, the drug cures ascites and jaundice."

PERIOSTRACUM SERPENTIS

It is defined in *Pharmaceutical Property* that: "The drug is sweet and salty in taste, mild and toxic in nature, curing pharyngitis."

The drug is the dry slough from *Elaphe taeniurus Cope.*, *Elaphe carinata (Günther)*, and *Zaocys dhumnades (Cantor)* of the *Colubridae* family. The slough is about a meter in length and looks like a membrane with scales, silvery color, lustre and grassy texture. The abdominal side of the slough is covered with scales in cuboid shape and arranged like tiles. The slough is felt slippery with foul smell.

ANTICANCER PHARMACOLOGICAL FUNCTIONS

The drug inhibits transplanted tumor on animals.

EXPERIMENTAL FORMULAS

For salivary gland tumor:

        Periostracum Serpentis 30g

        Scorpio 30g

        Nidus Vespae 30g

The herbs are ground into powder and taken 3 grams a time and twice a day. (*Diagnosis and Treatment of Tumor*)

For labiocancer:

        Periostracum Serpentis

        Nidius Vespae

        Cirinis

        Cirinis Animalis

        Holotrichia

Equal portion of the above herbs is ground into powder, blended with lard for rubbing on the lesion. (*Theoretical Essays of Medicine*)

For ameloblastoma:

        Periostracum Serpentis 9g

        Fructus Forsythiae 9g

        Nidus Vespae 9g

        Radix Vespae 9g

        Flos Carthami 9g

        Radix Scrophulariae 15g

        Radix Adenophorae 15g

        Flos Lonicerae 15g

        Herba Dendrobii 15g

        Herba Violae Yedoensis 15g

        Radix Glycyrrhizae 1g

The prescription is taken in decoction. (*Journal of New Traditional Chinese Medicine*, Vol. 6, 1978)

HISTORICAL COMMENTS

It is said in *Records of Famous Doctors* that: "The drug indicates for stubborn diseases in adults and rave, improves eyesight and heals various malignant sores when burnt."

It is reported in *Materia Medica* that: "The drug expels pathogenic foul and wind, kills parasites when burnt, ground and taken orally, cures female mammary abscess, acute pharyngitis in adults, phlyctenular keratitis with rigid tongue, sublingual swelling and swollen palate in infants."

It is recorded in *Yang Kong's Prescriptions* that: "The drug, when burnt moderately, ground into fine powder for blowing into the ear with a feather, cures acute unbearable otalgia with bleeding."

It is suggested in *Essential Prescriptions Worth a Thousand Gold* that: "To treat malignant boils lingering for ten years, a slough, is burnt and mixed with lard for external application to the lesion, and another slough is burnt and taken with wine."

It is mentioned in *Holy Prescriptions* that: "Tumors with a hard mass and no pus can be treated with a paste made from the drug for application every night."

It is believed in *Key Prescriptions* that: "For carbuncle, furuncles and boils, the drug is decocted in 160ml of water and the broth is either for oral administration or application."

It is also held in *Wai Tai Prescriptions* that: "Pyogenic naval sore can be cured with the drug when calcined, ground and mixed with egg white for external application."

THE AUTHOR'S NOTE

It is said in *Drugs Obtained from Animals in Northeast China* that: "The prescription for mammalgia can be applied to the treatment of early mastadenocancer. The prescription is composed of Periostracum Serpentis, Cornu Cervi and Nidus Vespae (9 grams each, calcined together, ground into powder and taken with millet wine twice a day)."

HERBA DUCHESNEAE

It is defined in *Records of Famous Doctors* that: "The drug is very cold in nature, eliminating severe pathogenic heat accumulated in the thorax and the abdomen."

The drug is obtained from *Duchesnea* of the *Rosaceae* family, the whole herb is for medical use, containing saponins, especially in the juice. The drug is produced all over China.

ANTICANCER PHARMACOLOGICAL FUNCTIONS

1. Experiments in vitro with Bacillus coil and ultraviolet ray showed that the drug has a function against sudden cytiovariation.
2. The drug inhibits the activation of ascites cancer and mice sarcoma-180.
3. The drug inhibits JTC-26 with an effective rate of 90%.

EXPERIMENTAL FORMULAS
For cystoma:

      Herba Duchesneae 15g
      Herba Solani Nigri 30g
      Rhizoma Smilacis Glabrae 30g
      Herba Aristolochiae Mollissimae 30g
      Spora Lygodii 10g
      Medulla Junci 10g

The prescription is taken one dosage a day in decoction, one dosage every other day after the disappearance of tumor, and stopped to use if there is no recurrence after one and a half year. The prescription can be taken one dosage every third week for the purpose of prevention. (*Shanghai Medical Journal*, Vol. 7, 1979)

For various cancers:

9-30g of the drug is decocted for oral administration. (*Dictionary of Chinese Materia Medica*)

For thoracic cancer:

      Herba Duchesneae 15g
      Cormus Iphigeniae 15g
      Spica Prunellae 15g
      Herba Arisitolochiae Mollissimae 30g
      Herba Solani Nigri 30g
      Rhizoma Smilacis Chinae 30g
      Radix Codonopsis Lanceolatae 30g
      Semen Coicis 30g
      Concha Ostreae 30g
      Bulbus Fritillariae Thunbergi 10g

The prescription is taken one dosage a day in decoction. (*Oncology of Traditional Chinese Medicine*)

HISTORICAL COMMENTS

It is said in *Materia Medica* that: "The drug relieves pain caused by scald and burn with instant effect."

It is reported in *Major Prescriptions for Exogenous Febrile Diseases* that: "Aphtha and acute dermatopathy can be cured with the juice of the drug when sipped."

It is suggested in *Zhou Hou Prescriptions* that: "Exogenous febrile disease complicated with boils can be treated with 60ml of juice of the drug blended with Fructus Mume and taken three times a day."

It is mentioned in *Textual Research on Plants and Their Nomenclature* that: "Carbuncle and sore were cured with the drug when pounded and applied to the lesions with miraculous effect."

It is recorded in *Guide to Crude Herbal Property* that: "The drug subsides swelling to relieve pain and eliminates stasis to promote hemopoiesis."

It is advised in *Materia Medica in the East of Fujian* that: "The drug is used to treat carbuncle in the head, mammary abscess, back sore and furuncle when pounded freshly with honey and applied to the lesions. While treating the unpyogenic lesion, the drug is pounded with Herba Taraxaci into juice to be blended with 30g of millet wine for oral administration, and the remaining of the drug is applied to the lesions."

RADIX AMPELOPSIS ACONITIFOLIAE

It is defined in *Jiangxi Herbal Medicine* that: "The drug is bland in nature and sweet-sour in taste, activating tendons to promote blood circulation and subsiding swelling to remove toxic materials."

The drug is obtained from *Ampelopsis brevipedunculata (Maxim.) Trautv.* of the *Vitaceae* family, its vine and radix are for medical use. *A. delavayana (Franch.) Planch.* of the same family is used as a substitute for the drug. The chemical elements contained in the drug are flavonoid glycosides, phenols, amino acid and saccharides. Its fruit contains invert sugar, organic acid, tannins, fats, pigment and vitamins.

ANTICANCER PHARMACOLOGICAL FUNCTIONS
1. The drug inhibits mice sarcoma-180.
2. Bacteriophagic screening tests showed that *A. delavayana (Franch.) Planch.* resists bacteriophage, and this suggests that the drug inhibits carcinocytic activation.
3. The inhibiting rate of the drug on mice sarcoma-180 is 36% for the hot water extract and 17.4% for the ethanol extract.

EXPERIMENTAL FORMULAS
For nephrocancer:

> Radix Ampelopsis Aconitifoliae 30g
> Herba Dioscoreae Bulbiferae 9g
> Herba Lobeliae Chinensis 15g
> Rhizoma Imperatae 15g
> Semen Coicis 15g

The prescription is taken in decoction. (*Diagnosis and Treatment of Tumor*)
For mammary cancer:

1>.   Radix Ampelopsis Delavayanae 60g
> Radix Actinidiae Chinensis 60g
> Radix et Rhizoma Diphylleiae 9g
> Rhizoma Arisaematis 9g
> Herba Taraxaci 30g
> Folium Citri Reticulatae 15g

The prescription is taken one dosage a day in decoction. (*Selected Therapies with Chinese Medicinal Herbs*)

2>.   Radix Ampelopsis Aconitifoliae 30g

Radix Actinidiae Chinensis 30g

Rhizoma Dysosmae 3g

Rhizoma Arisaematis 3g

The prescription is taken one dosage a day in decoction. (*Selected Data from a National Display of Herbal Therapies*)

For lung cancer:

1>.   Radix Ampelopsis Delavayanae 30g

Herba Scutellariae Barbatae 30g

Herba Lobeliae Chinensis 30g

Radix Adinae 30g

Radix Actinidiae Chinensis 60g

Radix Sophorae Tonkinensis 15g

Rhizoma Paridis 15g

Herba Pteridis Multifidae 25g

Rhizoma Imperatae 25g

Rhizoma Atractylodis Macrocephalae 10g

The prescription is taken one dosage a day in decoction. (*Oncology of Traditional Chinese Medicine*)

2 . 60g of Radix Ampelopsis Delavayanae (dried) is decocted and taken frequently as tea. (*Food Commonly Used for Medical Purpose*)

HISTORICAL COMMENTS

It is said in *Materia Medica* that: "The drug relieves pain in the waist, the foot, the arm and the leg through washing with its decoction, and the juice of the drug can promote urination, activate the small intestine and subside swelling when taken orally."

It is reported in *Dietetic Materia Medica* that: "Vomiting can be stopped by sipping the strong juice of the drug."

THE AUTHOR'S NOTE

In *Selected Data on Tumor Prevention and Treatment from a Symposium Held in Hubei* in 1971, it is said that one case of rectocancer was successfully cured with Herba Duchesneae, Herba Artemisiae Annuae and Radix Sanguisorbae (60 grams each) when put into a thermos bottle for 12 hours and taken as tea. The therapy was repeated daily and 15 days constituted a course of treatment.

RADIX RANUNCULI TERNATI

It is defined in *Dictionary of Chinese Materia Medica* that: "The drug is sweet and hot in taste and warm in nature, curing scrofula."

The drug is the radix of *Ranunculus ternatus Thunb.* of the *Ranunculaceae* family. The whole drug contains amino acid, organic acid, flavonoid glycosides and saccharides. The drug is mainly produced in Henan, Jiangsu, Zhejiang and Guangxi provinces.

ANTICANCER PHARMACOLOGICAL FUNCTIONS

Experiments with animals showed that the drug inhibits mice sarcoma-180, sarcoma-37 and ascites cancer.

EXPERIMENTAL FORMULAS

For malignant lymphosarcoma, thyroid tumor and mammary tumor:

1>. The drug is prepared into an injection containing 2 grams of the crude drug per milliliter and is administrated intramuscularly 2ml a time and once or twice a day.

2>.　　Radix Ranunculi Ternati 9g

　　　　Concha Ostreae 30g

　　　　Spica Prunellae 9g

The prescription is taken one dosage a day in decoction. (*Anticancer Preparations of Traditional Chinese Medicine*)

For carcinoceliascietes:

30-60g of the drug is decocted with 9g of Semen Descurainiae and the broth is taken twice a day orally. (*Diagnosis and Treatment of Tumors*)

HISTORICAL COMMENTS

It is said in *Handbook of Chinese Herbal Medicine* that: "The drug cures scrofula and tuberculosis."

It is reported in *Handbook of Chinese Herbal Medicine* in Henan that: "Scrofula can be cured with a proper amount of the drug and Spica Prunellae, when decocted, filtrated and boiled into paste for application to the lesions."

It is suggested in *Anticancer Herbal Preparation* that: "The drug functions to remove toxic materials to eliminate stasis, and is mainly indicative for lymphocancer, thyroma and mammoma. Clinically it is now used for experiment and observation. So its curative effect still needs to be further confirmed."

POLYPORUS

It is defined in *Canon of Materia Medica* that: "The drug is sweet and bland in taste and mild in nature, promoting drainage."

The drug is obtained from *Polyporus* of the *Polyporaceae* family, the sclerotium is for medical use. The drug is perennial and parasitizes on the roots of the plants of the *Fagaceae* family. The chemical elements contained in the drug are ergosterol, crude protein, polysaccharides, soluble saccharides, and α- hydroxytetracosanoic acid. The polysaccharides are the effective anticancer element, pertaining to PGU.

ANTICANCER PHARMACOLOGICAL FUNCTIONS

1. The drug is dissolvable in water and with a dosage of 0.5 mg/kg inhibits mice sarcoma-180 with 100% effective rate. The tumor was eliminated completely in 25 mice out of 30.

2. PGU-1, administrated thoracically with a dosage of 0.1mg/kg, inhibits sarcoma-180 with 97.2% effective rate and ten mice out of 12 having their tumor eliminated within five weeks.

3. Mice with lung cancer-7423 were treated with polyporus polysaccharide (100mg/kg) with a 100% effective rate and the tumor mass became evidently reduced after seven weeks of administration of the drug and 50% of the tumors disappeared completely after 41 days.

4. The extract of polyporus can increase phagocapacity of macrophagocytes in the liver, the spleen and the abdominal cavity, promote generation of cells bearing antigen in the spleen of the animals with tumor and the hemolymphocytic reversion rate in the victims and increase the amount of cyclophosphamide contained in oncocytes. The extract itself is non-toxic and reacts to the necrotoxin generated by methotrexate.

5. The hot water extract inhibits JTC-26 with a 33.3% effective rate and does not affect fabroblastocytes in adults.

EXPERIMENTAL FORMULAS

For various cancers:

15g of the drug is decocted in 300ml of water and taken in three times. (*Traditional Chinese Medical and Pharmaceutical Research Materials*, Vol. 6, 1978)

For nephrocancer:

>   Polyporus 3g
>   Poria 3g
>   Talcum 3g
>   Rhizoma Alismatis 3g
>   Colla Corii Asini 3g
>   Semen Coicis 5g

The prescription is taken in decoction and modified in accordance with the patient's conditions. (*Elucidation on Clinical Prescriptions*)

HISTORICAL COMMENTS

It is said in *Access to Drug Usage* that: "The drug diminishes constipation with its bitter taste, reinforces *yang* with its sweet taste and activates the senses with its bland taste, therefore, eliminating dampness and promoting urination."

It is reported in *Properties of Materia Medica* that: "The drug focuses on expelling high fever of exogenous febrile diseases, promoting diaphoresis, subsiding swelling and abdominal fullness, and relieving acute abdominal pain."

It is mentioned in *Herbal Decoction* that: "The drug promotes urination to eliminate pathogenic heat accumulated in the urinary bladder."

It is recorded in *Materia Medica* that: "The drug is characterized by bland taste and the capacity to ascend as well as to descend, therefore promoting urination. It is similar to poria in this respect but inferior to poria in terms of tonic evaluation."

It is suggested in *Extension of Materia Medica* that: "The drug is most superior in promoting drainage, therefore chronic administration will affect renal function, resulting in poor eyesight."

THE AUTHOR'S NOTE

30 cases of lung cancer were treated with the capsules of Polyporus polysaccharide and satisfactory result was achieved. 300 cases of malignant tumor were treated with an extract from Polyporus (called 757), among which 32 were treated only with "757" and the improvement of their condition was found to be 62.5% and the stabilization of their condition was found to be 25%. The experiment shows that 757 inhibits mice sarcoma-180 with a 50-70% effective rate and 6-7% of the tumors disappeared completely. No recurrence of tumor would occur in those mice when inoculated with oncocytes one or six months later, this indicating that it bears immune effect on tumor. In addition, 757 can increase the amount of cAMP in the cancer cells of ascites sarcoma-180 and reduce the side effect caused by chemical drugs. It was also reported that chromium[51] releasing test proved that polyporus can reinforce the capacity of the splenocytes of mice with cervical cancer-14 to engulf oncocytes, indicating that the drug can reinforce the lymphoidocytic effect on tumor specific immunity. (*Journal of Traditional Chinese Medicine*, Vol. 9, 1980) For producing a sort of industrialized Polyporus liquid to substitute raw Polyporus for clinical purpose, study was made on the bacterionuclear separation. Chinese Pharmaceutical Institute, Beijing Traditional Chinese Medicine Academy studied the separation of the bacterial nucleus, the liquid culture of the vegetative mycelium and its anti-tumor effect. The studies showed that the crude

extract of the fermentative liquid and the extract of wild Polyporus all evidently inhibit mice sarcoma-180 and ascites carcinocytes.

HERBA GALII APRINIS

It is defined in *Dictionary of Chinese Materia Medica* that: "The drug is mild and slightly cold in nature, sweet and hot in taste, removing toxic material by clearing away pathogenic heat and activating the channels by promoting blood circulation."

The drug is obtained from *Galium aparine L.* of the *Rubiaceae* family. The whole herb is for medical use. The young seedlings can be used as vegetable. But pigs will become ill if they eat the seedlings. The drug is produced all over China. The chemical elements contained in the drug are asperuloside, rubiadinprimveroside, galiosin, and 2-2-Dimethyl naphthol(1, 2b) pyran.

ANTICANCER PHARMACOLOGICAL FUNCTIONS
1. Experiments in vivo with ethylene blue method showed that the drug inhibits the growth of oncocytes.
2. Tests in vivo showed that the drug inhibits mice sarcoma-180 and leukemia.

EXPERIMENTAL FORMULAS
For mammary cancer, submandibular adenocancer, thyrocanccer and cervical cancer:
30g of the drug is decocted in water with the addition of brown sugar and taken one dosage and 3 to 6 times a day for a long period (or 250g of the fresh drug is squeezed into juice, added with brown sugar and taken orally). (*New Medicine*, Vol. 9, 1972)

For glossocancer and gingival cancer:
The decoction of the drug is for gargling without any dosage restriction. External application of the decoction can also treat mammary carcinoulceration, vulva cancer and penis cancer. (*Anticancer Consultation*)

For anal cancer:
>Herba Galii Aprinis 45g
>Herba Scutellariae Barbatae 30g
>Caulis Lonicerae 30g
>Herba Oldenlandiae Diffusae 60g
>Herba Duchesneae 24g

The prescription is taken in decoction. (*Popularized Medicine and Hygiene*)

For leukemia:
>Herba Galii Aprinis 45g
>Caulis Lonicerae 30g
>Herba Scutellariae Barbatae 30g
>Herba Solani Nigri 30g
>Radix Salviae Miltiorrhizae 30g
>Radix Lycii Radicis 30g
>Herba Dichondrae 15g
>Rhizoma Polygonati 15g

The prescription is taken in decoction. (*Popularized Medicine and Hygiene*)

For malignant lymphoma:
>Herba Galii 60g
>Herba Solani nigri 120g
>Herba Oldenlandiae Diffusae 250g

The prescription is taken in decoction. (Tumor Prevention)

For visceral and mammary cancer:

150g of the drug is pounded into juice and taken orally, or 30g of the drug is taken in decoction. (*Handbook of Chinese Medicinal Herbs in Ningxia*)

HISTORICAL COMMENTS

It is said in *Pharmaceutical Discrimination* that: "The drug cures carbuncles, abdominal mass, tympanites and jaundice."

It is reported in *Handbook of Chinese Medicinal Herbs in Ningxia* that: "The drug removes toxic material by clearing away heat, cooling blood and promoting urination."

It is recorded in *Dictionary of Chinese Materia Medica* that: "To cure breast cancer, 120g of the drug is pounded and mixed with lard for application to the lesion, or decocted for oral administration."

THE AUTHOR'S NOTE

It is reported in *Reference Material for Prevention and Treatment of Cancer* compiled in Jiangsu (1972) that: "Its variation, *Galium aparine L. Var.t.R.* inhibits acute lymphocytic leukemia and acute granulocytic leukemia."

TREMELLA

It is defined in *New Reference of Medicine* that: "The drug is sweet and bland in taste, cold in nature, clearing the lung and nourishing its *yin*."

The drug is obtained from the sporphore of *Tremella fusiformis Berk* of the *Tremellaceae* family. The herb parasitizes on the decayed wood, containing, a part from the common nutritional elements, DNA, 16 kinds of amino acid, coenzyme Q and polysaccharides.

ANTICANCER PHARMACOLOGICAL FUNCTIONS

1. Polysaccharide extracted from Tremella produced in Fujian Province inhibits mice sarcoma-180 with a rate of 35.4%.

2. The acid and neutral isopolysaccharide separated from the water extract of the drug produced in China and Japan inhibits mice sarcoma-180 with a rate of 45-91.7% and the polysaccharide from the Japanese Tremella proves to be much superior.

3. Tremella polysaccharide is found to reinforce phagocapacity of mice celiomacrophagocytes, and this indicates that its anticancer function lies in its immune system.

4. Tremella polysaccharide reduces the reaction of mice and dogs to cobalt[60] rays and cyclophosphamide after radiotherapy and chemotherapy, promoting the rehabilitation of the affected hematopoietic system, reducing mortality of radiotherapy and evidently rehabilitating dogs with radiation diseases.

EXPERIMENTAL FORMULAS

For cough induced by lung cancer:

    Tremella 6g

    Rhizoma Tupistrae Chinensis 6g

    Herba Epimedii 3g

The first two ingredients are steeped in cold water for several hours before being mixed with the third ingredient, a proper amount of crystal sugar, lard and some water in a bowl for steaming. The residue of the third ingredient should be removed before eating the drugs and drinking the broth. (*Collection of Folk Remedies in Guizhou*)

For *yin* deficiency induced by chemicals and radiotherapy:

9g of the drug is simmered with crystal sugar and taken every day for 2-3 months. The prescription is also effective for febrile reactions caused by radiotherapy in the nose, the pharynx and the larynx and is also effective for renal deficiency at the middle or advanced stage of hepatoma, lung tumor, leukemia and myeloma. (*Journal of Integrated Chinese and Western Medicine*, Vol. 2, 1985)

HISTORICAL COMMENTS

It is said in *Renewed Materia Medica* that: "The drug moistens the lung to nourish its *yin*."

It is reported in *Revised Discrimination of Pseudodrugs* that: "The drug clears heat and dryness accumulated in the lung, and is indicative for tussiculation, cough due to phlegm retention, nasal bleeding, hemoptysis and phlegm with blood."

It is recorded in *Dictionary of Chinese Materia Medica* that: "The desirable drug is the one that is dry, yellowish white, large, light, lustrous and thick."

THE AUTHOR'S NOTE

As an anticancer drug, Tremella has been drawing more and more attention. In 1972, Japanese researchers separated, from Tremella, polysaccharide A, B, and C which inhibit mice sarcoma-180. Besides, polysaccharide A has a strong effect against the activation of cancer. Anticancer elements such as emitanins A, B, and C have been separated out from the bacterial filament of Tremella and the fermentative liquid by means of fermentation. It was reported in 1975 by Shenyang Pharmacological College that Polyporus polysaccharide could, when applied externally, invert normal human lymphocytes, with a function similar to that of lectin. It also increases the inversion rate of lymphocytes in patients with leukemia and works well on tumor patients suffering from leukocytosis after radiotherapy and chemotherapy.

PEDICELLUS MELO

Huang Gongxin in the Qing Dynasty said that: "The drug is bitter in taste, and cold and toxic in nature."

The drug is obtained from *Pedicellus* of the *Cucurbitaceae* family, the fruit peel, the root and the vine are for medical use. Citrullus Colocynthis of the same family is used to treat various cancers and leukemia in Greece.

The drug is produced all over China. The unripe fruit stem contains melotoxin, a kind of bitter principle. The whole herb contains curcubitacin. And from the fruit stem, curcubitacin B and E have been extracted.

ANTICANCER PHARMACOLOGICAL FUNCTIONS

1. Curcubitacins have a significant cytoengulfing function. Curcubitacin B showed a cellular toxic activation of 0.005 to nasopharyngeal carcinocytes and 0.005 to Hela cells and Curcubitacin E, 0.01 to nasopharyngeal carcinoma and 0.05-0.01 to Hela cells. Obviously, Curcubitacin B bears a stronger anticancer function.

2. Experiments in vitro showed that Curcubitacin B inhibits the growth of mice sarcoma-180 with an effective rate of 21-55% and prolongs the survival period of mice suffering from Ehrlich's ascites carcinoma with an effective rate of 30-38%.

3. Curcubitacin E inhibits mice sarcoma-180 with an effective rate of 40-42% and inhibits Ehrlich's ascites carcinoma with an effective rate of 39-73%.

EXPERIMENTAL FORMULAS

For dermatocarcinoma:

The juice squeezed from the fresh peel is blended with a little powder of the drug into a paste for external application twice a day.

For gastrocancer:

150g of the dried fruit peel is ground into powder and blended with 9-18g of water and taken orally 3 times a day.

For gastrocancer and cystocancer:

120g of the fresh root and vine is decocted with 60g of pine wood and taken orally one dosage a day.

The above two prescriptions are used as folk remedies in America and Canada. (*Correspondance of Chinese Medicinal Herbs*, Vol. 6, 1974)

HISTORICAL COMMENTS

It is said in *True Materia Medica* that: "Acute dysentery with pus, blood and unbearable pain can be cured with several of the drug after being soaked in water and taken orally."

It is recorded in *Materia Medica* that: "Amenorrhea can be treated with Fructus Quisqualis (15g) and Radix Glycyrrhizae (18g) when ground into powder and taken with wine 6 grams a time."

It is suggested in *Dietetic Materia Medica* that: "The leaf of the drug nourishes the middle *jiao*, cures infantile malnutrition and eliminates homeostasis when ground and taken with wine."

It is described in *Holly Prescriptions* that: "Nasal polyp can be cured with the base of the drug after being pounded and blown into the nose three times a day. An alternative prescription for this illness is: 2.5 grams of the powder of the drug and Alumen is blended with lard and wrapped for inserting into the nostrils once a day."

It is reported in *Materia Medica Decoction* that: "The drug together with Moschus and Herba Acari can cure anosmia."

RADIX ACTINIDIAE CHINENSIS

It is defined in *Dietary Canon* that: "The drug is sweet in taste and cold in nature, harmonizing the middle *jiao* and calming the liver."

The drug is obtained from *Actinidia* of the *Actinidiaceae* family, the radix is for medical use. *Actinidia arguta (Sieb. et Zucc) Planch* of the same family is used as a substitute for the drug. The fruit of the drug contains vitamin C and actinidine; the leaf contains quercetin, kaempfevol, caffeine, cumaric acid, leucodelphinidin and leucocyanidin; the seed contains oil and protein; and the flower contains volatile oil. The fruit of *Actinidia arguta (Sieb. et Zucc) Planch* contains vitamin C, saccharides, organic acid, fruit acid, tannins, protein and phytochromes; and the leaf contains vitamin C.

ANTICANCER PHARMACOLOGICAL FUNCTIONS

1. Bacteriophageal experiments in vitro showed that the drug is against bacteriophage, and this indicates that it resists cancer activation.

2. Experiments in vivo showed that the drug inhibits transplanted tumor in mice.

EXPERIMENTAL FORMULAS

For malignant ophthalmomelanoma:

250g of the drug is simmered with 500g of dog meat and taken first; then 120g of the root of the drug is simmered with two eggs or a proper amount of pork and taken every day. 30 days constitutes a course of treatment. (*Fujian Medical Journal*, Vol. 2, 1978)

For gastrocancer:

1>.   Radix Actinidiae Chinensis 90g
        Herba Solani Nigri 60g
        Herba Oldenlandiae Chrysotrichae 30g
        Lignum Suberalatum Evonymi 30g
        Fructus Fici 30g
        Coridius 9g

The prescription is taken in decoction. (*Exchange of Medical Information*, Vol. 9, 1974)

2>. 120g of the fresh vine and root of Actinida arguta (Sieb. et Zucc) Planch is decocted or made into extract for oral administration. The prescription is effective for gastric cancer and is taken one dosage a day. (*Handbook of Medicinal Herbs in Northeast China*)

3>. 5kg of Actinidia arguta (Sieb. et Zucc) Planch is decocted for three hours into 5ooml of strong broth to be mixed with some sugar for oral administration 25ml a time, twice a day. The prescription is also effective for lung cancer, liver cancer and esophageal cancer. (*New Chinese Herbal Therapies*)

For mammary cancer:

        Radix Actinidiae Chinensiszcbm 30g
        Radix Vitidis Romanetis 30g
        Rhizoma Dysosmae 3g
        Rhizoma Arisaematis 3g

The prescription is taken one dosage a day in decoction. (*Diagnosis and Treatment of Tumor*)

For cancer of the gastroenteric system and breast cancer:

75g of the radix of the drug is decocted in 1000ml of water for three hours and taken orally one dosage a day. 10-15 days constitute a course of treatment. Between courses, there is an interval of several days. The prescription is continued for 4 courses in all. (*Shaanxi Journal of Chinese Medicinal Herbs*)

For primary liver cancer:

        Radix Actinidiae Chinensis 30g
        Herba Oldenlandiae Diffusae 30g
        Concha Ostreae 30g
        Radix Codonopsis Pilosulae 9g
        Rhizoma Atractylodis Macrocephalae 9g
        Radix Paeoniae Alba 9g
        Poria 9g
        Radix Curcumae 9g
        Squama Manitis 9g

The prescription is taken in decoction one dosage a day. (*Shanghai Journal of Traditional Chinese Medicine*, Vol. 4, 1979)

HISTORICAL COMMENTS

It is said in *Supplementation to Materia Medica* that: "The drug regulates the stomach to keep the adverse energy downwards, cures osteomyelitis, paralysis and chronic leukotrichia." "Stranguria caused by urolithiasis and regurgitation can be treated with the juice of the vine of the drug when taken together with ginger juice."

It is reported in *Dictionary of Chinese Materia Medica* that: "The drug relieves extreme thirst, restless hotness, cholelithiasis, urolithiasis and heat accumulation." "The vine juice is sweet in taste, cold, slippery and non-toxic in nature, curing regurgitation."

Ancient people believed that: "This drug might, when used in a large dosage, cool the spleen and the stomach and cause diarrhea. Therefore, it fits for those with sthenic heat."

THE AUTHOR'S NOTE

It is reported in *Selected Folk and Experienced Remedies in Chinese Herbal Medicine in Zhejiang Province* (Second Volume) that 74 cases of esophageal cancer and gastric cancer were treated in Hangzhou Oncological Hospital with 2kg of the drug alone when prepared into 1000ml of syrup and taken in two weeks. It was found by follow-up visits that 15 cases of gastric cancer and 18 of the esophageal cancer showed immediate satisfactory curative effect. A few patients were seen with reactions such as rash and nausea after taking the drug.

HERBA CROTALARIAE

It is defined in *National Compilation of Chinese Medical Herbs* that: "The drug is bitter in taste and mild in nature, removing toxic material and resisting cancer."

The drug is obtained from *Crotalaria* of the *Liguminosae* family, the whole herb is for medical use. The drug is produced in South, Central and Southwest China, containing monocrotaline (0.4% in the seed). Plants of the same family, *C. assamica Benth.* and *C. spectabilis Roth.* are used as the substitutes of the drug.

ANTICANCER PHARMACOLOGICAL FUNCTIONS

1. Monocrotaline significantly inhibits Walker's carcinoma, sarcoma-180, sarcoma-37, adenocancer-775 and lymphocytic leukemia-615.

2. The drug inhibits sarcoma-37 with an effective rate of 54-75%. If oxygen atoms are added to the nitrogen atoms of the maternal nucleus of Monocrotaline, the toxin of the drug is reduced and so is its inhibiting effect on sarcoma-180.

3. Monocrotaline can reduce the absorption of phosphorus by cancer tissues, therefore inhibiting the metabolism of phosphorus. It not only controls the amount of DNA and RNA in carcinocytes but also inhibits its biosynthetic process.

4. *C. assamica Benth.* also contains monocrotaline. The preparation of its fruit shell inhibits tumor with an effective rate of over 80%. This is of statistical significance. It is found by tests that the amount of monocrotaline contained in *C. assamica Benth.* is ten times as much as that contained in Herba Crotalariae.

EXPERIMENTAL FORMULAS

For chronic granulocytic leukemia:

>Herba Crotalariae 15g
>Radix Sanguisorbae Carbonisatus 15g
>Radix Rehmanniae 15g
>Radix Codonopsis Pilosulae 30g
>Radix Asparagi 30g

The prescription is taken one dosage a day in decoction. (*Prevention and Treatment of Common Tumors in Qinghai*)

For cutaneous squamous epithelial carcinoma:

1>. The drug is ground into powder, sterilized under high temperature, blended with physiological saline to make a paste for external application 2-3 times a day.

2>. Iontherapy: The drug is pounded into paste, painted on a piece of gauze, applied to the lesion and connected to the negative pole of electricity with low current. The therapy is practiced once daily for 20-30 minutes each time. 12 days will constitute a course of treatment. There will be an interval of 7 days between two courses. (*Diagnosis and Treatment of Tumor*)

For acute and chronic leukemia:

1.5g of the drug is blended with 1.5g of pig spleen (calcined and ground), packaged into capsules and taken 2-3 capsules a time and three times a day. (*Diagnosis and Treatment of Tumor*)

For cervical cancer:

1>. The juice squeezed from the fresh drug is applied to the lesion, or decocted into a strong decoction for washing the lesion.

2>. Monocrotaline hydrochloride antiseptic injection is injected around the focus of the lesion 1-4ml each time, once a day or every other day. (*National Compilation of Chinese Medicinal Herbs*)

For esophageal cancer:

1>. Monocrotaline hydrochloride antiseptic injection is injected 4ml a time, three times a day.

2>. Tablets and syrup made from the drug: 4-10 tablets are taken each time, three times a day; 20-50ml of the syrup is taken each time, 3-4 times a day. (*National Compilation of Chinese Medicinal Herbs*)

HISTORICAL COMMENTS

It is said in *Research on Plants and Their Nomenclature* that: "The drug cures lung inflammation."

It is reported in *Newly Compiled Materia Medica in South Zhejiang* that: "The drug cures dysentery."

THE AUTHOR'S NOTE

This drug is toxic and impairs the liver, the kidney and the digestive track if over used. The dosage for decoction is 15-30g. It is reported that 21 cases of malignant tumor were treated with monocrotaline and it was significantly effective in two cases, and effective in one patient. The ways for administering the drug is: 1. External application of the powder 15-80mg a day; 2. Local injection into the tumor mass, 30-100mg a day; 3. Intramuscular injection, 15-50mg a day; 5. Arterio-intubation injection, 200mg a day. One or two of the above methods may be chosen according to the tumor and a course of treatment may last for two or three weeks. The toxin of the drug may affect hematopoiesis with general side effects such as nausea, vomiting, poor appetite, fatigue, dizziness and headache.

FLOS CHRYSANTHEMI INDICI

It is defined in *Comments on Materia Medica* that: "The drug is bitter and hot in taste, cold and slightly toxic in nature, removing hemostasis to activate the liver and to heal furuncle through removing toxic materials."

The drug is obtained from *Chrysanthemum indicum L., C. boreale Mak.,* and *C. lavandulaefolium (Fisch.) Mak.*. Its capitulum or the whole herbs are for medical use. The drug contains lactone, bitter principles, chrysanthemin, volatile oils, vitamin A and B. The decoction of the drug inhibits exanthem subitum, Staphylococcus aureus, Bucillus diphtheriae and Bucillus dysenteriae.

ANTICANCER PHARMACOLOGICAL FUNCTIONS

1. Experiments in vitro showed that the hot water extract of the herb inhibits JTC-26 with an effective rate of 90%.

2. Bacteriophagic tests showed that the drug resists bacteriophagia, indicating that it is against cancer activation.

EXPERIMENTAL FORMULAS

For thyroma:

1>. One portion of the flower or the leaf of the drug and two portions of *Piper migrum L.* are pounded, added with some salt for pounding again before being steamed and applied to the lesion once daily. (*Journal of New Traditional Chinese Medicine*, Vol. 1, 1980)

2>.   Flos Chrysanthemi Indici 9g
        Semen Plantaginis 9g
        Radix et Rhizoma Rhei 9g
        Bulbus Fritillariae Verticillatae 9g
        Herba Taraxiaci 9g
        Sargassum 9g
        Herba Oldenlandiae Diffusae 30g
        Concha Ostreae 12g
        Herba Solani Nigri 15g
        Meihua Dianshe Dan 1 pill

The prescription is decocted and taken with a pill of Meihua Dianshe Dan twice a day. (*Anticancer Prescription of Traditional Chinese Medicine*)

HISTORICAL COMMENTS

It is said in *Comments on Materia Medica* that: "The drug removes female hematocele and cures acute virulent furuncles and erysipelas."

It is suggested in *Rui Zhutang's Experienced Recipe* that: "Scrofula without ulceration can be cured by the drug root when pounded, decocted and taken with wine. The dregs are applied to the lesion."

It is reported in *Practical Experienced Folk Remedies* that: "The drug works very well in removing toxic material when used both internally and externally."

RADIX GOSSYPII HIRSUTI

It is defined in *History of Medicinal Herbs in Fujian* that: "The drug is sweet in taste and warm in nature, invigorating *qi* and relieving cough and asthma."

The drug is obtained from *Gossy pium herbaceum L.* and *G. hirsutum L.* of the *Malvaceae* family. The radix or the peel of the radix is for medical use. The peel contains gossypol, flavones, salicylic acid and betaine, while *G. hirsutum L.* contains gossypol, asparagine and arginine.

ANTICANCER PHARMACOLOGICAL FUNCTIONS

1. Experiments in vitro showed that cotton phenol significantly inhibits Yoshida's sarcoma and ulcerous melanoma, and bears certain curative effect on ascites cancer.

2. Experiments in vitro showed that the drug bears a remarkable effect on ascites cancer and transplanted tumor in mice, and also exerts certain effect on sarcoma-37 and sarcoma-180, ascites tumor in rats, Walker's sarcoma and mammoma in mice.

EXPERIMENTAL FORMULAS
For liver cancer:
        Radix Gossypii Hirsuti 30g
        Herba Lobeliae Chinensis 30g
        Carapax Trionycis 15g
        Radix Salviae Miltiorrhizae 15g
        Rhizoma Scirpi 12g
        Rhizoma Zedoariae 12g
        Hirudo 6g

Herba Ardisiae Japonicae 9g

Fructus Polygoni Orientalis 9g

The prescription is taken one dosage a day in decoction. (*Brief Introduction to Oncology*)

For lung cancer:

Radix Gossypri Hirsuti 30g

Radix Codonopsis Lanceolatae 30g

Fructus Psoraleae 15g

Radix Semiaquilegiae 15g

The prescription is taken in decoction. (*Handbook of Practical Anticancer Drugs*)

For spermatocytoma:

Radix Gossypii Hirsuti 30g

Semen Trigonellae 30g

Fructus Psoraleae 15g

Fructus Foeniculi 6g

The prescription is taken in decoction. (*Handbook of Practical Anticancer Drugs*)

HISTORICAL COMMENTS

It is said in *History of Medicinal Plants in Fujian Province* that: "Gastralgia can be cured with 15-30g of the radix when decocted."

It is reported in *Chinese Herbal Preparation for Resisting Cancer* that: "Tumors of the digestive system can be treated with the radix syrup which is made by heating the radix in an appropriate amount of water for 2-4 hours before being filtered, added with a moderate amount of sugar, condensed to a thick liquid, filtered again with gauze and added with enough distilled water. The preparation is taken orally 20-40ml a time, twice a day."

FRUCTUS CAMPTOTHECAE

It is defined in *Chinese Herbal Pharmacology* that: "The drug is bitter in taste and astringent in nature, resisting cancer and diminishing hematostasis."

The drug is obtained from *Camptotheca* of the *Nyssaceae* family, and its fruit, radix, radix peel, twig and leaf are for medical use. The chemical elements contained in the drug are camptothecine, hydroxycamptothecine and methoxycamptothecine. The camptothecine is contained most in the fruit, and least in the twig.

ANTICANCER PHARMACOLOGICAL FUNCTIONS

1. Camptothecine bears certain inhibiting effect on mouse lymphocytic leukemia-615, Yoshida's sarcoma, sarcoma-180 and sarcoma-37 and ascites cancer.

2. The decoction of the fruit and the alcohol preliminary extract showed satisfactory curative effect on mice ascites cancer and gastrocancer. The ethanol extract of the bark inhibits adenocarcinoma-775.

3. It has been proved by experiments that camptothecine is an agent inhibiting the synthesis of DNA, and exerts the greatest cytotoxicity to cells at S stage. Camptothetine, with a dose of $10\mu g/ml$, can completely degrade cellular DNA in lymphocytic leukemia-1210 in one minute, and it still works at a temperature of zero degree centigrade. At 37 degrees centigrade, DNA reaggregates rapidly, but slows down at zero degree centigrade. It is believed that its inhibition on the synthesis of RNA is reversible.

EXPERIMENTAL FORMULAS

For hepatocancer, gastrocancer, enterocancer and malignant tumor:

Tablets made of 50% of the drug, 25% of Caulis Banbusae in Taenian and 25% of Rhizoma Imperatae are taken 8 to 12 tablets each time, 3 to 4 times a day. (*Tianjin Medical Correspondance*, Vol. 12, 1971)

For chronic granulocytic leukemia:

1>. Radix Camptothecae Injection (made by blending together 25g of Radix Camptothecae extract, 2g of chloroprocaine hydrochloride, 2g of Tween-80, 0.1g of activated carbon, a proper amount of HCI and 100ml of distilled water) is injected intramuscularly 4-8ml a day (each milliliter contains 250mg of the crude drug).

2>. The bark of the drug is ground into powder, filled into capsules and taken 6g a day at the beginning. When the blood index returns normal, the drug should be ceased or administrated with a maintenance dose (2-3g a day). (*Data of New Medicine*, Vol. 3, 1972)

For gastrocancer, rectocancer, hepatocancer, and cystocancer:

The radix peel is ground into powder and taken 3g a time and three times a day. The fruit is ground into powder and taken 6g a time and once a day. The leaf is ground into powder and taken 15g a time and twice a day. Each of the powders also can be taken in decoction. (*Therapies Based on Differentiation of Symptoms and Signs*)

HISTORICAL COMMENTS

It is reported in *Newly Compiled Introduction to Traditional Chinese Medicine* that: "The drug removes hematostasis, cures chronic lympholeukemia and chronic lymphomyeloleukemia with a satisfactory curative effect, and alleviates the symptoms of acute leukemia."

It is said in *Chinese Herbal Pharmacology* that: "It is generally believed that the fruit, though superior to the bark in function, contains much more toxin."

THE AUTHOR'S NOTE

The drug is forbidden to be decocted or processed in iron vessels. It was reported in 1979 in *Research Reference of Traditional Chinese Medicine and Pharmacology* that the extract of the herb inhibits Walker's sarcoma-256, sarcoma-37 and sarcoma-180 and cervical cancer-14.

REALGAR

Li Shicai in the Ming Dynasty said that: "The drug, hot in taste, warm and toxic in nature, is distributed to the Liver Channel, removing chronic stagnation and various toxic materials."

The drug is a mineral containing arsenicum sulfide, irregular in shape, various in size, deep-red and orange-red in color, covered with tangerine powder on the surface, dying hands if touched, heavy in weight, soft and crisp in quality, undissolvable in water and hydrochloric acid but in nitric acid, easily melting into a purple liquid and sending out yellow and white stingingly gas with a smell like that of garlic. The fresh-coloured and lustrous ones are called "Bright Realgar", emitting foul smell. The drug is mainly produced in provinces such as Shaanxi, Gansu, Hunan, Sichuan, Guizhou and Yunnan, containing arenicum sulfide and a small amount of other heavy metals.

ANTICANCER PHARMACOLOGICAL FUNCTIONS

1. Experiments in vivo showed that the drug resists the activity of cancer in animals.

2. Experiments in vivo showed that the hot water extract inhibits JTC-26 with an effective rate of 90%.

EXPERIMENTAL FORMULAS

For encephaloma:

Anqing Tumor Diminishing Powder and *Anqing* Paste are always used together. The paste is heated to make it soft, then sprinkled with the powder for application to the lesion or the nearby acupoints every third day. 1-3 months constitute a course of treatment. This therapy is also effective for other cancers.

For liver cancer:

>Realgar
>Cinnabaris
>Galla Chinensis
>Cormus Iphigeniae

Equal portions of the above herbs are ground into fine powder for inhalation with a very small dosage each time. (*National Compilation of Chinese Medicinal Herbs*)

For gastrocancer:

>Realgar 1.2g
>Bufo 3g
>Scolopendra 4
>Scorpio 4
>Bungarus Minimus 12g
>Rhizoma Arisaematis 6g
>Semen Strychni 2.4g
>Calomelas 1.2g
>Arsenicum 1.2g
>Salmiacum 2.4g
>Rhizoma Zingiberis 30g
>Rhizoma Dioscoreae Bulbiferae 2.4g
>Cormus Iphigerriae 6g
>Nidus Vespae 4.8g
>Borneol 4.8g
>Mylabris 3g
>Radix et Rhizoma Rhei 3g

The above herbs are ground into powder and mixed with sesame oil for application to the navel. (*Newly Compiled Introduction to Traditional Chinese Medicine*)

For chronic granulocytic leukemia:

The powder of the drug is taken 0.3-0.9g orally once or twice a day. (*Practical Oncology*)

For ameloblastoma:

>Realgar 9g
>Rhizoma Zingiberis 6g

Realgar is filled into Rhizoma Zingiberis, calcined yellow, ground into powder and applied to the lesion with 0.6-0.9g each time. (*Journal of New Traditional Chinese Medicine*, Vol. 6, 1978)

For pain caused by liver cancer:

30g of the drug is filled into a live toad (stripped off the viscera) to be applied to the tender part of the liver area. The pain will be relieved within 15-20 minutes. The application is changed every 6-8 hours in summer and 24 hours in winter. After two hours of application, the toad will turn green. This therapy has no side effect. (*Journal of New Traditional Chinese Medicine*, Vol. 3, 1980)

For tumor complicated with herpes zoster:

30g of the drug and 1g of Borneol are ground, mixed and applied to the tumor lesion. (*Journal of Heilongjiang Traditional Chinese Medicine*, Vol. 4, 1984)

HISTORICAL COMMENTS

It is recorded in *Materia Medica* that: "The drug removes hemocelia."

It is said in *Prescriptions Worth a Thousand Gold* that: "Abdominal mass can be treated with 60g of the drug when refined with water into a powder, filled into a piece of fresh bamboo corked with a piece of steamed cake, steamed and mixed with flour and rouge before being made into pills of the size of mung bean. The pills are taken three times a day, each time 7 pills."

It is suggested in *Zhou Hou Prescriptions* that: "Scrotum swelling with unbearable pain can be cured with Realgar (60g), Alupcen (60g), Radix Glycyrrhizae (30g), when decocted in 200ml of water into a broth of 80ml. The decoction is used for washing the lesion."

It is reported in *Key Prescriptions for Exogenous Febrile Disease* that: "Lower abdominal mass and dysuria can be cured through filling the honey-coated pills of Realgar powder into the vagina."

It is described in *Luo's Medical Mirror* that: "Nasal polyp can be cured through blowing the powder into the nostrils. However, because the drug affects *qi* and blood, patients with malnutrition caused by the deficiency of the *ying qi* and the *wei qi* should not taken the drug."

MYLABRIS

It is defined in *Canon of Materia Medica* that: "The drug is hot in taste, cold and toxic in nature, removing the decayed muscles and curing urolithiasis."

The drug is obtained from *Mylarbris phalerata Pallas.* of the *Mylabridae* family. The whole insect is for medical use. When exposed to the skin, it will cause the skin to become red with stabbing pain or blisters. The insects are usually found in groups, living on soybean, peanut, eggplant, sesame and melon. The insect is found in most parts of China. *M. cichorrii L.* of the same family is used as the substitute of the drug. The drug contains 1-1.2% cantharidin, 12% fat, resin, formic acid and pigment.

ANTICANCER PHARMACOLOGICAL FUNCTIONS

1. Cantharidin evidently inhibits various kinds of tumors transplanted to the experimental animals, and inhibits sarcoma-180 with an effective rate of 35-46% and lymphocytic leukemia with an effective rate of 38-66%. Its mechanism lies in its inhibition on the carcinocytic synthesis of protein and nucleic acid.

2. The drug slightly inhibits mice sarcoma-180, causing the cancer tissues to decay or to break. The drug can prolong the survival period of mice suffering from ascites hepatocarcinoma with a rate of 65-208% and its curative effect is 43-71%.

3. Experiments in vitro showed that the water, alcohol and acetone extract inhibits Hela cells and the cellular metabolism of esophageal cancer, cardiac cancer, gastric cancer, liver cancer, lung cancer, and breast cancer.

4. The drug inhibits JTC-26 with an effective rate of 90%.

5. Screening tests in vitro with methylene blue method showed that the drug resists the activity of cancer.

EXPERIMENTAL FORMULAS

For liver cancer:

1>. An egg is punctured a hole, filled with 1 to 3 Mylabris (stripped off the head, legs and wings), sealed with paper, wrapped with mud and calcined over fire. The Mylabris is taken for medical purpose, but not the egg. This prescription, also effective for stomach cancer, is taken once a day. (*News Bulletin of Science and Technology*, Vol. 8, 1971)

2>. 2 Mylabris and 30g of Spora Lygodii are decocted into syrup for oral administration three times a day, each time 2ml, accompanied with 9g of the crude flour of mung bean to remove the toxicity.

If the side effect is very strong, the prescription should be stopped at once. (*News Bulletin of Science and Technology*, Vol. 3, 1973)

3>.   Mylabris 1mg

         Fructus Evodiae 50mg

         Rhizoma Pinelliae 50mg

         Rhizoma Dioscoreae 100mg

         Fructus Trapae Bispinosae 100mg

The ingredients are ground into fine powder, filled into capsules and taken one capsule a day after meal accompanied with green tea to remove the toxicity. The dosage may be increased to 2-3 times a day when the patient is adapted to the therapy. Totally 30mg of the drug is needed to reduce the size of the liver.

For breast carcinoma:

One fresh red-shelled egg is filled with 3 Mylabris, wrapped with paper and steamed. The Mylabris is removed before eating the egg. This prescription is taken once a day. (*Diagnosis and Treatment of Tumor*)

For stomach cancer:

One Fructus Ziziphi Inermis without stone and one Mylabris without head and wings are simmered and taken on an empty stomach after removing Mylabris. (*Full Medical Record*)

For lymphatic adenocarcinoma and lymphosarcoma:

One Mylabris without wings and legs is roasted together with one liter of millet. Then the roasted Mylabris is ground with 120g of Herba Menthae into a powder to be mixed with egg white of a black chicken for making pills of the size of mung bean. The pills are taken on an empty stomach with tea, with a dose of 3 pills a day at the beginning, and 5 pills a day later. After a few day, the dose is reduced by one pill a day to totally one pill is taken daily. And again the dose is increased to 5 pills a day and maintained till the disappearance of the tumor mass. (*Dictionary of Chinese Materia Medica*)

For esophageal cancer, stomach cancer and cervical lymphosarcoma:

The drug is ground into powder for application to *Zu San Li* Point to induce blister. One Mylabris and an egg are steamed and taken simultaneously three times a day. (*Journal of Shanghai Traditional Chinese Medicine*, Vol. 9, 1984)

HISTORICAL COMMENTS

It is said in *Simplified Hygienical Recipe* that: "Three Mylabris are roasted with 15 grams of polished glutinous rice and then pounded with one garlic for external application to the lesion. This preparation is very effective for wart, nevus and melanoma."

It is reported in *Wai Tai Secret Recipe* that: "To cure furuncle and swelling, the drug is crushed and applied to the lesion being scratched with a needle."

THE AUTHOR'S NOTE

The drug, when accompanied with chemotherapy, can control leukopenia in patients with leukemia. The drug is preferable to be taken with meal and accompanied with plenty of green tea or water or drugs for promoting drainage, invigorating the spleen and harmonizing the stomach during the administration. To eliminate its side effect, some pharmaceutical factories at home have used the flour of mung bean as an excipient to increase the curative effect and decrease the side effect, when producing tablets.

Chinese archaeologists have discovered *Wen Wu Bamboo Slip Medical Records*, the earliest medical book so far existing in China, bears a clinical prescription, saying that: "Abdominal mass creeping as insects in the abdomen can be cured with decoction of ten Mylabris, one Melve Coaractatus and 0.33m of Cortex Cinnamomi. The patient should not eat any thing at night, take the decoction the next morning and then have a rich meal. The therapy is repeated once daily and totally for ten days.

Abdominal mass will surely be eliminated." Obviously the prescription focuses on abdominal mass which is typical of the current visceral tumor. Taking the drug once ten days and then having a rich meal indicates that the drug is highly toxic. It was really amazing that people learnt to use the drug to treat cancer two thousand years ago.

To extend its indications, Tianjing Municipal Pharmaceutical Institute has synthesized hydroxylcatharamine which is similar to cantharidin in tumor resisting, but with little toxicity. The synthesizing process is quite simple: 100 grams of Hydroxylamini is added to 250ml of water for dissolving, and then mixed with 10N of sodium hydroxide solution to cause alkalinity; then 250g of cantharidin is added for flowing reversely in oil bath for 2 hours; then 5 grams of activated carbon is added for flowing half an hour before filter while it is hot. The very liquid is immediately acidified to high acidity (pH=3) and separated out the white substance deposited after cooling down. The white substance is filtrated the next day to get crystals, which is refined through being dissolved in the same amount of distilled water and dried under 80 degrees centigrade for 6 hours.

PLACENTA HOMINIS

It is defined in *Elucidation on Materia Medica* that: "The drug is bitter and salty in taste, warm in nature, curing various deficient syndromes and impairments."

The drug is obtained from healthy woman's placenta, the substances contained in which are complex and the known ones are interferon ß-inhibiting factor, various hormones and enzymes. Some animals' placenta also share the same function.

ANTICANCER PHARMACOLOGICAL FUNCTIONS

1. The autolysate of human placenta is effective in treating spontaneous tumor in cats and dogs, and in inhibiting AHe mice's T_4 lymphosarcoma.

2. The extract of human placenta is effective for treating Brown-Pearce cancer of the domestic rabbits and for increasing the absorption of tumor tissues.

3. From human placenta are separated two highly acid anticancer proteins, the isoelectric points of which are 10.6 and 9.8, and the molecular weights of which are 90 thousand and 108 thousands, with inhibiting rates of 37% and 60% on sarcoma-37 and ascites cancer respectively.

4. No. 1 Anticancer Injection prepared from umbilical cord inhibits the size of experimental sarcoma-180 with an effective rate of 50%.

5. In animal research, cat's placenta have been used in treating tumor. There are also reports that the albumin of the ova of birds and fowls resist experimental tumors.

EXPERIMENTAL FORMULAS

For leukopenia induced by radiotherapy and chemotherapy:

1.5 grams of the drug powder is taken orally each time, twice a day. The prescription is continued for at least 3 months. (*National Compilation of Chinese Medicinal Herbs*)

For uterine carcinoma:

No. I Anticancer Injection is administrated intramuscularly 2- 4ml a time and once a day. (*Journal of Zhejiang Traditional Chinese Medicine College*, Vol. 6, 1977)

For esophageal cancer:

The placenta of cat are calcined, ground into powder and taken 6-10g in the morning and in the evening with millet wine. (*Reference for Clinical Treatment of Tumor*)

HISTORICAL COMMENTS

It is said in *Luo's Medical Mirror* that: "The drug can be used to treat hectic fever due to *yin* deficiency, night sweat, lumbago, sourness of the knee joint, weak physique with seminal exhaustion."

It is reported in *Zhe Hong's Medical Records* that: "The drug is wrongly understood as being hot in nature. Actually it is an agent for nourishing the *yin* blood. As it is forceful in function, it is often combined with other drugs to moderate it."

RAMULUS ET FOLIUM TAXI CUSPIDATAE

It is defined in *Handbook of Medicinal Herbs in Northeast China* that: "The leaf promotes menstruation and urination and the twig subsides swelling to relieve pain."

The drug is obtained from *Taxus* of the *Taxaceae* family growing in Northeast China. *T. beceata* of the same family also contains anticancer elements. The leaf contains taxusin, sciadopitysin and tannins. The stalk bark contains taxol.

ANTICANCER PHARMACOLOGICAL FUNCTIONS

1. Taxusin significantly inhibits lymphocytic leukemia-338 and leukemia-1534 and Walker's carcinoma-256.

2. The drug shows certain inhibiting effects on sarcoma-180, lymphocytic leukemia-1210, Lemis lung cancer and epithelial carcinocytes of human nose and pharynx.

3. In abroad, a plant with short leaves pertaining to the same family is used to treat tumor and it is said to have certain effect.

4. Experiments with Taxius done at home indicated that the drug inhibits the internal tumors of animals.

5. Taxol from the bark of the plant resists leukemia and the activity of cancer.

EXPERIMENTAL FORMULAS

For all sorts of tumors and leukemia:

1000g of the stalk bark is steeped in 2500g millet wine for a week and the broth is taken 5-10ml a time, twice a day.

The recommended dosage for tumor is: 3 to 6 grams of the leaf and 9 to 15 grams of the twig (without bark) are decocted for oral administration. (*Dictionary of Chinese Materia Medica*)

HISTORICAL COMMENTS

It is reported in *Improved Materia Medica* that: "The drug promotes urination and menstruation, treats nephropathy and diabetes." "When the bark is administered, the drug may cause vomiting, but when its leaf and wood are used, the drug does not cause vomiting."

THE AUTHOR'S NOTE

The drug is not recorded in ancient *Materia Medica*, but used as a folk remedy. Much work has been done abroad on the study of the one with short leaves pertaining to the same family, and it has been proved that its function to resist the activity of cancer lies mainly in the leaves, with taxusin as the effective element. Taxusin was separated out in 1971 from plants of the same family in China such as *Taxus cuspidata Sieb. et Zucc.*.

In Japan, *Taxus cuspidata Sieb. et Zucc.* has been used as a natural drug. It is said that the drug promotes urination when cut into pieces before decocting. But much caution should be given to the use of its leaves because the leaves contain a certain kind of toxic material. In Europe, the leaves of the plants pertaining to the same family are used to produce the drugs for inducing abortion. In China, *Taxus cuspidata Sieb. et Zucc.* is used to promote menstruation and urination, cure nephritic edema, stranguria and diabetes with a dosage of 3 to 6 grams. Dyspepsia and ascariasis can be treated with 3 to 6 grams of the seeds of the plant when roasted, decocted and taken orally.

RADIX LITHOSPERMI

Mu Xiyong in the Ming Dynasty said that: "The drug is bitter in taste, and cold and non-toxic in nature, and is a special medicine for cooling blood."

The drug is obtained from *Lithospermum* of the *Boraginaceae* family, and the radix is for medical use. *Arnebia euchroma (Rogle) Johnst., Onosma paniculata Bur. et Fr., O. hookeri Clarke var. longiflorum Duthie* and *Arnebia thomosii clarke* of the same family are used as the substitutes for the drug.

ANTICANCER PHARMACOLOGICAL FUNCTIONS

1. The ethanol extract, when administered celiacally, and the decoction of the drug inhibit mice sarcoma-180 with an effective rate of 30%.

2. The drug also inhibits chorioepithelioma and the cells of leukemia.

3. The preparation of the drug can reduce the morbidity of mice with spontaneous mammocancer.

EXPERIMENTAL FORMULAS

For uterochorioepithelioma and uterocarcinoma:

60 grams of the drug powder is steeped in 500ml of distilled water for 30 minutes and then boiled in casserole and filtrated. The decoction is taken 100ml a time, four times a day. (*Collection of Experienced Prescriptions of Traditional Chinese Medicine in Shandong*)

For esophageal cancer:

Radix Lithospermi 30g
Herba Scutellariae Barbatae 30g
Herba Oldenlandiae Diffusae 30g
Rhizoma Dioscoreae 15g
Corium Stomachichum Galli 9g
Radix Adenophorae 9g
Poria 6g
Rhizoma Imperatae 30g
Flos Inulae 6g
Radix Codonopsis Pilosulae 6g
Rhizoma Pinelliae 6g
Pericarpium Citri Reticulatae 6g
Radix Aucklandiae 9g
Fructus Oryzae Germinatus 30g
Fructus Hordei Germinatus 30g
Spica Prunellae 30g
Flos Caryophylli 3g
Fructus Ziziphi Inermis 5

The prescription is taken in decoction. (*Collection of Papers from Chinese Medicinal Herbs Exhibition Held in Wuhan*)

For ulceration caused by radiotherapy:

Radix Lithospermi 60g
Radix Angelicae Sinensis 60g

Cera Chinensis 60g
Radix Angeliicae Duhuricae 15g
Calomelas 12g
Sangnis Draconis 12g
Radix Glycyrrhizae 36g
Sesame oil 500g

The prescription is applied to the affected part. (*Journal of Heilongjiang Traditional Chinese Medicine*, Vol. 4, 1984)

HISTORICAL COMMENTS

It is said in *Properties of Materia Medica* that: "The drug cures malignant sores and tinea."

It is recorded in *Materia Medica* that: "The drug cures eruptions and smallpox, activates and cools blood, and smooths the large intestine."

It is suggested in *Key Prescriptions* that: "Smallpox can be cured by the decoction of 3 grams of the drug, 1.5 grams of Pericarpium Citri Reticulatae, and 10cm of scallion stalk."

It is reported in *Thirty-Six Prescriptions for Jaundice* that: "The drug is used to cure jaundice with flaming fever in the morning, but not effective for those with red or black flecks on the body. For those with red and black flecks, the drug is used for fumigating the arch of feet, palms and acupoints such as *Baihui* and *Xialian*. The decoction of the following herbs is taken daily:

Radix Lithospermi 30g
Fructus Polygoni Tinctorii 30g
Radix Aucklandiae 30g
Rhizoma Coptidis 30g

THE AUTHOR'S NOTE

The drug is, when used together with Radix Semiaquilegiae, sensitive to cephaloma. Three cases of cephaloma (one glossocarcinoma, one lid adenocarcinoma and one hypoparotidean tumor of auricular lobule) had been treated with the drug and Radix Semiaquilegiae as the main ingredients and satisfactory result was achieved in Hunan Traditional Chinese Medicine Academy. Another nine cases of tonsil carcinoma, nasopharyngeal carcinoma, thyroid carcinoma, gastric carcinoma and metastatic squamous carcinoma had been treated by the drug in Fuzhou District Hospital and it was reported to have certain curative effect. It was reported that a case of malignant hydatidiform mole complicated by chorioepithelioma (pulmonary metastasis) had been treated with the prescription of 30g of the drug taken once a day in decoction. The prescription was continued for four courses, each of which was composed of ten days. Clinical symptoms were largely reduced and the X-ray examination indicated that most of the pulmonary metastatic focus became diminished.

RADIX ASTERIS

It is defined in *Elucidation on Drugs* that: "The drug is bitter and sweet in taste, cool and moist in nature, and coincidentally agrees with the nature of pulmonary hemophase."

The drug is obtained from a herb of the *Compositae* family, the radix is for medical use, containing epifriedelinol, friedelin, shionone, quercetin and volatile oil. It is said in *Ri Hua Zhi Materia Medica* in the Ming Dynasty that: "The one that looks like millstone with twisted roots, purple color and soft texture is the best."

ANTICANCER PHARMACOLOGICAL FUNCTIONS

1. The ethanol extract from the radix inhibits ascites sarcoma-180 in mice with an effective rate of 16.7%.

2. The epifriedelinol separated from the drug inhibits the activity of ascites cancer.

EXPERIMENTAL FORMULAS

For lung cancer:

      Radix 12g

      Rhizoma Anemarrhenae 12g

      Semen Armeniacae Amarum 9g

      Bulbus Fritillariae Thunbergi 9g

      Cortex Mori 15g

      Poria 15g

      Radix Glycyrrhizae 6g

      Radix Ginseng 6g

      Semen Coicis 24g

      Radix Codonopsis Lanceolatae 24g

The prescription is taken one dosage and three times a day in decoction. (*Therapies for Tumor Based on Differentiation of Symptoms and Signs*)

For hemoptysis caused by lung cancer:

The drug and Radix Rubiae are ground into powder, mixed with honey before being made into pills of berry-stone size and taken one pill a time, many times a day.

HISTORICAL COMMENTS

It is reported in *Annotation on Materia Medica* that: "It is active in dissipation with its hot taste as indicated by its function in subsiding sorethroat and draining detained phlegm, and cannot be used alone or in large quantity due to its warm nature. Therefore, it is usually preferable to use the drug together with drugs with bitter and cold nature such as Radix Asparagi, Radix Stemonae, Radix Ophiopogonis and Cortex Mori for safety."

It is said in *Renewed Materia Medica* that: "The drug is a special medicine for hemophlegm, metrorrhagia and dysuria."

It is recorded in *Annotation on Materia Medica* that: "The drug is hot without dryness, moist without coldness and tonic without stagnation, but unable to exert the effect if not used alone and in large dosage. Dysuria and hematuria can be cured instantly with 30 grams of the drug."

BLOOD ANSERINA

It is defined in *Dictionary of Chinese Materia Medica* that: "The drug is salty in taste, moderate and non-toxic in nature, curing dysphagia and regurgitation."

The drug is obtained from an animal of *Anseriformes* tribe and *Chordata* family. The meat, blood and feather are for medical use.

ANTICANCER PHARMACOLOGICAL FUNCTIONS

1. Feeding mice of ascites cancer with the whole blood of geese for seven days can prevent the formation of ascitic fluid with a rate of 40%, and can cause the cancer cells to dissolve and degenerate.

2. The AKP and the lactic dehydrogenase contained in goose blood, particular the blood of the old goose, are much lower than those in the blood of chicken and duck. But the globulin in goose blood is significantly higher and the thoracic gland tissues of goose are well developed, this indicating that its curative effect is through activating human anticancer immune factors.

EXPERIMENTAL FORMULAS

For stomach cancer:

1>. A goose (or a white duck) is beheaded alive and the warm blood is sucked by the patient. This therapy is taken 1 or twice a week.

2>. The feather on the tail of a white goose (or a white duck) is stripped off, calcined on a clay or porcelain pot, ground into fine powder, sprinkled into porridge or blended with lotus root powder for oral administration without dosage restriction.

3>. The meat of white goose (or white duck) is simmered and a small amount of it is taken daily with other drugs for invigorating the stomach.

The above three prescriptions can be used in combination and they contraindicate wine and food with spices such as hot pepper and chill. (*Journal of New Traditional Chinese Medicine*, Vol. 4, 1973)

For malignant tumor of the digestive system:

1>. Sugar-coated Blood Anserina Tablet: 5 to 7 tablets a time, 3 to 4 times a day, before meal.

2>. Intestinal Blood Anserina Tablet: The usage is the same as the above.

3>. Blood Anserina Syrup: 20ml a time and 3 times a day, taken before meal. (*Public Medicine*, Vol. 6, 1975)

For gastroreticulolymphosarcoma:

200ml of fresh goose blood and 100ml of the juice from 250g of chives are blended and taken once a day or once every other day. (*New Medicine*, Vol. 4, 1975)

HISTORICAL COMMENTS

Renewed Materia Medica says that: "The drug cures dysphagia and regurgitation."

Dietetic Materia Medica says that: "Goose meat relieves visceral heat."

Qiuquan Prescriptions says that: "Ulcerous sores, boils with pus, tinea capitis, urticaria all over the body, itching verruca, numbness, soreness of the hand and the foot caused by wind attack, skin ulcer, sorescrotum and pruritus vulvae can be treated with the prescription of Radix Sophorae Flavescentis (300g, in powder) and goose feather (180g, roasted in sesame oil), when blended with millet to roll into pills coated with Cinnabar. The pills are taken twice a day with vegetable soup and the dose is regulated in accordance with the patients condition."

Collection of Experienced Prescriptions says that: "Carbuncle can be cured with calcined goose feather (30g) and Alumen (60g), when ground, mixed with wheat flour and made into pills for oral administration 6 grams a time with wine."

Collection of Inherited Prescriptions said that membranous pharyngitis was cured with the following formula:

> Goose feather (burnt to ashes) 0.09g
> Catechu 6g
> Calculus Bovis 0.09
> Realgar 3g
> Calamitas Urinae Hominis 4.5g

All the above drugs are calcined, ground and mixed with some roasted pearl powder. The throat is cleaned with tung oil first and then applied with the prepared powder. The effect of the powder will be greatly reinforced if Alumen is added.

Dictionary of Chinese Materia Medica says that: "The drug cures stab wound caused by poisonous arrow when taken orally or applied to the lesion."

Materia Medica says that: "The drug neutralizes toxicity of medicinal herbs."

Dietetic Materia Medica says that: "Sweating and boils in the head can be cured with oral administration of the broth of goose meat simmered together with scallion stalk." "The drug is sweet in taste, cold and non-toxic in nature." "The drug is salty and cold and non-toxic."

Materia Medica says that: "The drug neutralizes the toxicity of gold, silver and cinnabar, and cures the drowned and sore due to earthworm-bite."

THE AUTHOR'S NOTE
334 cases of malignant tumors (gastrocancer, lymphoma, lung cancer and nasopharyngeal cancer) were treated with goose blood preparations, and the total curative rate was found to be 65%. The blood cells of other animals have also been found to resist cancer.

1. White goose or duck leukocytes can obviously prolong the survival period of mice if administrated before transplantation of ascites cancer. The experiment done in Tianjing shows that the immune blood of chicken can alleviate the symptoms of lung cancer.

2. 10 cases of acute granulocytic leukemia were treated with fresh pig blood in Changchou and the symptoms were improved in six cases and alleviated in one case. One case of acute monocytic leukemia and one case of acute granulocytic leukemia were alleviated in Wu County with fresh pig blood when accompanied with other herbs. In Jiangdu County, two cases of acute lymphatic leukemia and 5 cases of acute granulocytic leukemia were treated with fresh pig blood, and all patients in the former group were completely alleviated, but only one case was completely alleviated and one case partially alleviated in the latter group.

3. The blood cells of slug can dissolve or kill cancer cells of Krebs-11 and ascites cancer when put together.

HERICIUM

It is defined in *Records of Drugs for Sexual Activities* that: "The drug is sweet in taste and moderate in nature, nourishing the stomach to eliminate abdominal mass and protect gastric energy."

The drug is obtained from sporphore of *Hericium erinaceus (B.ex Fr.) Pers.* of the *Hydraceae* family, containing polysaccharides and polypeptide. The drug can be cultivated artificially.

ANTICANCER PHARMACOLOGICAL FUNCTIONS
1. Experiments showed that the drug inhibits mice sarcoma-180.

2. Tests in vitro showed that the drug inhibits the synthesis of DNA and RNA of ascites carcinoma and prevents the intervention of thymidine and uridylic acid, and its inhibiting intensity is related to the concentration of the drug.

3. The drug's toxicity is very low. It has been administered orally with a dosage of 30 gram per kilogram of the body weight of mouse and no toxic reactions turned up.

4. The drug increases lymphocytic reversion rate, leukocytes and human immune capacity.

EXPERIMENTAL FORMULAS
For recovery after operation of cancer:

150 grams of the dried drug is cut into pieces and simmered together with pork, chicken or duck for oral administration. (*Anticancer Consultation*)

For stomach cancer, esophageal cancer and cardiac cancer:

1>. Hericium Tablets (each weights 0.2g and contains 0.13g of the extract of the drug) is taken 3 or 4 tablets a time and three times a day.

2>. Sweet Hericium Powder (An mixture of the extract of the drug and sugar, each kilogram containing 0.25 gram of the extract) is taken 2 or 3 grams a time, 3 times a day. (*Handbook of Anticancer Medicinal Herbs*)

HISTORICAL COMMENTS

It is said in *Chinese Medical Fungus* that: "The drug activates viscera and promotes digestion."

THE AUTHOR'S NOTE
The drug has been used in China to treat tumors of the digestive tract since 1975 and the effective rate for stomach cancer is 68.6% and for esophageal cancer is 78.5%. It is also reported that the drug is evidently effective in treating malignant tumors of the digestive system such as stomach cancer and cardiac cancer. The total curative rate is 69.3% and the significant effect is 15%.

HERBA TARAXACI

It is defined in *Materia Medica in the Tang Dynasty* that: "The drug is sweet in taste, mild and non-toxic in nature, curing female breast abscess."

The drug is obtained from many herbs of the *Compositae* family and the *Taraxacum* genus. The whole herbs are for medical use. The drug is found growing in most parts of China, containing sterol, choline and inulin. In America, the drug has been processed into an extract or pills widely used for treating various sorts of cancer.

ANTICANCER PHARMACOLOGICAL FUNCTIONS
1. The hot water extract of the herb inhibits mice sarcoma-180 with an effective rate of 43.5%, whereas the alcohol extract showed no effect.
2. The drug evidently inhibits transplanted human pulmonary cancer cells.
3. Its hot water extract contains a kind of polyose substance, which enables the host to regulate the anticancer function and promotes his immunity.
4. The hot water extract shows an evident curative effect ($P < 0.01$) on mice ascites cancer (300mg/kg) when administrated celiacally once every other day at the later stage of the illness.
5. The herb promotes T-DHR.

EXPERIMENTAL FORMULAS
For chronic granulocytic leukemia:
> Herba Taraxaci 30g
> Radix Rehmanniae 30g
> Herba Scutellariae Barbatae 30g
> Radix Actinidiae Chinensis 30g
> Flos Lonicerae 24g
> Gypsum Fibrosum 24g
> Radix Angelicae Sinensis 12g
> Radix Isatidis 12g
> Radix Scorophulariae 12g
> Radix Sophorae Flavescentis 9g
> Radix Asparagi 6g
> Radix Ophiopogonis 6g

The prescription is taken in decoction. (*Diagnosis and Treatment of Tumor*)
For cancer of the hard palate:
> Herba Taraxaci 30g
> Flos Lonicerae 30g
> Cormus Iphigeniae 30g
> Fructus Forsythiae 15g
> Rhizoma Smilacis Glabrae 15g

Pollen 9g

The prescription is taken in decoction. (*Diagnosis and Treatment of Tumor*)

For gingival cancer:

    Herba Taraxaci 30g

    Spica Prunellae 30g

    Quartz Album 30g

    Herba Oldenlandiae Diffusae 30g

    Herba Violae Yedoensis 15g

The prescription is taken one dosage a day in decoction. (*Diagnosis and Treatment of Tumor*)

For cervical cancer with metastasis to the intestine:

    Herba Taraxaci 20g

    Flos Lonicerae 20g

    Caulis Lonicerae 20g

    Semen Benincasae 20g

    Radix Astragali 20g

    Herba Oldenlandiae Diffusae 15g

    Flos Sophorae Immaturus 15g

    Olibanum 10g

    Myrrha 10g

    Rhizoma Cyperi Carbonisatus 10g

    Massa Medicata Fermentata 10g

    Radix Angelicae Sinensis 12g

    Herba Violae Yedoensis 12g

    Radix Rehmanniae 12g

    Radix Ginseng 1g

    Sangnis Draconis 1g

    Lignum Aquilariae Resinatum 1g

(*Journal of Beijing Traditional Chinese Medicine College*, Vol. 3, 1983)

For antral gastric cancer:

    Herba Taraxaci 12g

    Rhizoma Cyperi 12g

    Radix Angelicae Sinensis 12g

    Herba Lobeliae Chinensis 12g

    Herba Scutellariae Barbatae 12g

    Herba Oldenlandiae Diffusae 12g

    Radix Paeoniae Latiflorae 9g

    Herba Violae Yedoensis 9g

    Rhizoma Paridis 9g

    Fructus Citri Aurantii 9g

    Radix Aucklandiae 9g

    Radix Linderae 9g

    Semen Persicae 9g

    Radix Curcumae 9g

    Rhizoma Corydalis 6g

The prescription is taken in decoction. (*Journal of Guangxi Traditional Chinese Medicine*, Vol. 3, 1980)

For breast cancer:

    Herba Taraxaci 9g

    Radix Angelicae Sinensis 15g

Fructus Trichosanthis 1
Olibanum 3g
Myrrha 3g
Radix Glycyrrhizae 6g
Folium Citri Reticulatae 10 sheets

The prescription is decocted in wine for oral administration. (*Newly Compiled Mei's Experienced Prescriptions*)

For nasopharyngeal cancer with metastasis to the cervical lymphonodes:

Same amount of Herba Taraxaci, Folium et Ramulus Biotae and Radix Rehmanniae are pounded, blended with honey and applied to the swelling on the neck.

For angioma:

The white juice from the leaf and the stalk of the drug is used for rubbing the surface of angioma 5 to 10 times a day. (*Dictionary of Chinese Materia Medica*)

HISTORICAL COMMENTS

Elucidation on Materia Medica says that: "The drug is sweet in taste, mild and non-toxic in nature, distributed to the liver and the stomach and used as the key drug for eliminating pathogenic heat and cooling blood. The drug cures female breast abscess and breast cancer because breast abscess is distributed to the Liver Channel which dominates all the body activities during menstruation. The drug is taken orally when raw."

Renewed Materia Medica says that: "If asked which one is superior, Herba Taraxaci or Flos Lonicerae, since both of them are effective in subsiding swelling and ulceration? The answer is that Herba Taraxaci only enters the *Yangming* and the *Taiyang* Channel, while Flos Lonicerae enters every channel. The former is different from the latter in function. However, the latter will not exert its full effect without the former."

General Introduction to Medicine says that: "The drug is quite effective in curing dysphagia."

Renewed Compilation of Mei's Experienced Recipe says that: "Herba Taraxaci, with only one stock about 0.3 meter high, two flowers and a root as large as a human fist, cures dysphagia with a miraculous effect if pounded and taken with wine."

SEMEN LIVISTONAE

It is defined in *Lu Chu Materia Medica* that: "The drug is bland in taste and mild in nature, stopping hemorrhage and bleeding caused by exogenous pathogenic factors."

The drug is obtained from a herb of the *Palmae* family, and the seed is for medical use. The drug is mainly found in the south of China, the seed of which contains phenol, reduced sugar, tannin and triglyceride.

ANTICANCER PHARMACOLOGICAL FUNCTIONS

1. The drug evidently inhibits mice encephaloma-22 and also relieves pain.
2. Caryota ochlandra Hance of the same family is also found resisting cancer.

EXPERIMENTAL FORMULAS

For nasopharyngeal cancer and esophageal cancer:

60g of the drug is decocted and taken orally one dosage a day, or added with 30-90g of lean pork, simmered and taken as food once a day. (*New Compilation of Basic Traditional Chinese Medicine*)

For malignant hydatidiform mole and leukemia:

30g of the drug is decocted with 6 Fructus Ziziphi Inermis for oral taking twice a day. The prescription is continued for 20 dosages as a course of treatment. (*Dietetic Medicinal Herbs*)

For lung cancer:

60g of the drug and 60g of Herba Scutellariae Barbatae are decocted for oral taking one dosage a day. (*Handbook of Materia Medica*)

For other cancers:

30g of the dried drug is decocted for 1 or 2 hours or simmered with lean pork for oral taking. (*Dictionary of Chinese Materia Medica*)

HISTORICAL COMMENTS

Supplementation to Materia Medica says that: "The drug diminishes hemostasis and cures abdominal mass caused by stagnation of energy."

Records of Herbal Collection in Lingnan says that: "The leaves and stalk of the herb cures metrorrhagia if calcined on a new tile into ashes and taken in water, or roasted and decocted for oral administration."

Handbook of Commonly Used Medicinal Herbs says that: "The drug is sweet in taste, astringent and mild in nature. Its seeds resists cancer."

SEMEN RICINI

It is defined in *Annotation on Materia Medica* that: "The drug is sweet and hot in taste, mild and slightly toxic in nature, and easy to be absorbed."

The drug is obtained from the seed of *Ricinus* of the *Euphorbiaceae* family and contains oleum ricini, ricin, ricinine and ricinolein.

ANTICANCER PHARMACOLOGICAL FUNCTIONS

1. The effective element is its ricin, the molecular weight of which is 6,5000. The growth of cancer cells can be completely inhibited if $7.5\mu g$ of ricini is injected celiacally per kilogram of body weight of mice one or three days after ascites cancer has been transplanted.

2. Studies with the drug proved that a ricin molecule is capable enough of killing an ascites cancer cell. Its mechanism lies in the fact that it indirectly reinforces the enzymatic activity of RNA by reducing polyribosome, decreasing amino acid combination, coarsening the liver cells and changing the ultrastructure of the endoplasmic reticulum. Therefore it is a powerful agent for inhibiting the protein synthesis of ascites cancer.

EXPERIMENTAL FORMULAS

For colocancer:

        Semen Ricini (pounded) 6g
        Radix Actinidiae Chinensis 60g
        Rhizoma Paridis 15g
        Auriallaria 24g
        Rhizoma Dryo..teris Crassirhizomae 1.2g
        Rhizoma Impe..atae 30g
        Radix Sopho..e Tonkinensis 30g
        Rhizoma Cyperi 12g

The prescription is taken in decoction or ground into powder and taken 6 grams a time. (*Diagnosis and Treatment of Tumor*)

For malignant lymphosarcoma:

1>. 3 Semen Ricini (without shell) and 1 crude Rhizoma Dioscoreae (without peel) are pounded, glued to a piece of cloth and applied to the lesion. (*Ancient and Modern Prescriptions*)

2>. The drug is roasted, peeled and taken 2 to 3 grains through chewing before sleep and the dose may eventually be increased to 10 grains. (*Extension of Materia Medica*)

For lymphatic adnocarcinoma and lymphosarcoma:

Same amount of the drug (without shell) and Radix Semiaquilegiae is decocted in casserole for some time. 15 to 21 grains of the decocted drug are taken each time on an empty stomach. (*Effective Prescriptions for Women*)

For infantile eryoma:

5 grains of the drug (without shell) are ground, blended with a spoonful of wheat flour in water and applied to the lesion. (*Secret Doctrine for Medicine*)

HISTORICAL COMMENTS

Explanation on Materia Medica says that: "The seeds of the drug cures scrofula when roasted, peeled and taken two or three by chewing every night before going to bed. The dose can be gradually increased to 10 grains."

Materia Medica says that: "The drug cures sorethroat, beriberi and dermatoma, relieves all sorts of pain, subsides swelling and draws out pus."

Du Rei Prescriptions says that: "Sorethroat can be cured with a castor bean and 3 grams of Natrii Sulfas when ground and taken with fresh water. The prescription is continued for 2-3 courses."

THE AUTHOR'S NOTE

The effective anticancer element contained in the drug is ricin which can be destroyed when heated. Hence, the drug is not eligible to be taken in decoction, but in powder. Ricin has been used to treat 10 cases of cervical cancer and it was found effective in 5 cases, and among the 9 cases of skin cancer received the drug, 4 cases were found effective. It was reported that an International Conference on Anticancer Drugs was held in Auslo, West Germany, and a study done by Norwegian Anticancer Institute had proved that a toxic substance extracted from the seeds of the plant was very powerful in killing carcinocytes. It was found in the experiment that this toxic substance was very easy to be absorbed by carcinocytes. Therefore, it was thought that the drug would come to be a desirable anticancer drug.

RHIZOMA AMORPHOPHALLI

It is defined in *Dictionary of Chinese Materia Medica* that: "The drug is hot in taste, cold and non-toxic in nature, subsiding abscess, swelling and inflammation caused by pathogenic wind."

The drug is obtained from *Amphophallus rivieri Durieu* of the *Araceae* family and the *Amorphophallus* genus, and its rhizoma is for medical use, containing glucomannan, protein, starch, glucose, fructose, manneotriose and sucrose. The flower contains great quantity of vitamin B_1. *Amorphophallus dunnii Tutch.* of the same family is used as the substitute for the drug.

ANTICANCER PHARMACOLOGICAL FUNCTIONS

1. Pharmaceutical sensitivity test shows that the drug is sensitive to the cells of cardiac cancer and colocancer.

2 The mannan from Amorphophallus rivieri Durieu interferes with carcinocytic metabolism.

3. The hot water extract inhibits mice sarcoma-180 with an effective rate of 49.8%.

EXPERIMENTAL FORMULAS

For encephaloma:

1>.   Rhizoma Amorphophalli 30g
       Herba Xanthii 30g
       Rhizoma Dryopteris Crassirhizomae 30g
       Radix Typhae 15g
       Rhizoma Paridis 15g

The prescription is taken one dosage a day in decoction. (*Basic Knowledge of Traditional Chinese Medicine*)

2>. 30 grams of the drug is decocted for 2 hours first, then added with 9 grams of Rhizoma Paridis and 6 grams of Radix Glycyrrhizae and decocted again for ortal administration. For vomiting, 9 grams of Rhizoma Piinelliae is added; for stuffed nose, 9 grams of Herba Centipedae is added; and for haemorrhagia, 15 grams of Fructus Gardeniae is added. (*Basic Knowledge of Traditional Chinese Medicine*)

For thyroid cancer:

30 grams of the drug is decocted for 2 hours first, then added with Sargassum, Radix Typhae, Radix Scorophulariae (15 grams each), Herba Xanthii and Rhizoma Dryopteris Crassirhizomae (30 grams each). If the tumor is hard, 60 grams of Concha Ostrea is added. The prescription is administered in decoction for oral taking twice a day. (*Diagnosis and Treatment of Tumor*)

For tumors of the lymphatic system:

30 grams of the drug is decocted for 2 hours first, and then added with Rhizoma Amorphophalli, Rhizoma Dioscoreae Bulbiferae, Radix Semiaquilegiae, Radix Aucklandiae and Rhizoma Paridis (15 grams each). The prescription is taken in decoction.

For nasopharyngeal cancer:

30 grams of the drug is decocted for 2 hours first and then added with Rhizoma Amorphophalli, Radix Lycii Radicis, Herba Commelinae (30g each) and 15 grams of Rhizoma Paridis for further decoction. The broth is taken orally. (*Dictionary of Chinese Materia Medica*)

For malignant lymphonode tumor:
       Herba Duchesneae 30g
       Rhizoma Amorphophalli 30g
       Caulis Polygoni Multiflori 30g
       Concha Ostreae 30g
       Herba Oldenlandiae Diffusae 30g
       Bulbus Bolbostemmae 9g
       Radix Scrophulariae 9g
       Spica Prunellae 15g
       Sargassum 15g
       Cormus Iphigeniae 9g

The prescription is taken in decoction one dosage a day. Before decocted together, Rhizoma Amorphophalli is boiled for one hour and Concha Ostreae is boiled for 15 minutes. (*Journal of Shanghai Traditional Chinese Medicine*, Vol. 9, 1984)

For carcinoma of parotid gland:
       Rhizoma Amorphophalli 30g
       Radix Isatidis 30g
       Flos Lonicerae 15g
       Radix Sophorae Tonkinensis 15g

The prescription is taken in decoction. (*Anticancer Preparations of Traditional Chinese Medicine*)

HISTORICAL COMMENTS

San Yuan Longevity says that: "A person was suffering from consumptive disease and he tried to eat anything that caught his eyes. One day he saw Amorphophalli in his neighbor's home and asked to have a taste. Allowed, he found the plant was tasty and ate a great deal. Spontaneously his disease healed. It was also recorded that some people had their parotid abscess healed after having eaten a lot of the drug."

Major Toxic Plants in the North says that: "Dermatoposioning can be cured through washing the lesion with water or diluted vinegar and tannic acid. Poisoning caused by taking toxic plants accidentally can be relieved by taking diluted vinegar, strong tea or egg white."

HERBA PATRINIAE HETEROPHYLLAE

It is defined in History of Medicinal Herbs in Guangxi Province that: "The drug is hot in taste and warm in nature, diminishing stasis and subsiding swelling."

The drug is obtained from Patrinia heterophylla Bge. of the Patrinia genus and the Valerianaceae family. P. scabra Bge. and P. scabiosaefolia Fisch. of the same family are also used for the treatment of cancer, but P. scabra Bge. is used as the substitute of the drug.

ANTICANCER PHARMACOLOGICAL FUNCTIONS
1. Anticancer experiments in vitro with methylene blue method, eosin staining method, and the external and the internal cytomorphological method showed that the extract from the drug destroys cells of ascites cancer.
2. The drug administrated orally evidently inhibits ascites cancer in mice.
3. The drug exerts an evident curative effect on ascites cancer of mice, inhibiting cancer with rates of 82% and 78% when injected celiacally, and inhibiting tumor with a rate of 64% when administrated subcutaneously.
4. Local injection of the drug would cause mice ascites cancer to become hard and dry locally and to come off finally. And rehabilitation of the ulcerous lesion will occur gradually.

EXPERIMENTAL FORMULAS
For stomach cancer:
30 grams of the drug is decocted with 3 sheets of Rhizoma Zingiberis and 30 grams of brown sugar for oral taking as tea. (Brief Introduction to Oncology)
For leukemia:
15 grams of the drug is decocted with 30 grams of Radix Rumicis for oral taking. The decoction is taken one dosage a day. (Handbook of Anticancer Drugs in China)

HISTORICAL COMMENTS
Origin of Materia Medica says that: "The radix of the drug is black in color and foul in taste, the dry and old ones are more effective."
Dictionary of Prescriptions says that: "The drug is growing in the mountains in Nanning, Guangxi Province, with flowers looking like a metal arrow-head, curing wind syndrome and osteoalgia on the four extremities when decocted and applied to the lesions."
Materia Medica says that: "The drug cures metrorrhagia and leukorrhagia when decocted together with Flos Carthami in water blended with wine."

THE AUTHOR'S NOTE
The water extract of the drug, if injected into tumor, inhibits mice sarcoma-180 with a rate of 62.5% and also directly kills sarcoma-180 as observed through lens during celiac injection.

FRUCTUS SOPHORAE JAPONICAE

It is defined in *Canon of Materia Medica* that: "The drug is bitter in taste and cold in nature, clearing away visceral heat and curing breast nodule."

The drug is obtained from the seed of *Sophora japonica* L. of the *Liguminosae* family, containing 9 kinds of flavonoids and isoflavones, and a large quantity of rufin (46% in the green seed). The seed contains fatty oil, mainly linoleic acid. The drug is produced i ı Hebei, Shandong, Jiangsu and Liaoning provinces.

ANTICANCER PHARMACOLOGICAL FUNCTIONS

1. Rufin inhibits some transplanted tumors.

2. The extract of the seed contains PHA which can increase the organic immunity and resist cancer activity.

3. Experiments in vitro showed that the hot water extract of the drug inhibits JTC-26 with a rate of over 90%.

EXPERIMENTAL FORMULAS

For tumor of the digestive system:

1>. Fructus Sophorae Japhonicae Syrup (containing 1.25g/ml of the drug): 100ml a day, taken in twice.

2>. Honey-coated Pills of Fructus Sophorae Japonicae (each pill weights 9g): 1 pill a time and three times a day.

3>. 30 grams of the drug is filled into a thermos bottle full of hot water, and steeped for some time before taking as tea.

4>. Fructus Sophorae Japonicae Injection: Administrated intramuscularly twice a day, each time 1 or 2 ampule. (*Collection of Data for Anticancer Research*, 1978)

For hematuria caused by cystocarcinoma:

Fructus Sophorae Japonicae 9g
Semen Plantaginis 6g
Poria 6g
Caulis Aristolochiae Manshuriensis 6g
Radix Glycyrrhizae 2.1g

The prescription is taken in decoction. (*Simple Prescriptions Developed by Doctor Yang*)

HISTORICAL COMMENTS

Extension of Materia Medica says that: "The drug, when simmered into a paste with honey, cures hemorrhoid and anal fistula and chronic defecation with blood caused by wind-heat factors."

Materia Medica says that: "Yu Jianwan always takes the drug, therefore he is still wearing black hair and able to read tiny Chinese characters even at the age of 70. It is recorded in ancient prescription that the seed of the drug can improve vision and turn white hair black when steeped in a cow gall-bladder obtained in winter, dried in shade for 100 days and chewed after each meal."

HERBA WEDELIAE

It is defined in *Chinese Medicinal Herbs in Fujian* that: "The drug is slightly salty in taste and cool in nature, and clears away heat and removing toxic materials."

The drug is obtained from a herb of *Compositae* family, growing by the ditches or on the damp land along the seacoast in Guandong, Guangxi and Fujian provinces. The whole herb contains volatile oils, flavonoides and glycosides.

ANTICANCER PHARMACOLOGICAL FUNCTIONS

1. Screening tests in vitro with bacteriophagia showed that the drug resists bacteriophagic activation.

2. Experiments in vivo proved that the water extract of the whole herb inhibits mice ascites cancer with a certain effect when injected celiacally.

EXPERIMENTAL FORMULAS

For laryngocancer:

       Herba Wedeliae 60g

       Lasiosphaera seu Calvatia 3g

       Rhizoma Belamcandae 9g

       Radix Sophorae Tonkinensis 9g

       Calyx seu Fructus Physalis 9g

       Semen Oroxyli 4.5g

       Fructus Chebulae 6g

       Radix Platycodi 6g

       Radix Glycyrrhizae 5g

The prescription is taken in decoction one dosage a day. (*Prevention of Tumor in Traditional Chinese Medicine*)

For colocarcinoma:

       Herba Wedeliae 30g

       Herba Oldenlandiae Diffusae 30g

       Semen Coicis 30g

       Caulis Sargentodoxae 15g

       Flos Hibisci 15g

       Radix Pulsatillae 9g

       Radix Sophorae Flavescentis 9g

       Flos Sophorae Immaturus 9g

       Herba Agrimoniae 12g

The prescription is taken in decoction one dosage a day. (*Brief Introduction to Oncology*)

For cancer of the parotid gland:

Radix Wedeliae and Bulbus Allii Bakeri are pounded and applied to the lesion. (*Collection of Chinese Medicinal Herbs for Tumor*)

HISTORICAL COMMENTS

Reference for Essentials of Properties of Medicinal Herbs says that: "The drug heals sores, clears away heat, draws out pus, promotes pyogenic procession of sores, and controls pestilence and fistula. Its radix removes the teeth."

History of Medicinal Herbs in Fujian says that: "The drug cures diphtheria, pharyngitis, tonsillitis, pneumonitis, pulmonary ulcer, whooping cough, nasorrhagia, hemoptysis caused by tuberculosis, hematuria, dysentery, measles, infectious hepatitis, rheumatic arthritis, insomnia caused by violent restlessness, gingivitis, carbuncle and furuncle."

CORTEX ARALIAE CHINENSIS

It is defined in *Folk Medicinal Herbs in Guizhou Province* that: "The drug is sweet in taste, cold and non-toxic in nature, clearing away heat to expel wind and relieving cough."

The drug belongs to the *Araliaceae* family, growing in the north of the Yellow River and the Changjiang River Basin. Its cortex, radix and folium are for medical use.

ANTICANCER PHARMACOLOGICAL FUNCTIONS

1. Experiments in vivo showed that the drug inhibits mice SAK and solid hepatocarcinoma.

2. Experiments with bacteriophagic method showed that the drug produced in Guangdong Province resists bacteriophagia, and this indicates that it is active against cancer cells.

EXPERIMENTAL FORMULAS
For gastrocancer:

1>.   Cortex Araliae Chinensis 15g
Radix Gentianae 4.5g
Cortex Moutan 4.5g
Radix et Rhizoma Rhei 4.5g
Radix Aucklandiae 3g
Herba Sonchi Oleracei 9g

The prescription is taken one dosage a day in decoction. (*Journal of Jiangsu Traditional Chinese Medicine*, Vol. 1, 1962)

2>.   Cortex Araliae Chinensis 20g
Herba Pteridis Multifidae 20g
Herba Melastomae 25g
Radix Angelicae Sinensis 17g
Placenta Hominis 10g
Herba Elsholtziae Blandae 8g

The above herbs are ground into fine powder for oral administration with water 6 to 9 grams each time and 3 times a day. (*New Medical Information*, Vol. 3, 1972)

3>.   30 grams of the drug is decocted for oral administration. (*Practical and Proved Prescriptions*)

For lung cancer:

500 grams of the drug and 500 grams of Herba Scutellariae Barbatae are packed into 16 packets and decocted for oral administration. (*New Medical Information*, Vol. 3, 1972)

HISTORICAL COMMENTS

Supplementation to Materia Medica says that: "The drug cures edema with its cortex decocted for orally taking. Its radix, when pounded into juice can relieve very serious edema. The drug also can be used to treat dental caries by filling the cavities on the decayed tooth with appropriate amount of the drug, and the tooth will come off spontaneously."

Newly Compiled Materia Medica says that: "The drug cures diarrhea and dysentery, and edema when cooked together with pork." "The cortex of the radix and the trunk invigorate the stomach, astringentizes and promotes urination and glycogenesis, therefore curing diabetes, nephropathy and gastric ulcer."

THE AUTHOR'S NOTE

It was reported in 1983 in *Hunan Medical Journal* (Vol. 5) that the water dissolvable substance contained in the drug inhibited cervical cancer-14 to a certain degree, and this is closely relative to the result of the external experiment on solid cancer transplanted on animals.

RADIX TRIPTERYGII

It is defined in *History of Medicinal Herbs in Hunan* that: "The drug is bitter in taste and highly toxic in nature, killing bacteria, abating inflammation and removing toxic materials."

The drug is the root, the leaf and the flower of the herb, *Tripterygium Wilfordii Hook. f.* of the family *Celastraceae*, growing in the south of Changjiang River. The root contains alkaloid, celastral, triptolide, glucose and tannins.

ANTICANCER PHARMACOLOGICAL FUNCTIONS
1. The alcohol extract of the drug evidently inhibits mice lymphocytic leukemia-1210 and leukemia-388.
2. Experiments in vitro on human nasopharyngeal cancer showed that the drug inhibits the activation of cancer. The effective substance is its epoxy diterpenoid.
3. The drug inhibits cervical cancer-14 with a rate of about 40%.

EXPERIMENTAL FORMULAS
For primary liver cancer, lung cancer and leukemia:
1>. Radix Tripterygii Syrup: 10ml each time and three times a day.
2>. Radix Tripterygii Powder: 5 to 10 grams each time and three times a day.

HISTORICAL COMMENTS
History of Medicinal Herbs in Hunan Province says that: "The drug, together with Radix Linderae, cures herpes zoster when ground and applied to the lesion."

Dictionary of Chinese Materia Medica says that: "The drug is severe in toxicity, especially its cortex. Hence, the cortex, including the second layer, must be stripped off completely before use."

ESCA REGIA APIS

It is defined in *Dictionary of Chinese Materia Medica* that: "The drug is sweet and sour in taste and mild in nature, building up health, invigorating the liver and the spleen."

The drug is the syrupoid material brewed from the secretion of the working bee's retropharyngeal gland and honey, and it is the food for the queen bees and the young bees. The drug is white or yellowish in colour, semi-transparent, semi-liquid and slightly sticky in property, slightly sweet and hot in taste (pH 3.8-4.5), sensitive to heat and light, and liable to be oxidized in air.

According to *Techniques for Food Procession and Package* (Vol. 2, 1983), the drug contains the following elements:

Water 65-68%
Protein 14-16%
Saccharides 9-18%
Fats 2.5-5.0%
Ash 0.8-1.2%
Vitamin (mg/100g):
Vitamin B_1 690
Vitamin B_2 1390
Nicotinic acid 5980
Pantothenic acid 22000
Vitamin B_6 1220
Biotin 114

folic acid 40

Acetglcholine 958000

Inositol 11000

The drug also contains multiple amino acids, organic acids and trace elements that are essential to human body.

ANTICANCER PHARMACOLOGICAL FUNCTIONS

W-hydroxy-Δ^2-decenoic acid and the dissolvable substance contained in the drug powerfully inhibit carcinocytoplasia of the transplanted leukemia, lymphocancer-6C3HED, mammocancer and multiple ascites cancers, and prolong the survival period of domestic mice with cancer to a year, whereas those in the control group can only live for 21 days.

Oral taking or injection of the syrup made from the young bees of *Apis mellifera L.* can prolong the survival period of mice with ascites cancer, defer the occurrence of ascites and cause carcinocytoplasia to retrograde degeneration.

EXPERIMENTAL FORMULAS

For various sorts of cancer:

Appropriate amount of the syrup made from the drug is taken every day. (*Data of Traditional Chinese Medicine*, Vol. 6, 1978)

For lung cancer:

Two capsules of the drug is taken each time and three times a day, or accompanied with other anticancer drugs. (*Reference for Clinical Treatment of Tumor*)

HISTORICAL COMMENTS

Drugs Obtained from Animals in Northeast China says that: "The drug contains many physically active substances and resists cancer and bacteria to certain degrees."

Common Medicinal Animals says that: "The drug can promote protein synthesis and the growth of tissues, reduce cholesterol in the blood, increase the amount of oxygen consumed by tissues and the oxidatin of sugar by tissues, boost cytoregeneration of the liver, the kidney, the nerve and the hematopoietic tissue, elevate endocrine function, and reinforce the organic defence capacity and endurance to the adverse circumstances."

XYLOTRUPES

It is defined in *Records of Famous Doctors* that: "The drug is salty in taste, cold and toxic in nature, treating cold hands and feet, osteonumbness, and syndrome caused by adversely ascending *qi* from the kidney or the liver accompanied with abdominal pain or alternative episodes of chills and fever."

The drug is obtained from *Scarabaeidae* of the *Coleoptera* family, the whole insect is for medical use. It contains 1% xylotrupestoxin and the effective element is dissolvable in water, ethanol and chloroform, but not in ether.

ANTICANCER PHARMACOLOGICAL FUNCTIONS

The alcohol extract of the drug inhibits the growth of human lever cells.

EXPERIMENTAL FORMULAS

For nasopharyngeal cancer:

Xylotrupes 9g

Herba Xanthii 15g

Otolithum Sciaenae 15g

Folium Cordylini Fruticosae 30g

Rhizoma Paridis 30g

The prescription is taken one dosage a day in decoction. (*Handbook of Practical Anticancer Drugs*)

For esophageal cancer:

Xylotrupes 7

Gryllotalpa 7

Radix Aucklandiae 9g

Radix Angelicae Sinensis 15g

The above herbs are ground into fine powder, blended with half a bowl of saliva from black cow (Sprinkle salt on the cow's tongue, then the saliva will come off spontaneously) and taken in three times with millet wine. The prescription is taken twice a day. (*Newly Compiled Introduction to Traditional Chinese Medicine*)

For cystocancer:

Xylotrupes 9g

Herba Oldenlandiae Diffusae 30g

Herba Scutellariae Barbatae 30g

Radix Vitidis Romanetis 30g

The prescription is taken one dosage a day in decoction. (*Exchange of Medical Information*, Vol. 9, 1974)

For esophageal and cardiac cancer:

Xylotrupes 1

Bulbus Fritillariae Cirrhosae 9g

Indigo Naturalis 6g

Natrii Sulfas 6g

Radix Aucklandiae 3g

Lignum Aquilariae Resinatum 3g

Cinnabaris 3g

Calculus Bovis 1.5g

The above herbs are ground into powder, pounded with Folium Fohdeae, mixed with old wine to make paste for rubbing on the chest several times a day. (*Prescriptions for Diaphragm Syndrome*)

HISTORICAL COMMENTS

Materia Medica says that: "The drug cures dysuria, constipation, bloody dysentery, proctoptosis, all sorts of anal fistula, carbuncle, tarsal ulcer, cervical scrofula, pyogenic infection, sores caused by scald, incessant hemorrhagia, nasopolyp and infantile double tongue."

Collection of Sun's Effective Prescriptions says that: "Eructation can be treated with the drug processed as the follows: Firstly put two earthspiders and two xylotrupes into a pot, wrap the xylotrupes with mud when they have eaten the earthspiders, stew the xylotrupes over fire for an appropriate period of time, then roast it with 10g Pericarpium Citri Reticulatae and Fructus Crotonis, and finally grind it together with Pericarpium Citri Reticulatae without Fructus Crotonis. The powder is blown into the pharynx 0.3-0.6 gram a time.

SCOLOPENDRA

It is defined in *Materia Medica in the Great Ming Dynasty* that: "The drug is hot in taste, toxic in nature, removing abdominal mass and relieving snake poisoning."

The drug is obtained from *Scolopendridae* of *Myriopoda* family, the whole insect is for medical use, containing histamioid material, hemolytic protein, tyrosine, leucine, formic acid, fatty oils and cholesterol.

ANTICANCER PHARMACOLOGICAL FUNCTIONS

1. The hot water extract of the drug inhibits JTC-26 with a rate of 90%.

2. The injection prepared with the drug and Hirudo can cause speratogonium in mice to necrose or disappear.

3. Experiments in vitro, based on the fact that dead cancer cells are liable to being stained by eosin, showed that the injection prepared with the drug and Hirudo appear to be positive to the staining of carcinocytes by eosin.

4. The drug and Hirudo inhibit liver cancer of white mice with a rate of 26%, and reinforce reticuloendocytic function, but chronic use will impair the liver.

5. Cancer-melting Pills (contains scolopendra) inhibits ascites cancer in mice. The best result can be achieved through gastroperfusion or feeding with fodder mixed with the pills.

6. Experiments in vitro showed that the drug inhibits the respiration of cells of liver cancer in human. Methylene blue method proved that the drug affects human liver cancer cells and gastric cancer cells.

7. The drug still inhibits transplanted sarcoma-180 in mice and Walker's cancer-256. The hot water extract from the drug inhibits sarcoma-180 with a rate of 51.4%.

8. Long term oral taking of the drug impairs liver to some extent. Taking ten pieces of the drug a time will cause red specks all over the body, especially on the elbow and the knee. But the specks may fade away when touched and will disappear spontaneously 2-3 days after stopping the drug.

EXPERIMENTAL FORMULAS

For laryngeal cancer and gastric cancer:

20 Scolopendra and 6 grams of Flos Carthami are steeped in 0.5kg of wine with 60% alcohol for 20 days, then filtered and diluted with cold boiled water to make a mixture of water and wine with a ratio of 6:4. The preparation is taken 0.5kg a week. (*Handbook of Chinese Medicinal Herbs In Northeast China*)

For cancer of the digestive tract:

7 Fructus Ziziphi Inermis (without stone) are filled with the powder of 7 Scolopendra and 7 Mylabris, calcined in casserole on fire made with Ramulus Mori, ground into fine powder and packed into 7 equal packets. The preparation is taken with boiled water, one packet a time and once every two or three days. 20 days constitutes a course of treatment. (*Journal of Guangdong Traditional Chinese Medicine*, Vol. 11, 1960)

For rhinocancer:

Equal portions of the drug and Scorpio are ground into powder for oral administration 3 grams a time, 3 times a day. (*Diagnosis and Treatment of Tumor*)

For skin scar cancer:

    Scolopendra 10
    Honey 180g
    Galla Chinensis 740g
    Black vinegar 2500g

The above herbs are made into a paste for external application. Exposure to metal during or after preparation should be avoided. (*Diagnosis and Treatment of Tumor*)

For osteosarcoma:

1>.   Scolopendra 9g
       Scorpio 9g

Minium 30g
Semen Gingko 9g
Mylabris 9g
Gypsum Fibrosum 15g
The prescription is ground into powder.
2>.   Alumen 15g
Gypsum Fibrosum 15g
Rhizoma Arisaematis 1.5g
Venenum Bufonis 1.5g
Cortex Cinnamomi 45g
The prescription is ground into powder.
3>.   Radix Rehmanniae 15g
Herba Salviae Chinensis 15g
Concha Ostreae 15g
Radix Scrophulariae 9g
Rhizoma Anemarrhenae 9g
Massa Medicata Fermentata 9g
Calcitum 30g
Cortex Lycii Radicis 30g
Herba Scutellariae Barbatae 30g
Cortex Moutan 4.5g

Usage: The powder of Prescription 1 is sprinkled on a small plaster and applied to the patient's buttocks; the powder of Prescription 2 is sprinkled on a large plaster and applied to the patient's buttocks one week later accompanied with oral administration of the decoction of Prescription 3 one dosage a day. (*Selected Papers from a National Exhibition on New Medical and Herbal Therapies*)

For encephalocancer:

1>. 100 grams of the drug and 100 grams of Scorpio are ground into powder and taken 3g a time and 2-3 times a day. (*Journal of Liaoning Traditional Chinese Medicine*, Vol. 3, 1978)

2>. 1 Scolopendra and 0.6g Borneol are ground into powder and an appropriate amount of it is inhaled every day. This prescription is especially effective for metastatic encephaloma and stuffed nose and headache caused by some sorts of tumor. (*Journal of Heilongjiang Traditional Chinese Medicine*, Vol. 4, 1984)

HISTORICAL COMMENTS

Materia Medica of All Schools says that: "The drug removes hypochondriac mass."

Prescriptions for Mothers and Babies says that: "Infantile stomatospasm with tiny sores on the tongue can be cured with the application of the juice of the drug."

Pillow Prescription says that: "Scrofula and ulcerous sores can be treated with the drug, after being roasted with tea and pounded into powder. The lesion is washed with Radix Glycyrrhizoae Decoction before the powder is applied."

Extended Prescriptions of Materia Medica says that: "Ulcer and tumor can be cured with 1 Scolopendra, a loaf of Alumen, 1 Omphalia and 6 grams of Radix Stemonae, when ground into powder and mixed with vinegar."

Selected Prescriptions says that: "For female dactylitis with protrusion of diabrotic polyp, the powder of the drug is applied to the lesion first and then covered with the mixture of the powder of Rhizoma Arisaematis and vinegar."

HERBA SEU RADIX PHYSALIS

It is defined in *Dictionary of Chinese Materia Medica* that: "The drug is sour and bitter in taste, cold in nature, clearing away heat to smooth pharynx, and diminishing phlegm to promote urination."

The drug is obtained from a herb of *Physalis* genus of the *Solanaceae* family, the radix or the whole herb is for medical use. *Nicandra Physaloides (L.) Gaertn.* of the same family is used as the substitute of the drug, which, originally produced in North America, has been cultivated in China, bearing the same taste, nature and function as the drug, and is commonly used as an anticancer drug in abroad.

The whole herb contains physalin A, B, and C, while the radix contains tigloidine and hystonin. The extract from *Nicandra physaloides (L.) Gaertn.* contains a sort of food refusal agent of insects known as nicandrenone.

ANTICANCER PHARMACOLOGICAL FUNCTIONS

1. Experiments in vitro with Physalin B showed that its inhibition on ED_{50} of nasopharyngeal carcinocytes and PS (mice lympholeukemia) is $3.1\mu g/ml$ and $0.89\mu g/ml$ respectively.

2. Experiments in vivo showed that the T/C value of Physalin B under a dose of 300mg/kg to 3PS is 137%.

3. The 5a-6a-epoxy physalin synthesized from physalin B remarkably activates nasopharyngeal carcinocytes and PS cytes.

4. The extract from *Nicandra Physaloides (L.) Gaertn.* inhibits the activation of Eagle's nasopharyngeal carcinoma, and its activating substance is nicandrenone, a kind of cytotoxic material.

5. Nicandrenone resists lymphocytic leukemia-388 in vitro with its ED_{50} being $0.74\mu g/ml$.

6. Experiments in vitro proved that the drug resists the activation of nasopharyngeal carcinocytes with ED_{50} being $2.0\mu g/ml$.

EXPERIMENTAL FORMULAS

For various cancers:

1500 grams of the drug's fruit is decocted in 200ml of water and the broth is divided into three portions for oral administration three times a day, each time a portion. (*Information on Traditional Chinese Medicine Research*, Vol. 6, 1978)

HISTORICAL COMMENTS

Pictorial Materia Medica says that: "The drug clears away pathogenic heat to relieve restlessness and promotes menstruation to stop metrorrhagia. The drug also can help discharge placenta when taken orally."

THE AUTHOR'S NOTE

The author has treated cystocancer with the following folk prescription: 90 grams of the fresh radix of the drug is sliced to be decocted in water, 1kg of red-shelled eggs and an appropriate amount of brown sugar are added when the water is boiling. The patient is required to eat the eggs and drink the decoction one or twice a day.

SEMEN ARECAE

Wang Ang in the Qing Dynasty said that: "The drug is bitter and hot in taste and warm in nature, removing stasis, dissipating pathogenic factors, driving the adversely ascended energy downward with great force and directing all sorts of drugs right to the downward direction."

The drug is obtained from the dried fruit of *Areca catechu L.* of the *Palmae* family, mainly produced in Hainan Island, Taiwan and Southeast Asia.

ANTICANCER PHARMACOLOGICAL FUNCTIONS

1. Experiments in vivo on white mice with ascites sarcoma showed that the ethanol extract of the drug inhibits tumor with a rate of 91.9% and the hot water extract with 93.9%.

2. The drug inhibits JTC-26 with a rate of 50-70%.

3. The drug inhibits mice sarcoma-180 with a rate of 50-70%.

4. Screening tests with monolayer culture of Hela cells indicated that the drug resists the activation of Hela cells.

EXPERIMENTAL FORMULAS

For esophageal cancer:

Semen Arecae 1.5g

Radix Glycyrrhizae 0.3g

Flos Carthami 0.3g

Radix Rehmanniae(roasted) 1.5g

Radix Rehmanniae(crude) 1.5g

Rhizoma Cimicifugae Foetidae 3g

Semen Persicae 3g

Radix Angelicae Sinensis 3g

The prescription is taken in decoction. (*Secret Home Recipes*)

For gastrocancer:

Semen Arecae 30g

Radix Aucklandiae 30g

Rhizoma Scirpi 30g

Pericarpium Citri Reticulatae Viride 30g

Radix Angelicae Sinensis 30g

Radix Peucedani 30g

Radix et Rhizoma Rhei 30g

Semen Longan 30g

Carapax Trionycis 45g

Rhizoma Pinelliae 45g

The above herbs are ground into powder and taken 9 grams a time with Rhizoma Zingiberis decoction. (*Prescriptions According to Pathogenic Factors*)

HISTORICAL COMMENTS

On *Properties of Herbs* says that: "The drug releases inhibited visceral energy, dissipates mass and hemostasis, cures edema and stomachache."

Guide to Materia Medica says that: "The drug expels abdominal mass, promotes digestion to remove phlegm and pathogenic wind, kills parasites, soberizes the drunk, diminishes phlegm-accumulation and cures dysuria and constipation."

Materia Medica says that: "People in Lingnan use the drug as tea to prevent miasma."

Daily Diet and Life says that: "The drug dissipates stagnation and stasis, relieves pain to regulates the stomach, smoothens the intestines to promote drainage, and neutralizes rich diet with much fat."

Newly Compiled Materia Medica says that: "The drug activates muscles to relieve pain."

Materia Medica of All Schools in the Great Ming Dynasty says that: "The drug expels all sorts of pathogenic wind, descends all sorts of adversely rising *qi*, invigorates the spleen, regulates the stomach and eliminates abdominal mass."

TAKYDROMUS AMURENSIS

It is defined in *Collection of Chinese Medicinal Herbs* that: "The drug is salty in taste, cold and slightly toxic in nature, promoting drainage and dissipating stasis."

The drug is obtained from *Lacertidae* of the *Reptilia* family, the whole body is for medical use. The insect, 20-24cm or 1-2m in length, is slim with four legs, similar to a snake in its body and tail. Its tongue is short and its tail is liable to break and to regenerate. The female is usually brown and the male bluish green. It often hides inside the cracks of stones and lives on small insects.

ANTICANCER PHARMACOLOGICAL FUNCTIONS
1. The ethanol extract of the drug inhibits the respiration of human liver cancer cells.
2. Methylene blue method proved that the water extract inhibits human liver cancer cells.
3. Experiments in vivo showed that the drug can prolong the survival period of animals transplanted with tumors.

EXPERIMENTAL FORMULAS
For cervical cancer:

The dried reptile is pounded, steeped in equal amount of ethanol for 20 days. Then filter out the deposit, and add in distilled water of the same amount as the filtrated liquid. An isotonic solution is prepared with potassium chloride, after ethanol being removed. 0.5% activated carbon is added to decolor the solution twice, and finally anodyne is added before being sealed for sterilization for 15 minutes. 1ml of the preparation contains 2 grams of the crude drug. The preparation is injected intramuscularly or cervically twice a day. (*Hebei New Medical Journal*, Vol. 3, 1974)

For mammary cancer:

The drug is ground and applied to the lesion. (*Research Information on Traditional Chinese Medicine*, Vol. 6, 1978))

HISTORICAL COMMENTS
Materia Medica says that: "The drug cures abdominal mass, edema, syncope, detained phlegm, erosion of the valva with its property of promoting drainage."

Drugs Obtained from Animals in Northeast of China says that: "The powder of the drug has been used to treat gastrocarcinoma in the recent years. The drug is also used to treat lupus erythematosus when roasted with sesame oil."

PERIOSTRACUM CICADAE

It is defined in *True Materia Medica* that: "The drug is sweet in taste and cold in nature, focusing on the treatment of the syndrome caused by the attack of wind-heat factors against the Liver Channel."

The drug is obtained from the slough of the young cicada of the *Cicadidae* family, mainly produced in Jinhua, Zhejiang Province, and also in Fujian. Ascomycetes is often found on the cicada as parasites. The stroma of the fungus seen on the ground is also for medical use. During the raining season, the drug is mostly found in Double-Dragon Hole and Ice-Pot Hole in Jinhua.

ANTICANCER PHARMACOLOGICAL FUNCTIONS
1. The drug inhibits JTC-26 with a rate of 100% and healthy human fibroembryocytes with a rate of 50%.
2. Clinical experiment showed that the drug indeed inhibits normal cells at the early stage of administration, but this inhibition will disappear five months after the use of the drug.

EXPERIMENTAL FORMULAS

For thyroid cancer:

        Periostracum Cicada

        Scolopendra

        Bombyx Batryticatus

        Scorpis

        Excrementum Vespertilii

        Squama Manitis

        Massa Medicata Fermentata

        Cinnabaris

Equal portions of the above herbs are ground into powder, rolled into pills of chestnut size and coated with Cinnabaris for oral administration during meal twice a day, each time 4.5g. (*Orthodox Surgery*)

For acute granulocytic leukemia:

        Periostracum Cicadae 1.5g

        Pulvis Glycyrrhizae Praeparatus 1.5g

        Radix et Rhizoma Rhei 3g

        Radix Scrophulariae 3g

        Folium Isatidis 3g

        Cortex Moutan 1g

        Radix Trichosanthis 2g

(*Medical Research Correspondance*, Vol. 7 and 8, 1973)

For meningoma:

        Periostracum Cicada 100g

        Scorpis 100g

        Magnetitum 100g

        Scolopendra 50g

The prescription is ground into powder and taken 7.5g a time, 2-3 times a day with boiled water. (*Journal of Liaoning Traditional Chinese Medicine*, Vol. 3, 1978)

HISTORICAL COMMENTS

Chinese Materia Medica says that: "The drug dissipates wind- heat, invigorates lungs, promotes the development of papule and cures convulsive diseases and heat-syndrome."

RADIX RHAPONTICI UNIFLORI

It is defined in *Canon of Materia Medica* that: "The drug is bitter and salty in taste and cold in nature, curing dermatopathy caused by heat and ulcerous sores."

The drug is obtained from *Rhaponticum uniflorum (L.) DC.* of the *Rhaponticum* genus of the *Compositae* family, the radix is for medical use. *Echinops latifolius Tausch.* of the same genus and family is used as a substitute of the drug. *Rhaponticum uniflorum (L.) DC.* contains 0.1% volatile oils and *Echinops latifolius Tausch.* contains echinopsine.

ANTICANCER PHARMACOLOGICAL FUNCTIONS

1. The drug helps to build up the physique of the patients suffering from vascular malnutrition accompanied with general deficiency.

2. The drug can promote reversion of lymphocytes, increase organic immunity and indirectly inhibit carcinocytoplasia.

EXPERIMENTAL FORMULAS

For glossocancer:

150 grams of the drug and 150 grams of Radix et Rhizoma Veratri Nigri are steeped in 500ml of 95% ethanol for 72 hours and then the remains of the drugs are filtrated out. The tumor lesion is washed with cotton balls or soft cloth immersed in the preparation. (*Mindong Medicine*, Vol. 1, 1976)

For cancer of the uterus:

24 grams of the drug and 18 grams of Semen Iridis are decocted for oral administration one dosage a day. (*Secret and Experienced Prescriptions*)

For mammary cancer:

> Radix Rhapontici Uniflori 15g
> Radix Semiaquilegiae 30g
> Rhizoma Dysosmae 9g
> Semen Brassicae Campestris 30g
> Eupolyphaga 9g
> Radix Ampelopsitis 30g
> Fructus Fici Pumilae 9g
> Nidus Vespae 9g

The prescription is taken in decoction. (*Medical Information*, Vol. 9, 1974)

HISTORICAL COMMENTS

Canon of Materia Medica says that: "The drug cures skin ulcer caused by heat, pyogenic sores and arthralgia caused by dampness, promotes lactation, invigorates *qi*, improves vision and prolongs life if taken for a long time."

Wei Tai's Secret Prescriptions says that: "The drug cures mammocancer and breast abscess (similar to breast tumor) with the prescription composed of Radix Rhapontici Uniflori, Bulbus Fritillariae Cirrhosae, Fructus Forsythiae, Radix Glycyrrhizae, Flos Lonicerae, Folium Citri Reticulatae, Faeces Trogopterore, Radix Angelicae Dahuricae, Radix Sophorae Tonkinensis, Cormus Iphigeniae and Spica Prunellae."

Ri Hua's Materia Medica of All Schools in the Great Ming Dynasty says that: "The drug smoothens the small intestine, cures emission, hematuria, hematodefecation, infantile high fever, breast abscess and scrofula, stops hemorrhagia to draw out pus and supplements the blood to nourish the muscles."

INDOCALAMUS

The drug is obtained from *Indocalamus tessellatus (Munro) keng f.* of the *Gramineae* family, the leaves are for medical use. The leaves of many plants in its family are active against cancer. The plant is perennial with stems similar to those of a small bamboo. Its leaves are blue, large and broad (20-24cm) and its lower side is tender in texture. The plant is green all year round with a height of 1.5-2m. The big ones can grow as high as 3m and is known as "Ghost Indocalamus", while the small ones can only reach 30cm and is called "Small Indocalamus". The stalk is thin and long and tough. The seed is edible. The plant is mainly produced in the southern provinces of China. The drug produced in Japan is widely used to treat cancer.

ANTICANCER PHARMACOLOGICAL FUNCTIONS

1. The extract from the leaves of the drug growing in Japan inhibits ascites liver cancer-AH36 with a rate of 100%.

2. The drug reduces the size of ascites tumor and solid sarcoma-180 when administrated every other day for about 30 days.

3. The hot lime extract of the leaves of the plant in Japan is processed with ether to obtain 1 to 5 portions of substance with DEAE cellulose acetate column chromatograph. The refined pErI-A from Portion 1 inhibits sarcoma-180 with a rate of 99.6% and cures seven out of nine tumors.

4. The bacteriophagic experiments in vitro shows that the radix and leaves of *Lophatherum gracile Brongn.* resist bacteriophagia and this indicates that they are active against cancer.

5. Experiments in vitro discovered that the polysacchraide of the radix and leaves of the herb inhibit tumor of animals.

6. The leaves of the herb are found inhibiting mice sarcoma-180 and ascites cancer, and increasing body immunity.

EXPERIMENTAL FORMULAS
For various sorts of cancer:
Juice of the leaves is taken as tea. (*Research Information of Traditional Chinese Medicine*, Vol. 6, 1978)

For hemorrhoid caused by enterocancer:
The leaves of the plant are burned into ashes, crushed to fine powder, mixed with a little Noschus and taken on an empty stomach with millet porridge. (*Selected Prescriptions*)

HISTORICAL COMMENTS
Dictionary of Chinese Materia Medica says that: "The drug, roasted and taken 3 to 5 grams a time with a warm broth, cures spitting blood, hemorrhagia, hemoptysis and defecation with blood. It also promotes urination, invigorates lungs, cures sorethroat, carbuncle and jaundice."

THE AUTHOR'S NOTE
Bamfolin, an extract from the drug, cures carcinoma of the maxillary sinus, laryngeal carcinoma, esophageal carcinoma, ovarian carcinoma, nasopharyngeal carcinoma and celiac carcinoma with remarkable curative effect. Bamfolin, a sort of polysacchraide, can be extracted from multiple sorts of bamboo. It is reported in *How to Prevent and Treat Cancer* published by World Publishing House in Hong Kong that: "A patient had oral cancer and underwent an operation. But three months after operation, the cancer returned with unbearable pain and a mass 5mm in diameter. He was in a dangerous condition and refused to take another operation. Therefore bamfolin was prescribed. Both the pain and the cancer were reduced one month after administration. The cancer completely disappeared four months later."

CORTEX AILANTHI

It is defined in *Supplementation to Materia Medica* that: "The drug is cold in nature, astringentizing blood."

The drug is the twig or the root bark of *Ailanthus altissima (Mill.) Swingle* of the *Simarubaceae* family. Its leaves and samara are also for medical use. The root bark contains margoside.

ANTICANCER PHARMACOLOGICAL FUNCTIONS
Animal experiment showed that the drug inhibits mice sarcoma-180, sarcoma-37, leukemia-16 and the Hela cells.

EXPERIMENTAL FORMULAS

For enterocancer:

The bark of the plant is washed, dried, ground and mixed with excipient to make powder (10g contains 9g of the root bark). The powder is taken 10 grams a time, 3 times a day. (*Anticancer Preparations of Traditional Chinese Medicine*)

For cervical cancer:

1>.   Cortex Ailanthi 15g

        Cortex Phellodendri 15g

        Radix Paeoniae Alba 15g

        Herba Scutellariae Barbatae 30g

        Herba Pteridis Multifidae 30g

The prescription is taken in decoction one dosage a day. (*Handbook of Practical Anticancer Drugs*)

2>. 1000 grams of the bark is decocted with 500 grams of wheat chaff in 300ml of water for oral administration 50ml each time 3 times a day. The decoction also can be applied locally. (*Dictionary of Chinese Materia Medica*)

HISTORICAL COMMENTS

Dietetic Materia Medica says that: "The drug cures infantile malnutrition complicated with dysentery and ascariasis."

Supplementation to Materia Medica says that: "The drug cures scabies and defecation with blood."

Ren Cuntang's Experienced Prescriptions says that: "Chronic bloody defecation can be cured with 9 grams of the drug decocted in an appropriate amount of water and taken with wine."

Dictionary of Chinese Materia Medica says that: "To cure hemodefecation, 120 grams of the sliced drug, the juice of 120 grams of green bean sprouts and 120 grams of turnip are blended and decocted in water. The broth is then filtrated and finally added with an appropriate amount of millet wine. The prepared decoction is warmed and taken orally before going to bed. For children, the dosage is reduced accordingly."

HERBA ECLIPTAE

It is defined in *Guide to Materia Medica* that: "The drug is sweet and salty in taste, black in juice, nourishing kidney to stop hemorrhagia."

The drug is obtained from *Eclipta prostrata L.* of *Compositae* family, the whole of which is for medical use. Since the leaves and the stalk become black when steeped in water, it was widely used in ancient time to restore the black color of the hair. The whole herb contains saponins, nicotine, tannins, vitamin A and ecliptine.

ANTICANCER PHARMACOLOGICAL FUNCTIONS

Experiments both in vivo and vitro showed that the drug inhibits oncocytoplasia.

EXPERIMENTAL FORMULAS

For uterocancer at the middle or the advanced stage:

        Herba Ecliptae 30g

        Radix Codonopsis Pilosulae 30g

        Radix Glycyrrhizae 3g

        Auricularia 6g

        Radix Glehniae 20g

Herba Dendrobii 20g
Radix Pseudostellariae Heterophyllae 20g
Fructus Ligustri Lucidi 20g
Radix Paeoniae Alba 20g
Flos Lonicerae 20g
Poria 20g

The prescription is taken in decoction. (*Journal of Shanghai Traditional Chinese Medicine*, Vol. 9, 1984)

For esophageal cancer:

250 grams of the drug is squeezed to get 100ml of juice for oral administration in three times rawly or after being simmered. (*Traditional Chinese Medical and Pharmacological Correspondance*, Vol. 3, 1972)

For giant dermatokeras at the earlier stage of dermatocancer:

Herba Ecliptae 20g
Radix Angelicae Sinensis 20g
Radix Paeoniae Alba 20g
Radix Scrophulariae 30g
Rhizoma Chuanxing 10g
Radix Cynanchi Atrati 10g
Rhizoma Dioscoreae 15g
Rhizoma Atractylodis Macrocephalae 15g
Radix Salviae Miltiorrhizae 15g
Cortex Moutan 15g
Poria 15g

The above herbs are taken in decoction twice a day, and at the same time is given the external application of Effective Paste, which is composed of:

Talcum 500g
Calamina 150g
Cinnabaris 50g
Semen Setariae 100g

(*Journal of Liaoning Traditional Chinese Medicine*, Vol. 3, 1979)

HISTORICAL COMMENTS

Guide to Properties of Raw Medicinal Herbs says that: "Violent spitting of blood can be cured with the decoction of the drug, young boy's urine, pounded inkstick and joints of lotus root."

Medical Stories says that: "Infantile hematuria can be cured with the natural juice of Folium Plantaginis Asiaticae and Folium Ecliptae, taken on an empty stomach."

Proved Secret Prescriptions says that: "Hemodefecation caused by visceral inflammation can be cured with an oral administration of 6 grams of the powder of the drug each time, after being calcined on tile and pounded."

General Collection of Holy Prescriptions says that: "Migraine and over-all headache can be cured by dropping the sweet juice of the drug into the nose."

SEMEN COICIS

It is defined in *Canon of Materia Medica* that: "The drug is sweet in taste and slightly cold in nature, curing the syndrome characterized by stiffness of muscles, arthralgia and immobility of joints."

The drug is obtained from a plant of the *Coix* genus of the *Gramineae* family. The kernel of the seed is for medical use, containing coixenlide, amino acid, saccharides and alkaloids.

ANTICANCER PHARMACOLOGICAL FUNCTIONS

1. The acetone and the ethanol extract from the seed inhibits ascites cancer.

2. The extract of the herb is found inhibiting Yoshida's sarcoma.

3. The alcohol extract can change the nature of oncocytoplasm, and the other substances of the herb can stop the nucleodivision at the middle stage.

4. The ester of the drug has already been synthesized and is widely used to resist cancer.

EXPERIMENTAL FORMULAS

For chorioepithelioma:

> Semen Coicis 30g
> Herba Houttuyniae 30g
> Semen Phaseoli 30g
> Herba Patriniae Scabiosaefoliae 15g
> Radix Astragali 9g
> Radix Rubiae 9g
> Semen Benincasae 9g
> Radix Angelicae Sinensis 9g
> Colla Corii Asini 9g
> Radix Glycyrrhizae 9g

The prescription is taken in decoction.

For chorioepithelioma with metastasis:

The following prescription is given in decoction one dose a day:

> Semen Coicis 30g
> Poria 6g
> Radix Codonopsis Pilosulae 6g
> Radix Curcumae 6g
> Radix Glycyrrhizae 6g
> Colla Corii Asini 9g
> Rhizoma Cyperi 9g
> Radix Angelicae Sinensis 9g
> Crinis Carbonisatus 1.5g
> Pollen Typhae 6g
> Faeces Trogopterore 3g

(*Diagnosis and Treatment of Tumor*)

For gastrocancer, laryngocancer, Yoshida's sarcoma and malignant reticular cellular hyperplasia:

30 to 59 grams of the drug is simmered with japonica rice or glutinous rice and taken all year round. (*Reading Is Beneficial*, Vol. 6, 1984)

For uteromyoma:

1>. 500 grams of the drug is ground with 150 grams of Radix Notoginseng and taken 15g each time three times a day with boiled water. (*Journal of Jiling Traditional Chinese Medicine*, Vol. 3, 1983)

2>. *Guizhi Fulin Pill* is taken together with 15 grams of the drug all the year round. This is an experienced prescription developed by a Japanese doctor. (*Elucidation on Prescriptions for Clinical Application*)

For mammary cancer:

15 grams of the drug and 15 grams of Rhizoma Corydalis are decocted in millet wine and taken on an empty stomach. (*Prescriptions for Mammary Cancer*)

HISTORICAL COMMENTS

Materia Medica says that: "The drug invigorates the spleen and the stomach, supplements the lung to clear away pathogenic heat, expels pathogenic wind and wetness, descends *qi* to harmonize the *ying qi* and cures severe arthralgia."

Wang Yan's Prescriptions says that: "Cough due to pulmonary abscess and pathogenic dryness and the disorder of the thorax can be cured by the drug boiled in bitter millet wine into a strong decoction for oral administration while it is warm. If there is stasis of blood in the lung, it will be vomited out immediately after taking the decoction."

Effective Prescriptions for Women says that: "Abscess seen during pregnancy can be cured with the decoction of the drug taken frequently."

Wai Tai Secret Prescriptions says that: "Acute laryngeal abscess can be cured with two Semen Coicis when swallowed."

THE AUTHOR'S NOTE

Gastric carcinoma was treated with the decoction of 15 grams of Semen Coicis, 6 grams of Caulis Wisteriae Sinensis, 6 grams of Fructus Chebulae and 6 grams of Fructus Trapae Bispinosae during the 1950s in Japan. It was said to be effective.

FRUCTUS FICI PUMILAE

It is defined in *Guangdong Chinese Medicinal Herbs* that: "The drug is bland in taste and slightly cool in nature, promoting drainage to expel dampness and dissipating toxic material."

The drug is obtained from *Ficus Pumila L.* of the *Ficus* genus in the *Moraceae* family, the flower and the seed are for medical use. The drug contains inositol, rutin, ß-sitosterol, taraxeryl acetate and ß-amyrin acetate; the seed contains mucilage; the stalk, the twig, the leaf and the juice of the fruit contains rubber.

ANTICANCER PHARMACOLOGICAL FUNCTIONS

1. Experiments in vitro showed that the drug resists the activation of cancer and significantly inhibits ascites and subcutaneous lymphosarcoma-I, cancer-256, sarcoma-180 as well as ascites and subcutaneous reticulocytic sarcoma.

2. The drug can remarkably reduces cell division of ascites reticulocytic sarcoma.

3. It has been proved that ß-sitosterol resists cancer.

EXPERIMENTAL FORMULAS

For liver cancer at the earlier stage:

Fructus Fici Pumilae 30g

Rhizoma Pinelliae Cordatae 30g

Massa Medicate Fermentata 30g

Fructus Hordei Germinatus 30g

Fructus Crataegi 30g

Herba Ardisiae Japonicae 30g

Concha Ostreae 30g

Hippocampus 3g

Radix Actinidiae Valvatae 60g

Carapax Trionycis 12g

The prescription is taken in decoction. (*Anticancer Consultation*)

For cavernous hemangioma:

Fructus Fici Pumilae 30g

Herba Aristolochiae Mollissimae 30g

Rhizoma Smilacis Glabrae 30g

Radix Astragali 30g

Radix Codonopsis Pilosulae 12g

Radix Paeoniae Alba 12g

Radix Arneliae 9g

Cortex Moutan 9g

The prescription is taken one dosage a day in decoction. (*Journal of Shanghai Traditional Chinese Medicine*, Vol. 6, 1979)

For mammary cancer:

Fructus Fici Pumilae 30g

Sargassum 30g

Semen Vaccariae 12g

The prescription is taken in decoction. (*Handbook of Practical Anticancer Drugs*)

For cervical cancer, gastrocancer, enterocancer and liver cancer:

15 to 30 grams of the drug is decocted for oral taking. (*Therapies Based on Differentiation of Symptoms and Signs*)

HISTORICAL COMMENTS

Materia Medica says that: "The drug prevents emission, subsides swelling to dissipate toxic material, stops hemorrhagia, promotes lactation, cures perianal abscess due to chronic dysentery, stomachache, and loss of pudendal hair." "Painful hemostranguria can be cured with 90g of the drug and 0.3g of roasted Radix Glycyrrhizae, when decocted together and taken orally."

Pictorial Materia Medica says that: "The leaves cure back abscess and the powder cures dysentery."

Chinese Materia Medica says that: "A seventy year old man cured his carbuncle on the back with the juice squeezed from the leaves of the drug and applied to the lesion by himself because there was no doctor in his village."

Textual Research On Plants and Their Nomenclature says that: "Wood lotus is another name for the drug which is also called by people in the south of the Changjiang River as Wood Bread. The seed of the drug is ground and deposited in water and the sediment is locally made into bean jelly for summer enjoyment."

Pharmacology of Chinese Medicinal Herbs says that: "The juice from the vine stimulates sexual desire, reinforces kidney function to prevent emission, diminishes inflammation and subsides swelling."

Chinese Materia Medica says that: "The plant, to some extent, resists cancer."

GECKO CHINENSIS

Li Shizhen in the Ming Dynasty said that: "The drug is salty in taste, cold and slightly toxic in nature, cures paralysis caused by apoplexy and abdominal mass due to hemodetention."

The drug is obtained from *Geckonidae* in the *Reptilia* family, the whole body of which is for medical use.

ANTICANCER PHARMACOLOGICAL FUNCTIONS
The drug dissolved in liquid inhibits the respiration of hepatocarcinocytes.

EXPERIMENTAL FORMULAS

For mediastinal tumor:

15 grams of the drug is ground together with 9 grams of Lumbricus and 6 grams of Bombyx Batryticatus, rolled into honey-coated pills (each weights 1.5-3g) and taken one pill a time, twice a day. (*Diagnosis and Treatment of Tumor*)

For mammary cancer:

2 Gecko Chinensis are steeped in sesame oil for 2 months and applied to the affected lesion with gauze. The prescription is eligible for ulcerous mammary cancer. (*Experienced Prescriptions*)

For esophageal and cardiac cancer:

1>. 10 whole live Gecko Chinensis are steeped in 500ml of white spirit of excellent quality for 7 days and then 10ml of the wine is taken each time, three times a day. (*Prescriptions Selected from the Pharmaceutical Exhibition Held in Wuhan*)

2>. 1 Gecko Chinensis and some rice are calcined, ground and taken in 2-3 times with a little millet wine each day. (*Dictionary of Chinese Materia Medica*)

For cervical cancer:

Gecko Chinensis Injection is administrated intramuscularly 4 to 6ml every day or every other day. (*Hebei New Medical Journal*, Vol. 3, 1974)

For multiple malignant tumor:

A hole is drilled on an egg, through which a Gecko Chinensis is inserted, wrapped with rough straw paper, covered with mud, calcined over coal fire, ground into powder and taken with boiled water. (*New Traditional Chinese Medicine Journal*, Vol. 1, 1976)

HISTORICAL COMMENTS

Materia Medica says that: "The insect is named after tiger because it is good at hiding to catch scorpions and flies. It is characterized by a flat head, long neck, fine scales and four paws. It is usually about two decimeters long and never bites human beings."

Qing Nang Zha Zhuan says that: "Scrofula can be cured with one Gecko Chinensis calcined and ground into powder for oral administration with wine 0.3g each time."

Precious Inspection into Hygiene says that: "Pestilence can be cured with one Gecko Chinensis (calcined), 75g of Faeces Bombyx (washed twice in water and dried in the sunshine) and 2-2.5kg wheat flour, when blended together. The mixture is dried and ground into powder for oral administration with 15-30g each time, three times a day, with Folium et Ramulus Biotae decoction before each meal."

History of Chinese Medicinal Herbs in Sichuan says that: "The drug diminishes hemostasis and cures tumor."

Collection of Comments on Materia Medica says that: "In treating diseases caused by blood deficiency and asthenic *qi* (not by wind-phlegm and exogenous pathogenic factors), the drug should be carefully used."

THE AUTHOR'S NOTE

50 cases of advanced esophageal carcinoma were treated with significant effect in Wuhan No.1 Hospital. The prescription contained Gecko Chinensis (10%), Semen Coicis, Herba Euphorbiae Hirtae and Rhizoma Dioscoreae Bulbiferae (30% for each). All the above drugs are steeped and sealed in wine for two weeks. Then 15-20ml of the wine is taken each time, three times a day on an empty stomach or during the meal. For those with alcohol addiction, the dosage could be slightly larger, but no more than 150ml a day.

In Wengzhou City, 4 cases of esophageal carcinoma were treated with oral administration of the powder of the drugs, twice a day and the focus of the cancer was found disappeared completely.

BLATTELLA ORIENTALIS

Canon of Materia Medica says that: "The drug is salty in taste and cold in nature, diminishing hemostasis and abdominal mass, and curing sore-throat."

The drug is obtained from *Blattella Orientalis* of the *Blattidae* family, the whole of which is for medical use. The insect is often found in the kitchens, hiding during daytime and coming out at night, and likes to eat vegetables, foods and liquids. It secretes a foul substance when it defecates. The insect is found all over China. For medical purpose, it is killed in boiling water, washed and calcined for use.

ANTICANCER PHARMACOLOGICAL FUNCTIONS

1. The alcohol extract of the drug without wings and paws evidently inhibits mice sarcoma-180, and directly kills carcinocytes of sarcoma-180 when used externally.

2. The alcohol extract can significantly increase the macrophagic index of celiac macrophagocytes on mice safely without much toxicity.

EXPERIMENTAL FORMULAS

For spitting blood caused by cancer:

Five Blattella Orientalis without wings are calcined on clean tile and ground into powder to be wrapped with wet bean curd sheet, boiled and swallowed. This formula is continued for five days without any interval.

For primary liver cancer:

The AT-2 extract from the drug is made into capsules or tablets for oral administration 3 to 6 tablets each time, three times a day.

HISTORICAL COMMENTS

Materia Medica in the Tang Dynasty says that: "The drug is hot in taste and foul in smell, is effective for moving *qi* downwards."

Luchuan Materia Medica says that: "The drug expels wind to clear away pathogenic heat and activate blood circulation."

Zhou Yisheng's Private Prescriptions says that: "Abdominal distention can be cured with one Blattella Orientalis (calcined) and a pinch of Semen Raphani, after being roasted, ground and taken with wine."

THE AUTHOR'S NOTE

It was reported, by a coalition research group on the treatment of liver cancer with AT-2, that among the 37 cases who took AT-2, the condition of 22 became stabilized, subjective feeling of improvement of symptoms was 87.3.87%, reduction of severity of tenderness was 81.8%, and reduction in the size of the liver was 39.39%. The follow-up visit to 30 cases indicated that the effective rate was 66.7% and the average survival period was 8.25 months (*Fujian Medical Journal*, Vol. 5, 1981). One case of nephrocarcinoma was treated by the author with satisfactory result with a prescription composed of 40 grams of Rhizoma Dioscoreae, 20 grams of Scolopendra and 30 grams of Hippocampus, when calcined and ground into powder for oral administration 3 grams a time, twice a day, accompanied with 3 pills of vitamin C and 3 pills of vitamin B. This prescription was taken for 15 days and renewed after four days' interval.

EUPOLYPHAGA SEU STELEOPHAGA

It is defined in *Properties of Medicinal Herbal* that: "The drug is bitter and salty in taste, diminishing hemostasis and abdominal mass."

The drug is obtained from female *Eupolyphaga Sinensis Walker* of the *Polyphaginae* family or *Opisthoplatia orientalis (Burm.)* of the *Phyllodromiidae* family.

ANTICANCER PHARMACOLOGICAL FUNCTIONS
1. Experiments in vivo with methylene blue method showed that the bathing paste of the drug inhibits leukocytes.
2. The drug inhibits cellular inspiration of liver cancer and stomach cancer.

EXPERIMENTAL FORMULAS
For uteromyoma, ovarian cancer and salpingioma:

> Eupolyphaga seu Steleophaga 9g
>
> Semen Persicae 9g
>
> Radix et Rhizoma Rhei 6g

The herbs are decocted in the liquid composed of half water and half wine for oral administration. This prescription is quite effective in removing hematostasis. (*Prescriptions of Gynecology in Modern Times*)

For glossocancer:

1>. 7 pieces of Eupolyphaga seu Steleophaga are decocted with 45 grams of salt in a large cup of water for a short period of time and the broth is only for gargling 3 to 5 times a day without being swallowed. (*Prescriptions for Infants by Dr. Bao*)

2>. The drug is pounded with Herb Menthae to get juice for application to the lesion with a piece of cloth. (*Prescriptions for Infants by Dr. Bao*)

HISTORICAL COMMENTS
Canon of Materia Medica says that: "The drug diminishes hemostasis and abdominal mass and cures amenorrhea due to hemostasis."

Extended Materia Medica says that: "Lactostagnation can be cured with one piece of the drug, after being ground, melted in water and taken after filtration.

THE AUTHOR'S NOTE
The drug has been clinically used by some people to treat thick phlegm and gastrocancer when stewed and taken twice a day; it is also used by some doctors to treat nasopharyngeal carcinoma when pounded with Herba Oxalitis and applied to the lesion. 10 cases of hepatocarcinoma were treated with Five Insect Pill (containing the drug) and a remarkable curative effect was achieved in Shanghai. Based on the clinical observation, it is inferred that the drug may function to stabilize the patient's immune condition, or to inhibit the multiplication of liver cells. The decoction of the drug has been used to treat nasopharyngeal carcinoma in Hunan and the total effective rate is 66.7%.

GUTTI CAMBOGIA

It is defined in *Origin of Materia Medica* that: "The drug, being toxic in nature, removes toxic materials."

The drug is obtained from the resin of *Garcinia Morella Desv.* of the *Guttiferae* family. Before blossoming, the bark 3 meters above the earth is cut spirally and the resin will come off spontaneously. The dried resin is for medical use.

ANTICANCER PHARMACOLOGICAL FUNCTIONS

1. The extracted liquid 736-1 inhibits human hepatocarcinocytes when administered with a dose over 16μg/ml. Its function is superior to that of camptothecine, lycorine and colchicine.

2. The Morellic acid contained in its acid resin directly kills cancer cells of rat breast cancer-737 and cervical cancer-14.

3. Isomorellic acid is also against cancer.

4. The extract administrated celiacally inhibits mice ascites hepatocarcinoma and ascites cancer, especially inhibits sarcoma-180 and sarcoma-37 with a rate of 35.6-80%.

5. Animal toxicity tests showed that the dosage and the administration method of the drug do not affect much the hematopoietic system of mice and domestic rabbits. This indicates that the drug can be safely used clinically in proper dosage.

EXPERIMENTAL FORMULAS
For cervical cancer:
Apply the suppository of the drug to the cervix and change every other day. (*Chinese Oncology*)
For dermatocancer:
The paste of the drug is applied to the lesion. (*Chinese Oncology*)

HISTORICAL COMMENTS
Supplementation to Materia Medica says that: "The drug cures carbuncle and stops hemorrhagia to eliminate toxic materials."

Dictionary of Chinese Materia Medica says that: "The pills are taken orally 0.03-0.06 gram each time. Patients with weak physique are forbidden to take the drug. A large dosage will cause dizziness, nausea, abdominal pain, diarrhea or even death."

HERBA DIANTHI

It is defined in *Canon of Materia Medica* that: "The drug is bitter in taste and cold in nature, and is effective for obstruction syndrome characterized by frequent vomiting accompanied with difficulty in defecation or urination, and all sorts of mass and distention."

The drug is obtained from a herb of *Dianthus* genus of the *Caryophyllaceae* family, the whole herb or the radix is for medical use. *D. Chinensis L.* of the same family is used as a substitute for the drug. The drug contains saponins, volatile oils, saccharides, substance like vitamin A, and alkaloids.

ANTICANCER PHARMACOLOGICAL FUNCTIONS
1. The hot water extract inhibits JTC-26 with a rate of 90%.

2. The hot water extract of the radix inhibits JTC-26 with a rate of 100%. The extract also inhibits JTC-Helas$_3$ as well as the normal cells with a rate of 66.7%.

3. Experiments in vitro with the hot water extract of the radix showed that it inhibits mice sarcoma-180 with a rate of 35.9%. Among the 24 herbs tested together, its activation is just next to Herba Agrimoniae.

4. The alcohol preparation of Radix Dianthi Chinensis of the same family inhibits cancer cells of human cardiac cancer and cystocancer as indicated by pharmaceutical sensitivity test.

EXPERIMENTAL FORMULAS
For cystocancer:
        Herba Dianthi 30g
        Radix Rubiae 30g
        Herba Solani Nigri 30g

Radix Citidis Romanetis 30g

The prescription is taken in decoction. (*Handbook of Practical Anticancer Drugs*)

For rectocancer:

The drug is dried in sunshine, ground into powder and sprinkled over the lesion. (*Surgery of Traditional Chinese Medicine*)

For esophagocancer and rectocancer:

1>. The fresh root (30 to 60 grams for the fresh and 24 to 30 grams for the dried) of the drug is washed with rice swill, decocted and taken twice orally.

2>. The extract is taken half a spoonful each time with boiled water and twice a day.

3>. The root of the drug is dried in sunshine, ground into powder and sprinkled over the lesion.

The above prescriptions can be accompanied with Si Jun Zhi (Four Ingredients) Decoction if the patient is weak. (*Traditional Chinese Medical and Pharmacological Correspondance*, Vol. 3, 1972)

HISTORICAL COMMENTS

Canon of Materia Medica says that: "The drug treats obstruction syndrome, all sorts of mass, carbuncles and amenorrhagia."

Chinese Materia Medica says that: "The leaves of the drug cures anal fistula, hemodefecation and ascariasis, neutralizes toxicity of the mineral drug and cures ophthalmia and female tinea sores."

Cui's Prescriptions says that: "Carbuncle on the tip of the thumb can be treated with the ashes of the drug blended with vegetable oil and applied to the lesion."

Wai Tai Prescriptions says that: "Sorethroat can be cured with a satisfactory result by the powder taken orally."

HISTORICAL COMMENTS

The paste or the decoction of the drug was administered alone to treat a patient with esophageal cancer and a patient with rectal cancer in Hefei Chinese Medicinal Herbal Processing Factory in Anhui Province and it was reported to have achieved satisfactory result.

VENENUM BUFONIS

Miao Xiyong in the Ming Dynasty said that: "The drug is hot in taste and cold in nature, dissipating toxic materials and clearing away heat."

The drug is obtained from *Bufo bufo gargarizans Cantor* of the *Bufonidae* family, its skin, viscera, glands behind the ear and the secretion from the dermatoglands are for medical use. *Bufo melanostictus Schneider* and others of the same family all can be used medically. The drug contains bufotalin, cinobufagin, desacetylcinobufagin, cinobufotalin, sterols, 5-indoxylcholine, arginine, ouabain, suberic acid, bufotenine and bufotenidine.

ANTICANCER PHARMACOLOGICAL FUNCTIONS

1. The drug dissolved in water inhibits JTC-26 with a rate of 90% in experiments in vivo.

2. The drug inhibits the cytes of human ovarian cancer and hepatocancer as indicated by methylene blue test.

3. Bacteriophagic screening tests showed that the drug induces bacteriophagia, and this indicates that it is against the activity of cancer.

4. The extract of the whole drug inhibits, when used externally, the carcinocytic respiration of ovarian adenocancer, the undifferentiated inferior and superior jugomaxillary cancer, intracutaneous cancer, gastrocancer and splenosarcoma.

5. The alcohol and the water extract of the drug inhibits cancer cells of human gastric cancer as indicated by methylene blue method.

6. The extract from the skin of the drug inhibits mice sarcoma-180 and rabbit tumor B and P, prolongs the survival period of mice with seminoma, ascites cancer and hepatocarcinoma, and also inhibits the cells of leukemia in tube.

7. The skin of the drug inhibits the activation of cervical cancer-14 and ascites hepatocarcinoma in mice.

8. The drug can also inhibits the growth of Hela cells and the cellular respiration of human hepatocarcinoma and leukemia.

9. The cardiac glycosides and aglycone contained in the skin of the animal inhibits cancer cells of Hela-S_3, and ouabain inhibits cells of ascites cancer.

10. The tryptic hydrolytic liquid of the drug inhibits solid tumor in mice.

EXPERIMENTAL FORMULAS

For stomach cancer:

12.5kg of the drug is stewed, blended with 6kg of wheat flour to make a paste for oral administration 2 to 3 grams a day. (*Basic Knowledge of Traditional Chinese Medicine*)

For gastrocancer, pulmonary cancer and cystocancer:

Live Bufos are stripped off their skin, cut off their heads, got rid of their liver, gallbladder and heart, boiled in water three times as much as the drug for 30 minutes and then filtered. The decoction is added with water twice as much and filtrated again. The decoction after three times of filtration is stewed to a volume one third of the original and then cooled. The cooled decoction is mixed with 95% alcohol (2 to 3 times) and then the protein of the broth is removed. 3% alcohol benzylis is added and the pH value is adjusted to 6 or 7. A little Tween-80 can be added. The preparation is finally packaged into individual containers and sterilized before use. The preparation is injected intramuscularly or at acupoints or locally 2ml a time and twice a day. (*Diagnosis and Treatment of Tumor*)

For chronic granulocytic leukemia:

500g of the drug and 9g of Fructus Arnomi. The drug is filled with Fructus Arnomi in the mouth, wrapped with mud, calcined over fire, ground into powder for oral administration 3 grams each time and 3 times a day. (*Diagnosis and Treatment of Tumor*)

For liver, pulmonary and esophageal cancer, nasopharyngeal cancer and multiple myeloma:

500mg of the drug, 100mg of pancreatin, 50ml of phosphate (with 0.2 gram of Na_2SO_3) and 1ml of benzyl alcohol are hydrolysed for six hours, boiled for 10 minutes, filtrated (pH=6.4), added with 100mg pancreatin, hydrolysed again for 22 hours under 87 degrees centigrade (pH=8), boiled again, added with a little diatomite, filtrated with filter paper, kept in refrigerator for a night, filtrated with routine method the next day (pH=6.3), added with 5g of glucose (pH is adjusted to 7.2-7.5 with sodium hydroxide), filtrated again and sterilized for 30 minutes under 100 degrees centigrade. An ampule contains 2ml and each milliliter contains 5mg of the drug. The preparation is injected intramuscularly 10-20mg a time and twice a day.

For various tumors, sarcomas and unbearable pain:

Vaseline is warmed first, then blended with powder of the drug (1:10) and applied to the lesion. Rashes will appear in a few patients but will vanish spontaneously a few days later when washed with water. This prescription is indicative for liver cancer, lung cancer, thyroid cancer, lymphosarcoma fibroma and pain caused by tumor.

For esophageal cancer:

50 live toads are starved for three days, then washed, put into 5kg of river water, heated and then stewed for 3-4 hours into a thin paste, which is filtrated with gauze, taken off the residual, decocted for 1 or 2 more hours into a semi-liquid paste (about 500ml), blended with 1kg of roasted corn flour and

packaged in a pot. The preparation is taken 10g a time (with boiled water or millet porridge mixed with a spoonful honey), twice a day for three days and renewed after one day's interval.

For acute granuloleukemia:

The toad is cut open along the abdominal mid-line (without removing the skin and the viscera), filled with a duck egg in the abdomen, sewed up and boiled in 300-400ml of water for 30-40 minutes. The duck egg is taken orally.

For tumor complicated with chronic and radiant pneumonia:

A toad is filled with 20 grains of Fructus piperis in the mouth, calcined after three days, then ground into powder and taken 1g a time, twice a day.

For exezematoid papillary carcinoma:

A big toad is pounded and applied to the lesion daily with gauze dress. The wrappage should be changed timely because the pounded toad is easy to go bad.

For stomach and liver cancer:

1>. Seven toads are boiled for six hours and stripped off the bones. Both the meat and the decoction are taken for treatment.

2>. Three live toads are boiled in 0.5kg of millet wine for half an hour and the broth is taken, after it become cool, 10ml a time, three times a day for 30 days in secession. The therapy is renewed after three days interval and three months make up a course of treatment.

For cancerous hemorrhagia:

A piece of inkstick 0.3cm long) is inserted into a live toad and after five days, the toad is roasted and ground into powder for application to the lesion.

HISTORICAL COMMENTS

Materia Medica of All Schools says that: "The drug cures infantile malnutrition, diminishes abdominal mass, and treats pyogenic sores when burned into ash and blended with dietetic oil for application to the lesion."

Dictionary of Chinese Materia Medica says that: "The skin of the toad removes severe poison when applied to the lesion."

Materia Medica says that: "The drug cures carbuncle on the back and all sorts of pyogenic swelling."

Life Preserving Prescription says that: "All sorts of carbuncle and swelling can be cured with the drug (3g) and Moschus (3g), when ground, blended with human milk and kept in a pot for drying. The prepared drug is mixed with a little liquid before application, and covered with other paste after application."

Key Prescriptions for Emergency says that: "Pyogenic or ulcerous suppurative osteomyelitis can be treated with a big toad, a handful of hair and 120g of lard, when decocted, filtered and condensed into a paste for application to the lesion which has been washed with the decoction of Cortex Mori and Radix Aconiti and applied with Fossilia Ossis Mastodi."

Sun Shimiao's Prescriptions says that: "All sorts of dermatopathy can be cured with toad ash when blended with vinegar and applied 3 to 5 times a day."

CARAPAX TRIONYCIS

It is defined in *Annotation to Canon of Materia Medica* that: "The drug is salty in taste, mild and non-toxic in nature, curing abdominal hard mass."

The drug is obtained from the shell of *Trionyx Sinensis Weigmann* of the *Trionychidae* family. The drug is found almost all over China, especially in the Changjiang River Basin. For medical purpose, the drug is usually roasted with vinegar.

ANTICANCER PHARMACOLOGICAL FUNCTIONS

1. Tests with methylene blue method showed that the drug is effective in inhibiting cells of hepatocancer, gastrocancer and acute lympholeukemia.

2. The drug inhibits respiration of hepatocarcinocytes and gastrocarcinocytes.

EXPERIMENTAL FORMULAS

For variant cancer:

        Carapax Trionycis 50g

        Herba Solani Nigri 50g

        Herba Solani Lyrati 50g

        Herba Oldenlandiae Diffusae 50g

        Herba Scutellariae Barbatae 50g

The prescription is taken one dosage a day in decoction. (*Diagnosis and Treatment of Tumor*)

For celiac tumor:

        Carapax Trionyci

        Cortex Chebulae

        Rhizoma Zingiberis

Equal portions of the above herbs are put together, ground into powder and made into pills for oral administration, 30 pills each time on an empty stomach. (*Properties of Medicinal Herbs*)

For vomiting blood caused by lung cancer:

        Carapax Trionycis 30g

        Gecko 30g

        Radix Rehmanniae 45g

The herbs are ground into powder and taken 6 grams each time after meal with tea. (*Collection of Holy Prescriptions*)

HISTORICAL COMMENTS

Properties of Medicinal Herbs said that: "The drug diminishes undigested food, abdominal hard mass, leukorrhagia and hemostasis."

True Materia Medica says that: "This is a drug for clearing away pathogenic heat accumulated in the liver, not for tonifying the liver. Therefore, it is contraindicative for patients only with liver deficiency and without heat accumulation."

Enlightenment of Materia Medica says that: "The drug is the key ingredient in Carapax Trionycis Pills for treating accumulated liver-*qi*, key ingredient in Rhizoma Pinelliae Powder for abdominal mass and key ingredient in Carapax Trionycis Pills for splenic mass."

THE AUTHOR'S NOTE

In Japan, the whole turtle, including the meat and shell, is decocted to treat various cancer.

NIDUS VESPAE

Li Shizhen in the Ming Dynasty said that: "The drug is sweet in taste, mild and toxic in nature, removing toxic materials."

The drug is obtained from honeycomb of *Polistes mandarinus Sanssure* belonging to *Vespidae* family in *Hymenoptera* class, containing myricin and resin. The volatile oil contained in the drug is toxic and can kill cestode and earthworm.

ANTICANCER PHARMACOLOGICAL FUNCTIONS

1. The drug has been proved to inhibits cells of gastric cancer by methylene blue method.
2. Experiments in vivo showed that the drug inhibits cells of liver cancer.

EXPERIMENTAL FORMULAS

For uterochorioepithelioma:

> Nidus Vespae 6g
> Radix Angelicae Sinensis 9g
> Poria 12g
> Radix Salviae Miltiorrhizae 15g
> Squama Manitis 9g
> Fructus Crataegi 18g

The prescription is taken one dosage a day in decoction and 5 dosages constitutes a course of treatment. (*Data of Medicine and Drugs*, Vol. 3, 1974)

For gastrocancer:

3 grams of Semen Strychni is steeped in water for 24 hours first. Then get the drug out and immerse it in fresh water for 7 to 10 more days before being peeled, dried, roasted with sesame oil and ground into powder; 1.5 grams of honeycomb, 4.5 grams of Solopendra and 0.9 gram of Scorpio are roasted yellow and ground into powder; 0.5 gram of snail is pounded, dried in sunshine and ground into powder. The powders are blended with 0.3 gram of Olibanum powder and made into small pills (20 pills weigh 3 gram) for oral administration twice a day, each time 10 pills. (*Diagnosis and Treatment of Tumor*)

HISTORICAL COMMENTS

Records of Famous Doctors says that: "The drug cures bee stings and subsides pyogenic swelling when burned into ashes with baby hair and snake slough and taken 2 grams a day with wine. The drug can also be used to treat suppurative osteomyelitis and all sorts of pyogenic carbuncles, furuncles and sores."

Recipes for Saving Civilians says that: "The drug cures breast cancer and galactostasis when burned into ashes and decocted (6 grams each time) in a small cup of water for 6 minutes."

Prescriptions for Emergencies says that: "The drug cures pyogenic acne rosacea when roasted, ground and taken 1g a time and three times a day."

Yun Tai Prescriptions says that: "Glossorrhagia can be cured with 30g of the top hard part of the drug, 12g of Bulbus Fritillariae Cirrhosae and 9g of Aloë when ground and rolled with honey into pills of the size of Omphalia. Each time one of the pills is decocted mildly in a bowel of water and taken orally. The pills also cure spitting blood and nasal hemorrhage."

MOSCHUS

It is defined in *Properties of Medicinal Herbs* that: "The drug is bitter and hot in taste, curing gastralgia."

The drug is the dried substance secreted from the scented bladder of male *Moschus berezovskii Flerov* of the *Cervidae* family. The animal has a adenobladder between the umbilicus and the penis, full of secretion known as Moschous. Moschus is shaped oval or round, oblately flat on the top, depressed on the bottom, and covered with hair. There is a tiny hole on the center with radiant thick hair. The outer skin is similar to leather and the cyctomembrance is very thin, composed of two layers between which is kept the scent liquid which is as thick as paste when it is fresh and turns into grains of different size when dried. Moschus is dissolvable in water, but not in ethanol, and contains muscone, steroidal hormone, androsterone, 5-ß-androsterone, fat, resin, protein and inorganic salts.

ANTICANCER PHARMACOLOGICAL FUNCTIONS

1. The drug, implanted in the abdomen of a healthy sheep, has been found to promote lymphocytic hyperplasia, improve microcirculation and dredge lymph duct. Therefore, the drug is thought to be able to increase the immunity against tumor, destroy the defence factors around carcinocytes and eliminate the remaining carcinocytes.

2. *Xihuang* Pill, made from Moschus, Calculus Boris, Olibanum and Myrrha, evidently inhibits fusocellular sarcoma in mice.

3. It has been observed through scanning that natural Moschus kills Hela cells and ascites cancer with a strong effect.

EXPERIMENTAL FORMULAS

For esophagocancer, gastrocancer, hepatocancer, colocancer and rectocancer:

1. The sterilized drug is embedded preperitoneally, retroperitoneally and subcutaneously with excellent efficacy. (*Research Reference of Traditional Chinese Medicine and Pharmacology*, Vol. 4, 1975)

2. The 50% or 100% injection made from the drug is administered intramuscularly 2ml a time and once or twice a day. (*Research Reference for Traditional Chinese Medicine and Pharmacology*, Vol. 4, 1975)

For maxillary sinus cancer and ovarian cancer:

Moschus 0.6g
Sanguis Draconis 6g
Cow gallbladder (dried) 30g

The above ingredients are ground into powder to make 100 capsules for oral administration 1 capsule a time, twice a day. (*Diagnosis and Treatment of Tumor*)

For cervical cancer:

1>. Moschus 1.2g
Fructus Cnidii 4.5g
Sanguis Draconis 7.5g
Olibanum 10.5g
Myrrha 15g
Olibanum 10.5g
Borneol 10.5g
Borax 10.5g
Salmiacum 10.5g
Catechu 9g
Realgar 13.2g
Stalactitum 13.2g
Minium 10.8g
Alumen 58g

The above ingredients are ground into powder and applied to the lesion twice a week. (*Exchange of Medical Information*, Vol. 8, 1974)

2>. Fructus Ziziphi Inermis (without stone) 20
Indigo Naturalis 3g
Borneol 3g
Alumen 3g
Realgar 2g
Olibanum 2g
Myrrha 2g
Calamina 6g

Moschus 1g

Each Fructus Zizipi Inermis is filled with 0.9g of Arsenicum, roasted with bean shaft and ground into powder. Then grind the rest of the herbs into powder. The two powders are mixed and rolled with honey into pills, each weighing 3 grams. One of the pills is inserted into the vagina every 3 to 4 days. (*Journal of Shanghai Traditional Chinese Medicine*, Vol. 9, 1984)

For malignant lymphosarcoma:

Moschus 0.3g
Borax 3g
Indigo Naturalis 0.9g
Borneol 0.9g
Venenum Bufonis 0.6g

The prescription is ground into powder and applied externally. (*Journal of Shaanxi Traditional Chinese Medicine*, Vol. 1, 1980)

HISTORICAL COMMENTS

Dietetic Materia Medica says that: "The drug cures all sorts of diseases and eliminates all sorts of foul smell."

Materia Medica says that: "The drug activates all senses and channels, penetrates all muscles and bones and cures all sorts of detention and abdominal mass."

Miraculous Prescriptions for Pestilence says that: "Stomatoma can be cured with 3 grams of the drug when ground and taken with water. The tumor will disappear spontaneously in three days."

Recipes for Saving Life says that: "All sorts of abscess, carbuncle, furuncle and swelling can be cured with the powder of Moschus, Rhizoma Bletillae, Radix Ampelopsitis, Radix Polygoni Cillinerve, Realgar, Os Galli, Olibanum, Myrrha and Borneol."

SCAPTOCHIRUS SEU MOGERA

It is defined in *Records of Famous Doctors* that: "The drug is salty in taste, cold and non-toxic in nature, curing abscess, carbuncle, fistula and pyogenic sores."

The drug is obtained from *Scaptochirus moschatus M.* and *Mogera robusta N.* of the *Talpidae* family. Its whole body or meat is for medical use. *Scaptochirus Moschatus M.* mainly grows in Hebei, Shandong and Inter Mongolia, while *Mogera robusta N.* in the Northeast of China. These animals live underground all their life, digging very long underground channels, pushing the dug soil above the earth and seldom creeping out. They live on insects, worms and wild plants, and do not resort to hibernation. Their eyesight is poor but audibility is good.

ANTICANCER PHARMACOLOGICAL FUNCTIONS

The drug inhibits transplanted tumor on animals.

EXPERIMENTAL FORMULAS

For gastrocancer:

A Scaptochirus seu Mogera is stripped off the viscera, calcined yellow on tile and ground into powder for oral administration with wine 2 grams each time and twice a day.

HISTORICAL COMMENTS

Supplementation to Materia Medica says that: "The meat controls pathogenic wind and cures sores and fistula if taken for a long period of time; and its paste cures all sorts of pyogenic sores when applied to the lesion."

Illustrated Materia Medica says that: "The drug cures sores and carbuncle due to pathogenic wind-heat accumulation and hemostasis, and infantile ascariasis."

Drugs Obtained from Animals in the Northeast says that: "The drug removes toxic material, regulates *qi*, cures carbuncle, fistula, stranguria, asthma and gastrocancer."

THE AUTHOR'S NOTE

In *New Edition of Experienced Prescriptions for Men* (written by Men Qizhao in the Qing Dynasty), it is recorded such a prescription called Breast Cancer Powder composed of 90 grams of male mouse drippings, 90 grams of Fructus Meliae Toosandan and 90 grams of Nidus Vespae. The herbs are ground into powder for oral administration with old wine 9 grams each time, once every other day. The prescription can be regarded as a sort of reference in the treatment of cancer. There was also a report that patients with esophageal cancer who could not eat and drink could be helped by the pills made from new-born mouse. Two cases of breast cancer were treated with the drippings of mouse decocted or calcined, ground and rolled into pills. It was reported that the tumor mass disappeared in one patient and contracted in another.

I. FOR BREAST CANCER:

Jiawei Guipi Powder

    Rhizoma Atractylodis Macrocephalae 3g
    Radix Ginseng (baked) 3g
    Poria 3g
    Radix Bupleuri 1.5g
    Rhizoma Chuanxiong 1.5g
    Fructus Gardeniae (baked) 1.5g
    Radix Paeoniae (baked) 1.5g
    Radix Glycyrrhizae (baked) 1.5g
    Radix Rehmanniae 240g
    Radix Angelicae Sinensis 240g

The prescription is effective for breast cancer at early stage and is taken in water decoction. (*Xuan's Medical Record*)

Jiawei Xiaoyiao Powder

    Radix Glycyrrhizae 3g
    Radix Angelicae Sinesis (baked) 3g
    Radix Paeoniae Alba 3g
    Poria 3g
    Rhizoma Atractylodis Macrocephalae 3g
    Radix Bupleuri 1.5g
    Cortex Moutan 1.5g
    Fructus Gardeniae 1.5g

The above herbs are taken in water decoction daily and it is effective for breast cancer at early stage. (*Xuan's Medical Record*)

Yiqi Yangrong Decoction

    Radix Ginseng 3g
    Poria 3g
    Pericarpium Citri Reticulatae 3g
    Bulbus Fritillariae Cirrhosae 3g
    Rhizoma Cyperi 3g
    Radix Angelicae Sinensis 3g
    Rhizoma Chuanxiong 3g
    Radix Paeoniae Latiflorae 3g
    Radix Rehmanniae 3g
    Radix Paeoniae Alba 3g
    Radix Glycyrrhizae 1.5g
    Radix Platycodi 1.5g
    Rhizoma Atractylodis Macrocephalae 6g
    Rhizoma Zingiberis 3g
    Fructus Ziziphi Inermis 2g

The above herbs are decocted with 2 pieces of ginger and 2 pieces of red date in 2 cups of water and the broth is taken daily. The prescription is effective for breast cancer at early stage. (*Orthodox Surgery*)

Lianqiao Jinbei Decoction

    Flos Lonicerae 9g

Bulbus Bolbostemmae 9g
Herba Traxaci 9g
Spica Prunellae 9g
Caulis Sargentodoxae 24g
Fructus Forsythiae 21-30g
Radix Trichosanthis 6g

The above herbs are decocted in two bowls of good wine to a broth of one bowl for oral administration daily. The patient is suggested to take a rest after taking the broth. (*Jinyuan's Complete Works of Medicine*)

Shiliuwei Liuqi Yin
Radix Angelicae Sinensis
Radix Paeoniae Alba
Radix Ginseng
Radix Astragali
Rhizoma Chuanxiong
Radix Ledebouriellae
Folium Perillae
Radix Angelicae Tonkinensis
Fructus Citri Aurantii
Radix Platycodi
Semen Arecae
Radix Linderae
Cortex Magnoliae
Cortex Cinnamomi
Caulis Aristolochiae Manshuriensis

The above herbs are decocted in water and taken daily.
Radix Aucklandiae
Radix Rehmanniae

The above two herbs are smashed to powder and heated for hot application to the lesion.
Radix Glycyrrhizae
Pericarpium Citri Reticulatae Viride

The above two herbs are decocted in Rhizoma Zingiberis soup into a thick broth for frequent oral administration. (*Orthodox Surgery*)

Yongquan Powder
Squama Manitis is ground to powder and taken twice daily, each time one gram. (*Danxiang's Prescriptions*)

Danxi Fang
Pericarpium Citri Reticulatae Viride 12g is decocted in one and a half cup of water to a broth of a cup for oral administration slowly. (*Compendium of Materia Medica*)

Jian Fang
Herba Taraxaci is smashed for application to the lesion and this herb has a marvelous effect for breast cancer.

II. PRESCRIPTIONS FOR DYSPHAGIA AND REGURGITATION:

Dabanxia Tang
Rhizoma Pinelliae 1000g
Radix Ginseng 90g
Honey 489 ml

The three ingredients are decocted in 480ml of water to a broth of 100ml for oral administration daily, each time 40ml. (*Materia Medica of the Golden chamber*)

Wu Yi Yuan

        Rhizoma Zingiberis 1.5g

        Pericarpium Zanthoxyli Bungeani 1.5g

        Fructus Corni 1.5g

        Semen Longan 1.5g

        Radix Ginseng 1.5g

        Herba Asari 1.2g

        Rhizoma Atractylodis Macrocephalae 1.2g

        Poria 1.2g

        Radix Aconiti Lateralis Preparata 1.2g

        Pericarpium Citri Reticulatae 1.8g

The above herbs are ground into powder and rolled with honey into pills of the size of Semen Firmianae for oral administration with wine, three pills each time, three times a day. The dosage can be increased to 10 pills if the illness is stubborn. (*Prescriptions Worth a Thousand Gold*)

Hua Tuo Fang

        Margarita 90g

        Realgar 90g

        Cinnabaris 90g

        Magnetitum 150g

        Rhizoma Zingiberis 10

The above herbs are ground into fine powder for rolling with honey into pills of the size of Semen Firmianae for oral administration three pills each time. The patient may feel upset after taking the drug, but this will disappear by itself after drinking some hot water. And 30 grams Semen Longan can be taken alone and it has a fantastic effect. (*Record of Medicine*)

Dingchen Touge Tang

        Rhizoma Cyperi 30g

        Fructus Amomi 30g

        Radix Ginseng 30g

        Flos Caryophylli 15g

        Fructus Hordei Germinatus 15g

        Radix Aucklandiae 15g

        Semen Myristicae 15g

        Fructus Amomi Rotundus 15g

        Pericarpium Citri Reticulatae Viride 15g

        Lignum Aquilariae Resinatum 25g

        Cortex Magnoliae 25g

        Herba Pogostemonis 25g

        Pericarpium Citri Reticulatae 25g

        Rhizoma Atractylodis Macrocephalae 60g

        Radix Glycyrrhizae 45g

        Massa Medicata Fermentata 7.5g

        Rhizoma Pinelliae 7.5g

        Fructus Tsaoko 7.5g

        Rhizoma Zingiberis 3

        Fructus Ziziphi Inermi

The above herbs are mixed together and 12 grams is decocted in a cup of water with 3 pieces of ginger and a piece of date for oral administration. (*Mediating Recipe*)

Wuge Kuanzhong San
        Fructus Amomo Rotundus 60g
        Radix Glycyrrhizae 150g
        Radix Aucklandiae 90g
        Cortex Magnoliae 500g
        Rhizoma Cyperi 500g
        Flos Caryophylli 120g
        Fructus Amomi 120g
        Pericarpium Citri Reticulatae Viride 120g
        Pericarpium Citri Reticulatae
        Rhizoma Zingiberis

All the above herbs are ground into powder and 6 grams is decocted with 3 pieces of ginger and a little bit of salt for oral administration. (*Mediating Recipe*)

Kunbu Wan
        Thallus Laminariae seu Eckloniae 4g
        Radix Ophiopogonis 4g
        Radix Asparagi 4g
        Fructus Chebulae 4g
        Caulis Aristolochiae manshuriensis 30g
        Radix et Rhizoma Rhei 30g
        Magnetitum 30g
        Semen Pruni Japonicae 30g
        Cortex Cinnamomi 30g
        Bulbus Lilii 15g
        Cornu Saigae Tataricae 15g
        Fructus Perillae 15g
        Rhizoma Belamcandae 15g
        Semen Armeniacae Amarum 15g
        Radix Bupleuri 7.5g
        Aloë 7.5g
        Pericarpium Citri Reticulatae 7.5g
        Semen Arecae 7.5g

The above herbs are ground to powder and rolled with honey into pills of the size of Semen Firmianae for oral administration 30 pills with hot wine.

Yige Fanwei Fang

1 >. 6 grams of Salmiacum is wrapped in the mixture of Rhizoma Fagopyri Cymosi with water and baked over fire. 3 grams of the center of the baked dough is calcined, mixed with 6 grams of Semen Arecae and 2 pieces of Flos Caryophylli and ground into powder for oral administration with wine, tree times a day, each time 1 gram. (*Compendium of Materia Medica*)

2 >. Slamiacum 30g and Arsenicum 30g are boiled for three hours and then added with Minium 30 grams for further boiling to make an extract to be dried and ground into powder. 30 grams of the powder is mixed with 30 grams of Lignum Mori Carbonisatus and ground into powder for oral administration 0.9g each time with hot wine. (*Collections of Song Tianren's Prescriptions*)

Runchang Gao

Radix Clematidis 120g and Rhizoma Zingiberis 120g are smashed to get a juice to be mixed with 60 grams of sesame oil and 120 grams of white sugar and decocted for oral administration one time a day when it becomes cool.

Ali Duoming Wan

Testa Setariae 250g, Radix Clematidis 250 and rice 250g are ground into powder, rolled with ox saliva into pills of the size of Arillus Longan, and boiled in water for taking as a food after being mixed with 30 to 60 grams of sugar. (*Orthodox Medicine*)

For stubborn cases, Calculus Canitis 0.3g and Radix Clematidis 60g and salt 6g are smashed and mixed with water for oral administration twice a day, no more than three days in all. Tonics are given after the administration of the drugs.

III. PRESCRIPTIONS FOR STAGNATION AND STASIS:

1. Prescriptions for the five kinds of stagnation:
Guangzhu Kuijian Tang

    Cortex Magnoliae 1.5g
    Radix Scutellariae 1.5g
    Rhizoma Coptidis 1.5g
    Fructus Alpiniae Oxyphyllae 1.5g
    Semen Alpiniae Katsumadai 1.5g
    Radix Angelicae Sinensis 1.5g
    Rhizoma Pinelliae 2.1g
    Rhizoma Atractylodis Lanceae 6g
    Rhizoma Cimicifugae Foetidae 6g
    Flos Carthami 6g
    Fructus Evodiae 6g
    Radix Glycyrrhizae 0.9g
    Radix Bupleuri 0.9g
    Rhizoma Alismatis 0.9g
    Massa Medicata Fermentata 0.9g
    Pericarpium Citri Reticulatae Viride 0.9g
    Pericarpium Citri Reticulatae 0.9g
    Radix Puerariae 1.2g

The above herbs are sliced into small pieces and decocted with 3 pieces of Rhizoma Zingiberis in two cups of water for oral administration on an empty stomach when it is warm. No wine, vinegar and noodle soup during the administration. Usually after taking two doses, the abdominal fullness is half reduced and the patient is asked to take the following formula. (*Dongyuan's Prescriptions*)

Banxia Houpo Tang

    Flos Carthami 0.15g
    Lignum Sappan 0.15g
    Radix Aucklandiae 0.6g
    Pericarpium Citri Reticulatae Viride 0.6g
    Fructus Evodiae 0.3g
    Rhizoma Zingiberis 0.3g
    Rhizoma Coptidis 0.3g
    Semen Myristicae 0.9g
    Rhizoma Atractylodis Lanceae 0.9g
    Poria 0.9g
    Rhizoma Alismatis 0.9g
    Radix Bupleuri 0.9g
    Pericarpium Citri Reticulatae 0.9g
    Radix Scutellariae 0.9g
    Semen Alpiniae Katsumadai 0.9g

                Radix Glycyrrhizae 0.9g
                Rhizoma Scirpi 1.2g
                Radix Angelicae Sinensis 1.2g
                Polyporus 1.2g
                Rhizoma Cimicifugae Foetidae 1.2g
                Massa Medicata Fermentata 1.8g
                Cortex Magoliae 2.4g
                Rhizoma Pinelliae 9g
                Semen Persicae 7
                Thallus Laminariae seu Eckloniae 1.5g
                Radix Puerariae 0.9g
        The above herbs are sliced into small pieces and decocted in three cups of water to a cup of
broth for oral administration when it is still hot. After taking the formula, the remaining abdominal
fullness is cured and the previous formula is prescribed through modification.

        2. Prescriptions for lump at the right hypochondrium:
        Xipen Wan
                Cortex Magnoliae 24g
                Rhizoma Coptidis 39g
                Rhizoma Zingiberis 4.5g
                Pericarpium Zanthoxyli Bungeani 4.5g
                Poria 4.5g
                Radix Asteris 4.5g
                Radix Ginseng 6g
                Cortex Cinnamomi 3g
                Radix Platycodi 3g
                Rhizoma Scirpi 3g
                Radix Asparagi 3g
                Pericarpium Citri Reticulatae 3g
                Radix Aconiti 3g
                Fructus Amomi Rodundus 3g
                Pericarpium Citri Reticulatae Viride 1.5g
                Fructus Crotonis Pulveratum
        The above herbs are ground into fine powder and rolled with honey into pills of the size of
Semen Firmianae for oral administration on an empty stomach two pills for the first day. The dose is
increased by one pill daily. In winter Cortex Magnoliae is increased by 12 grams to 36 grams totally and
Rhizoma Coptidis is decreased to 18 grams. (*Dongyuan' Prescriptions*)
        Xipen Tang
              . Rhizoma Pinelliae 4.5g
                Semen Longan 4.5g
                Radix Ginseng 4.5g
                Semen Descurainiae 4.5g
                Fructus Evodiae 4.5g
                Cortex Mori 4.5g
                Radix Glycyrrhizae 4.5g
        All the above herbs are decocted with 5 pieces of Rhizoma Zingiberis and 2 pieces of Fructus
Ziziphi Inermis in two cups of water into a cup of broth for oral administration before meal.
(*Prescriptions Based on Three Categories of Pathogens*)
        Banxia Tang

Herba Asari 45g

Rhizoma Pinelliae 45g

Radix Platycodi 45g

Cortex Mori 45g

Radix Peucedani 45g

Bulbus Fritillariae Cirrhosae 30g

Fructus Chebulae 30g

Radix Bupleuri 30g

Radix Glycyrrhizae 30g

Radix Ginseng 6g

Rhizoma Atractylodis Macrocephalae 6g

The above herbs are mixed together and each time 9 grams of the mixed herbs is decocted in a cup of water with 3 pieces of Rhizoma Zingiberis and 3 pieces of Fructus Ziziphi Inermis. The broth is taken before the patient goes to bed. (*Prescriptions Based on Three Categories of Pathogens*)

3. Prescriptions for mass in the upper or lower abdomen:

Fulian Wan

Rhizoma Coptidis 45g

Cortex Magnoliae 6g

Radix Ginseng 6g

Radix scutellariae 3g

Cortex Cinnamomi 3g

Poria 3g

Radix Salviae Miltiorrhizae 3g

Rhizoma Zingiberis 1.5g

Rhizoma Acori Graminei 1.5g

Fructus Crotonis Pulveratum 1.5g

Radix Aconiti 1.5g

Fructus Alpiniae Galangae 1.5g

The above herbs are ground into powder and rolled with honey into pills of the size of Semen Firmianae for oral administration two pills for the first day. The dose is increased by one pill daily or two pills every three days, and is reduced by one pill gradually when the stool becomes loose. (*Dongyuan's Prescriptions*)

Ganqi Wan

Lacca Sinica Exsiccata 30g

Flos Genkwa 30g

Carapax Trionycis 30g

Salmiacum 30g

Radix Aucklandiae 15g

Semen Persicae 15g

Radix Aconiti 15g

Realgar 7.5g

Moschus 7.5g

All the above herbs are ground to powder and rolled with flour paste into pills of the size of mung bean for oral administration 10 pills with warm wine before meals. (*Prescriptions Based on Three Categories of Pathogens*)

Banxia San

Rhizoma Pinelliae 45g

Carapax Trionycis 45g

Semen Longan 30g

Pericarpium Chebulae 30g

Radix Peucedani 30g

Radix Angelicae Sinensis 30g

Pericarpium Citri Reticulatae Viride 30g

Semen Arecae 30g

Radix Aucklandiae 30g

Rhizoma Scirpi 30g

The above herbs are ground to powder for oral administration 3 grams each time with a cup of water. At the same time, 0.15g of Rhizoma Zingiberis is decocted and taken frequently. (*Prescriptions Based on Three Categories of Pathogens*)

Fuliang Wan

Poria

Radix Ginseng

Cortex Magnoliae

Fructus Citri Aurantii

Rhizoma Scirpi

Rhizoma Pinelliae

Rhizoma Atractylodis Macrocephalae

Equal portions of the above herbs are ground into powder and rolled with flour paste into pills of the size of Semen Firmianae for oral administration 50 pills each time with rice porridge. (*Prescriptions Based on Three Categories of Pathogens*)

IV. PRESCRIPTIONS FOR MASS IN THE ABDOMEN:

Piqi Wan

Cortex Magnoliae 15g

Rhizoma Coptidis 24g

Fructus Evodiae 9g

Radix Scutellariae 6g

Rhizoma Atractylodis Macrocephalae 6g

Herba Artemisiae Capillaris

Fructus Amomi 4.5g

Rhizoma Zingiberis 4.5g

Poria 3g

Radix Ginseng 3g

Rhizoma Alismatis 3g

Radix Aconiti 1.5g

Pericarpium Zanthoxyli Bungeani 1.5g

Fructus Crotonis Pulveratum

Cortex Cinnamomi 15g

All the above herbs are ground to powder and rolled with honey into pills of the size of Semen Firmianae for oral administration 3 pills for the first day. The dose is increased by one pill daily till the patient's stool becomes loose. Then two pills are taken with the decoction of Radix Glycyrrhizae. The formula is continued till the size of the mass becomes half of it original size. (*Dongyuan's Prescriptions*)

Suanhong Wan

Flos Caryophylli 30g

Radix Aucklandiae 30g

Lignum Aquilariae Resinatum 30g

Fructus Amomi 30g

Pericarpium Citri Reticulatae Viride 30g

Semen Arecae 30g

Exocarpium Citri Rubrum

Rhizoma Zedoariae 30g

Fructus Tsaoko 30g

Semen Pharbitidis

Calomelas

Semen Myristicae 3g

Poria 25g

Radix Ginseng 25g

All the above herbs are ground into powder and rolled with garlic juice into pills of the size of Semen Firmianae for oral administration 5 to 7 pills daily at the beginning. The dose can be increased to 15 pills. The pills are taken with salt water and the patient can only eat rice porridge during the period of administration. (*Prescriptions Based on Three Categories of Pathogens*)

Bijia Wan

Radix Aconiti Lateralis Preparata 30g

Rhizoma Scirpi 30g

Lacca Sinica Exsiccata 30g

Radix Aucklandiae 30g

Radix et Rhizoma Rhei 60g

Fructus Evodiae 15g

Carapax Trionycis 90g

Salmiacum 30g

The above herbs are ground into powder to be rolled with flour paste into pills of the size of Semen Firmianae for oral administration 20 pills each time with wine on an empty stomach. (*Prescriptions Based on Three Categories of Pathogens*)

V. PRESCRIPTIONS FOR STONY GOITER:

Huangyaozi Wine

15 grams of Rhizoma Dioscoreae Bulbiferae is immersed in 80ml of wine for oral administration a small cup every morning and evening. (*Doumen's Prescriptions*)

Wuying Fang

Sargassum 90g

Radix Gentianae 90g

Gecko 90g

Medulla Tetrapanacis 90g

Thallus Laminariae seu Eckloniae 90g

Alumen 90g

Usnea 90g

Massa Medicata Fermentata 1.2g

Rhizoma Pinelliae 0.6g

The above herbs are ground into powder and taken with wine 6g each time, three times a day. No fish, pork, hot pepper or raw vegetables during the period of the administration. (*Prescriptions Worth a Thousand Gold*)

Haizao Yuhu Tang

Sargassum 3g

Pericarpium Citri Reticulatae 3g

Bulbus Fritillariae Cirrhosae 3g
Fructus Forsythiae 3g
Thallus Laminariae seu Eckloniae 3g
Pericarpium Citri Reticulatae Viride 3g
Radix Angelicae Pubescentis 3g
Rhizoma Chuanxiong 3g
Radix Angelicae Sinensis 3g
Radix Glycyrrhizae 3g
Thallus Laminariae 1.5g

The above herbs are decocted in two cups of water and taken either before or after meals according to the location of the disease.

LIST OF DRUGS FOR DIFFERENT TYPES OF CANCER

FOR CANCER OF THE MOUTH CAVITY: Caulis Aristolochiae Manshuriensis, Herba Sedi

FOR CANCER OF THE LIPS: Herba Artemisiae Capillaris, Herba Sedi, Fructus Gardeniae, Cortex Phellodendri, Periostracum Serpentis, Venenum Bufonis

FOR CANCER OF THE TONGUE: Herba Solidaginis, Rhizoma Cimicifugae Foetidae, Radix Glycyrrhizae, Herba Sedi, Cortex Phellodendri, Rhizoma Dioscoreae Bulbiferae, Lumbricus, Herba Galii Aprinis, Flos Chrysanthemi Indici, Radix Rhapontici Uniflori, Eupolyphaga seu Steleophaga

FOR LARYNGEAL CANCER: Herba Solidaginis, Radix Sophorae Tonkinensis, Radix Codonopsis Lanceolatae, Rhizoma Cimicifugae Foetidae , Fructus Arctii, Herba Solani Glabrae, Borneol, Herba Geranii, Fructus Chebulae, Radix Scutellariae, Herba Wedeliae, Semen Coicis

FOR GINGIVAL CANCER: Lumbricus, Herba Galii Aprinis, Herba Taraxaci

FOR CANCER OF THE VOCAL FOLD: Herba Solani Glabrae, Herba Solani Lyrati, Herba Oldenlandiae Chrysotrichae

FOR CANCER OF THE GNATHIC SINUS: Moschus

FOR CANCER OF THE SALIVARY GLAND: Periostracum Serpentis

FOR CANCER OF THE PAROTID GLAND: Sargassum, Rhizoma Amorphophalli, Herba Wedeliae

FOR CANCER OF THE HARD PALATE: Herba Taraxaci

FOR CANCER OF THE EYE REGION: Radix Actinidiae Chinensis

FOR CANCER OF THE EAR: Rhizoma Atractylodis Macrocephalae, Agkistrodon, Fructus Bruceae, Radix Scutellariae, Rhizoma Coptidis

FOR NASOPHARYNGEAL CANCER: Periostracum Serpentis, Radix Zanthoxyli, Folium Pruni Daridianae, Semen Strychni, Radix Trichosanthis Cucumeroidis, Rhizoma Arisaematis, Herba Hydrocotyli Sibthorpioiditis, Radix Semiaquilegiae, Fructus Crotonis, Herba Conyzae, Herba Lobeliae Chinensis, Folium Artemisiae Argyi, Herba Salviae Chienesis, Rhizoma Imperatae, Alumen, Spina Gleditsiae, Rhizoma Paridis, Radix Stephaniae Tetrandrae, Herba Scutellariae Barbatae, Fructus Xanthii, Herba Selaginellae, Flos Lonicerae, Arsenicum, Herba Faxilli, Herba Taraxaci, Folium et Semen seu Radix, Livistonae, Rhizoma Amorphophalli, Xylotrupes, Scolopendra, Bufo

FOR CANCER OF THE THYROID GLAND: Herba Solidaginis, Rhizoma Scirpi, Fructus Polygoni Orientalis, Polium Artemisiae Argyi, Radix Paeoniae Latiflorae, Thallus Laminariae seu Eckloniae, Spica Prunellae, Radix Euphorbiae Ebracteolatae, Radix Codonopsis Lanceolatae, Cormus Iphigeniae, Fructus Tritici Levis, Concha Meretricis, Rhizoma Arisaematis, Radix Semiaquilegiae, Flos Chrysanthemi Indici, Rhizoma Amorphophalli, Periostracum Cicadae

FOR CANCER OF THE THYMUS GLAND: Radix Salviae Miltiorrhizae

FOR CANCER OF THE MEDIASTINUM: Gecko Chinensis

FOR CANCER OF THE SOFT TISSUES: Herba Solani Nigri

FOR CANCER OF THE PLEURA: Herba Scutellariae Barbatae

FOR LUNG CANCER: Folium Ilecis, Radix Ginseng, Rhizoma Dysosmae, Radix Wikstroemae, Bulbus Allii, Rhizoma Arisaematis, Radix Semiaquilegiae, Herba Pteridis Multifidae, Herba et Radix Ranunculi Japonici, Herba Scutellariae Barbatae, Herba Salviae Chinenesis, Herba Agrimoniae, Rhizoma Atractylodis Macrocephalae, Herba Geranii, Herba Aristolochiae Mollissimae, Agkistrodon, Herba Solani Lyrati, Cortex Dictamni, Bulbus Lilii, Semen Armeniacae Amarum, Herba Ainsliaeae, Bittern, Concha Ostreae, Herba Sedi, Herba Ecliptae, Herba Artemisiae Annuae, Herba Houttuyniae, Herba Patriniae Scabiosaefoliae, Sargassum, Radix Euphorbiae Ebracteolatae, Radix Cynanchi Paniculati, Herba Duchesneae, Radix Ampelopsis Aconitifoliae, Tremella, Radix Gossypii Hirsuti, Realgar, Radix Asteris, Folium et Semen seu Radix Livistonae, Ramus Araliae Chinensis, Radix Triptergii, Mel, Bufo

FOR MALIGNANT LYMPHOMA: Rhizoma Dysosmae, Radix Wikstroemae, Rhizoma Smilacis Glabrae, Herba Cephalanoploris, Radix Asparagi, Radix Semiaquilegiae, Caulis Aristolochiae

Manshuriensis, Radix Adinae, Radix Aconiti, Fructus Arctii, Rhizoma Pinelliae, Agkistrodon, Herba Oldenlandiae Diffusae, Cortex Dictamni, Bombyx Batryticatus, Flos Genkwa, Concha Ostreae, Herba Euphorbiae Lunulatae, Radix Sophorae Flavescentis, Thallus Laminariae seu Eckloniae, Squama Manitis ,'Herba Saginae Japonicae, Rhizoma Thphonii, Fructus Lagenaria, Radix Berberidis, Caulis Marsdeniae, Fructus Cassiae Occidentalis, Lumbricus, Radix Rannunculi Ternati, Herba Galii Aprinis, Mylabris, Semen Ricini, Moschus, Rhizoma Amorphophalli

FOR ECZEMATOID CANCER: Squama manitis, Bufo

FOR CANCER OF THE DIGESTIVE SYSTEM: Herba Sarcandrae, Semen Strychni, Cortex Acanthopanacis, Flos Hibisci Mutabilis, Radix Adinae, Radix Cudraniae, Bulbus Lycoridis Radiatae, Caulis Marsdeniae, Radix Gossypii Hirsuti, Blood Anserina, Hericium, Fructus Sophorae, Scolopendra

FOR ESOPHAGEAL CANCER: Radix Ginseng, Radix Notoginseng, Radix Sophorae Tonkinensis, Cormus Iphigeniae, Radix Asparagi, Radix Trichosanthis, Radix Semiaquilegiae, Fructus Fici, Hydrargyrum, Fructus Mumi, Calculus Bovis, Radix Salviae Miltiorrhizae, Radix Glycyrrhizae, Caulis Sacchari Sinensis, Radix Kansui, Herba Solani Glabrae, Rhizoma Pinelliae, Herba Scutelleriae Barbatae, Herba Agrimoniae, Agkistrodon, Herba Oldenlandiae Diffusae, Rhizoma Imperatae, Herba Solani Lyrati, Herba Chelidonii, Bombyx Batryticatus, Testa Oryzae, Flos Carthami, Fructus Chebulae, Ganoderma, Semen Armeniacae Amarum, Concho Ostreae, Herba Sedi, Corium Stomachichum Galli, Herba Euphoribae Lunulatae, Indigo Naturalis, Thallus Laminariae seu Eckloniae, Herba Patriniae Scabiosaefoliae, Herba Bideni Bifinatae, Semen Impatientis, Arsenicum, Semen Juglandis, Fructus Bruceae, Radix Rubiae, Herba Isodi, Rhizoma Paridis, Radix Stephaniae Tetrandrae, Rhizoma Heleocharidis, Caulis Marsdeniae, Cortex Mori, Fructus Trapae Bispinosae, Rhizoma Smilacis Chinae, Salmiacum, Rhizoma Coptidis, Rhizoma Dioscoreae Bulbiferae, Radix Actinidiae Chinensis, Herba Crotalariae, Placenta Hominis, Radix Arnebiae, Folium et Semen seu Radix Livistonae, Xylotrupes, Scolopendra, Semen Arecae, Herba Ecliptae, Gecko Chinensis, Herba Dianthi, Bufo, Moschus, Scaptochirus seu Mogera

FOR GASTRIC LYMPHOSARCOMA: Semen Juglandis, Blood Anserina

FOR STOMACH CANCER: Radix Ginseng, Fructus Akebiae, Fructus Ziziphi Inermis, Lignum et Radix Acronychiae, Cormus Iphigeniae, Fructus Crataegi, Concha Meretricis, Radix Trichosanthis Cucumeroidis, Herba Hydrocotyli Sibthorpioiditis, Fructus Fici, Cortex Acanthopanacis, Radix Bombai, Fructus Polygoni Orientalis, Radix Aconiti, Semen Phoenix Dactyliferae, Fructus Mume, Radix Salviae Miltiorrhizae, Radix Glycyrrhizae, Caulis Sacchari Sienesis, Herba Solani Glabrae, Rhizoma Pinelliae, Herba Scutellariae Barbatae, Agkistrodon, Herba Oldenlandiae Diffusae, Alumen, Herba Chelidonii, Bombyx Batryticatus, Radix Helianthi Annui, Lignum Aquilariae Resinatum, Semen Armeniacae Amarum, Concha Ostreae, Herba Sedi, Corium Stromachichum Galli, Herba Euphorbiae Lunulatae, Semen Sophorae Alopecuroiditis, Herba Artemisiae Annuae, Herba Patriniae Scabiosaefoliae, Rhizoma Polygoni Cuspidati, Semen Dolichoris Album, Herba Bideni Bipinatae, Semen Impatientis, Semen Juglandis, Poria, Herba Gelsemii, Herba Isodi, Radix Stephaniae Tetrandrae, Cortex Mori, Herba Taxilli, Radix Euphorbiae Ebracteolatae, Fructus Trapae, Bispinosae, Mylabris, Rhizoma Smilacis Chinae, Salmiacum, Herba Oldenlandiae Chrysotrichae, Rhizoma Dioscoreae Bulbiferae, Blood Anserina, Pedicellus Melo, Radix Actinidiae Chinensis, Fructus Camptothecae, Realgar, Herba Taraxaci, Herba Patriniae Heterophyllae, Ramus Araliae Chinensis, Xylotrupes, Scolopendra, Semen Arecae, Semen Coicis , Gecko Chinensis, Eupolyphaga seu Steleophaga, Bufo, Nidus Vespae, Moschus, Scaptochirus seu Mogera

FOR PANCREATIC CANCER: Herba Sarcandrae, Caulis Aristolochiae Manshuriensis, Herba Conyzae, Flos Carthami, Herba Sedi, Concha Ostreae

FOR LIVER CANCER: Folium Ilecis, Fructus Akebiae, Radix Wikstroemae, Rhizoma Scirpi, Herba Hydrocotyli Sibthorpioiditis, Fructus Polygoni Orientalis, Radix Adinae, Semen Phoenix Dactyliferae, Calculus Bovis, Herba Lobeliae Chinensis, Herba Scutellariae Barbatae, Agkistrondon, Scorpio, Herba Lycopi, Herba Selaginellae, Herba Artemisiae Annuae, Squama Manitis, Semen Juglandis, Herba Sedi,

Herba Gelsemii, Rhizoma Alpiniae Officinarum, Fructus Akebiae, Radix Euphorbiae Ebracteolatae, Lumbricus, Mylabris, Radix Actinidiae Chinensis, Radix Gossypii Hirsuti, Fructus Campothecae, Fructus Fici Pumilae, Blattella Orientalis

FOR INTESTINAL CANCER: Radix et Rhizoma Rhei, Fructus Fici, Fructus Crotonis, Hirudo, Herba Pteridis Multifidae, Fructus Arctii, Herba Scutellariae Barbatae, Semen Benincasae, Herba Oldenlandiae Diffusae, Herba Geranii, Lignum Aquilariae Resinatum, Aloë, Herba Sonchi Arvensis, Radix Sophorae Flarescentis, Semen Sophorae Alopecuroiditis, Herba Patrimiae Scabiosaefoliae, Arsenicum, Fructus Bruceae, Rhizoma Smilacis Chinae, Rhizoma Dioscoreae Bulbiferae, Radix Ampelopsis Aconitifoliae, Fructus Camptothecae, Semen Ricini, Herba Chebulae, Cortex Ailanthi, Fructus Fici Pumilae, Herba Dianthi, Bufo

FOR CANCER OF THE APPENDIX: Herba Houttuyniae, Herba Patriniae Scabiosaefoliae

FOR CANCER OF THE ABDOMINAL CAVITY: Rhizoma Scirpi, Fructus Chaenomelis, Fructus polygoni Orientalis, Radix Salviae Miltiorrhizae, Radix Kansui, Alumen, Testa Oryzae, Semen Armeniacae Amarum, Concha Ostreae, Semen Dolichoris Album, Herba Gelsemii, Herba Leonuri, Rhizoma Zedoariae, Salmiacum, Lumbricus, Carapax Trionycis

FOR BLEEDING OF INTESTINAL CANCER: Fructus Cannabis, Radix et Rhizoma Rhei, Radix Trichosanthis Cucumeroidis, Bombyx Batryticatus, Bulbus Lilii, Scorpio, Fructus Chebulae, Radix Scutelariae, Folium Indocalami Tessellati

FOR BREAST CANCER: Radix Ginseng, Radix Wikstroemae, Bulbus Bolbostemmae, Cormus Iphigeniae, Semen Strychni, Radix Asparagi, Fructus Trichosanthis, Fructus et Folium Solani Indici, Radix Semiaquilegiae, Flos Hibisci Mutabilis, Herba Pteridis Multifidae, Semen Phoenix Dactyliferae, Herba et Radix Ranuculi Japonici, Herba Solani Glabrae, Rhizoma Cimicifugae Foetidae, Calculus Bovis, Bulbus Fritillariae Cirrhosae, Radix Glycyrrhizae, Agkistrodon, Herba Oldenlandiae Diffusae, Borneol, Bulbus Lilii, Herba Geranii, Herba Aristolochiae Mollissimae, Flos Trifolii, Concha Ostreae, Spina Gleditsiae, Herba Artemisiae Annuae, Flos Lonicerae, Squama Manitis, Arsenicum, Radix Salix Babylonicae, Semen Juglandis, Poria, Herba Isodi, Herba Leonuri, Sargassum, Radix Scutellariae, Periostracum Serpentis, Radix Ampelopsis Aconitifoliae, Herba Galii Aprinis, Radix Actinidiae Chinensis, Mylabris, Herba Taraxaci, Takydromus amurensis, Radix Rhapontici Uniflori, Semen Coicis, Fructus Fici Pumilae, Gecko Chinensis, Scaptochirus, seu Mogera

FOR UTERUS CANCER: Radix Ginseng, Rhizoma Dysosmae, Radix Notoginseng, Rhizoma Scirpi, Fructus Cannabis, Radix et Rhizoma Rhei, Folium Bretschaeiderae, Semen Strychni, Semen Iridis, Herba Cephalanoploris, Rhizoma Arisaematis, Fructus Crotonis, Hirudo, Hydrargyrum, Herba Pteridis Multifidae, Semen Phoenix Dactylifera, Herba et Radix Ranunculi Japonici, Fructus Mume, Fructus Arctii, Bulbus Fritillariae Cirrhosae, Herba Solani Glabrae, Rhizoma Pinelliae, Herba Salviae Chinensis, Rhizoma Acori Graminei, Herba Oldenlandiae Diffusae, Herba Geranii, Herba Aristolochiae Mollissimae, Flos Carthami, Semen Armeniacae Amarum, Flos Genkwa, Herba Sonchi Arvensis, Herba Euphorbiae Lunulatae, Radix Sophorae Flavescentis, Semen Sophorae Alopecuroiditis, Indigo Naturalis, Flos Lonicerae, Herba Patriniae Scabiosaefoliae, Squama Manitis, Arsenicum, Fructus Bruceae, Poria, Radix Rubiae, Herba Leonuri, Rhizoma Zedoariae, Radix et Rhizoma Podophylli, Caulis Marsdeniae, Fructus Trapae Bispinosae, Rhizoma Coptidis, Cortex Phellodendri, Pedicellus Melo, Herba Crotalariae, Placenta Hominis, Radix Arnebiae, Herba Taraxaci, Fructus Trachycarpi, Semen Ricini, Rhizoma Amorphophalli, Takydromus amurensis, Radix Rhapontici Uniflori, Cortex Ailanthi, Herba Ecliptae, Semen Coicis, Fructus Fici Pumilae, Gecko Chinensis, Gutti, Cambogia, Moschus

FOR OVARIAN TUMOR: Rhizoma Scirpi, Radix et Rhizoma Rhei, Fructus Crataegi, Hirudo, Herba Solani Glabrae, Herba Scutellariae Barbatae, Radix Cudraniae, Fructus Akebiae, Herba Taxilli, Eupolyphaga seu Steleophaga, Moschus, Carapax Trionycis

FOR CHORIOEPITHELIOMA: Fructus Crataegi, Radix Trichosanthis, Herba Pteridis Multifidae, Radix Glycyrrhizae, Herba Solani Glabrae, Agkistrodon, Herba Houttuyniae, Radix Arnebiae, Herba Andrographitis, Herba Patriniae Scabiosaefoliae, Fructus Akebiae, Nidus Vespae

FOR MALIGNANT MOLE: Radix Trichosanthis, Hydrargyrum, Herba Pteridis Multifidae, Herba Scutellariae Barbatae, Flos Genkwa, Herba Patriniae Scabiosaefoliae, Fructus Akebiae, Herba Houttuyniae, Herba Andrographitis, Folium et Semen seu Radix Livistonae

FOR CANCER OF THE BILIARY TRACT AND GALLBLADDER: Herba Cephalanoploris, Caulis Aristolochiae Manshuriensis, Herba Conyzae

FOR MALIGNANT RETICULOSIS: Fructus Mume, Herba Selaginellae, Arsenicum, Rhizoma Typhonii, Semen Coicis

FOR MALIGNANT PELVIC TUMOR: Herba Lycopi

FOR CHORIOCARCINOMA: Herba Solani Lyrati, Herba et Semen Sophorae Alopecuroiditis

FOR LEUKEMIA: Bulbus Allii, Radix et Rhizoma Rhei, Semen Strychni, Fructus Tritici Levis, Agkistrodon, Herba Geranii, Flos Carthami, Aloë, Herba et Semen Sophorae Alopecuroiditis, Radix Asparagi, Herba Catharanthi, Radix Rumei Crispi, Calculuc Bovis, Indigo Naturalis, Caulis Millettiae, Herba Senecio Integrifolii, Radix Daucis Carotae, Realgar, Fructus Gardeniae, Rhizoma Smilacis Chinae, Herba Crotalariae, Fructus Camptothecae, Radix Salix Babylonicae, Semen Juglandis, Herba Galii Aprinis, Ramulus et Folium Taxi Cuspidatae, Taraxaci, Herba Patriniae Heterophyllae, Periostracum Cicadae, Bufo

FOR TUMOR OF THE BLOOD VESSELS: Herba Solani Lyrati, Radix Tinosporae, Sargassum, Spica Prunellae, Radix Astragali, Cortex Phellodendri, Herba Taraxaci, Fructus Fici Pumilae

FOR MALIGNANT TUMOR OF THE NERVE SYSTEM: Rhizoma Arisaematis
Herb Scutellariae Barbatae

FOR AMELOBLASTOMA: Realgar

FOR MELANOSARCOMA: Concha Ostreae

FOR SEMINOMA: Rhizoma Zedoariae, Radix Gossypii Hirsuti

FOR PROSTATIC CANCER: Herba Geranii

FOR KIDNEY CANCER: Herba Lobeliae Chinensis, Fructus Lagenaria, Rhizoma Smilacis Chinae, Salmiacum, Radix Astragali, Radix Scutellariae, Polyporus, Blattella Orientalis

FOR CARCINOMA OF URINARY BLADDER: Rhizoma Smilacis Glabrae, Herba Cephalanoploris, Herba Hydrocotyli Sibthorpioiditis, Radix Semiaquilegiae, Rhizoma Arisaematis, Fructus Fici, Caulis Aristolochiae Manshuriensis, Fructus Crotonis, Herba Solani Glabrae, Radix Sophorae Flavescentis, Arsenicum, Poria, Rhizoma Zedoariae, Herba Duchesneae, Pedicellus Melo, Fructus Camptothecae, Fructus Sophorae Japonicae, Xylotrupes, Herba seu Radix Physalis, Herba Dianthi, Bufo

FOR CANCER OF THE VULVA: Cortex Dictamni

FOR CANCER OF THE PENIS: Radix Aconiti, Fructus Mume, Realgar

FOR SKIN CANCER: Radix Zanthoxyli, Rhizoma Dysosmae, Radix Wikstroemae, Rhizoma Smilacis Glabrae, Prospirobolus, Semen Strychni, Rhizoma Arisaematis, Herba Hydrocotyli Sibthorpioiditis, Hirudo, Hydrargyrum, Semen Phoenix Dactyliferae, Herba et Radix Ranunculi Japonici, Radix Rumei Crispi, Herba Salviae Chinensis, Semen Armeniacae Amarum, Radix Paeoniae Latiflorae, Flos Genkwa, Rhizoma Alpiniae Officinarum, Bulbus Lycoridis Radiatae, Arsenicum, Semen Abri, Cortex Mori, Cortex Phellodendri, Pedicellus Melo, Herba Crotalariae, Scolopendra, Gutti, Cambogia

FOR OSTEOCARCINOMA AND OSTEOSARCOMA: Herba Aristolochiae Mollissimae, Bittern, Concha Ostreae, Fructus Crataegi, Herba Agrimoniae, Cortex Dictamni, Scolopendra, Squama Manitis, Sargassum, Salmiacum, Radix Astragali, Periostracum Serpentis

FOR CANCER OF THE ANUS: Radix Sophorae Tonkinensis, Semen Strychni, Aloë, Squama Manitis, Herba Galii Aprinis, Herba Sonchi Arvensis, Herba Houttuyniae

FOR CEREBRAL CANCER: Rhizoma Smilacis Glabrae, Semen Strychni, Fructus Tritici Levis, Herba Solani Glabrae, Rhizoma Imperatae, Bombyx Batryticatus, Fructus Xanthii, Semen Juglandis, Rhizoma Paridis, Rhizoma Heleocharidis, Realgar, Rhizoma Amorphophalli, Scolopendra, Periostracum Cicadae

FOR CARCINOMATOUS THORACO-ABDOMINAL EDEMA: Radix Wikstroemae, Bulbus, Fructus Arctii, Radix Kansui, Bulbus Lycoridis Radiatae, Semen Dolichoris Album, Radix Ranunculi, Ternati

FOR CARCINOMATOUS LOW FEVER: Herba Artemisiae Annuae

FOR CARCINOMATOUS HEMOPTYSIS: Radix Notoginseng, Fructus Ziziphi Inermi, Herba Agrimoniae, Herba Houttuyniae, Radix Rubiae, Radix Astragali, Radix Asteris, Blattella Orientalis

FOR CARCINOMATOUS ULCER: Fructus Crotonis, Radix Glycyrrhizae, Alumen, Bittern

FOR CARCINOMATOUS PAIN: Cormus Iphigeniae, Radix Trichosanthis Cucumeroidis, Herba Agrimoniae, Herba Aristolochiae Mollissimae, Radix Polygoni Ciliinerve, Spina Gleditsiae, Indigo Naturalis, Rhizoma Paridis, Rhizoma Alpiniae Officinarum, Radix Cynanchi Paniculati, Realgar

FOR CARCINOMATOUS WHITE SPOTS: Bulbus Allii

FOR REACTIONS TO RADIOTHERAPY AND CHEMOTHERAPY: Radix Ginseng, Radix Trichosanthis, Cortex Acathopanacis, Cordyceps, Ganoderma, Rhizoma Polygoni Cuspidati, Semen Julandis, Rhizoma Coptidis, Tremella, Placenta Hominis, Radix Arnebiae, Bufo

FOR KERATODERMIA AT THE EARLY STAGE OF CANCER: Caulis Millettiae, Herba Ecliptae

FOR ALL VARIOUS CANCER: Radix Wikstroemae, Ramulus et Folium Cephalotaxi Fortunei, Bulbus Allii, Radix Sophorae Tonkinensis, Hydrargyrum, Radix Aconiti, Fructus Mume, Herba Solani Glabrae, Herba Agrimoniae, Lignum et Radix Acronychiae, Herba Cephalanoploris, Coriolus, Fructus Chaenomelis, Herba et Radix Ranunculi Japonici, Fructus Arctii, Herba Scutellariae Barbatae, Flos Carthami, Flos Trifolii, Ganoderma, Fructus Xanthii, Herba Artemisiae Annuae, Thallus Lamnariae seu Eckloniae, Herba Houttuyniae, herba Isodi, Caulis Marsdeniae , Cortex Mori, Ramulus et Folium Taxi Cuspidatae, Herba Salviae Chinensis, Rhizoma Acori Graminei, Herba Oldenlandiae Diffusae, Herba Geranii, Herba Elephantopi, Semen Julandis, Poria, Glossogyne, Herba Taxilli, Fructus Gardeniae, Fructus Trapae Bispinosae, Herba Oldenlandiae Chrysotrichae, Herba Duchesneae, Polyporus, Flos Chrysanthemi Morifolii, Fructus Camptothecae, Folium et Semen seu Radix Livistonae, Mel, Herba seu Radix Physalis, Folium Indocalami Tessellati, Gecko Chinensis, Bufo, Carapax Trionycis

Appendix Three: INDEX OF ANTICANCER MEDICINAL HERBS

Int Reg Or Medicine
Gu Hedges House
"   "   Ave
East Grinstead
E. Sussex RH19 1DZ
0342

Reg Trad Chinese Med
7 a Thorndean St
London SW18 4HE
01